ALL ABOUT SEX

Books by Planned Parenthood Federation of America, Inc.:

The Planned Parenthood Women's Health Encyclopedia

All About Sex: A Family Resource on Sex and Sexuality

ALL ABOUT SEX

A Family Resource on Sex and Sexuality

Edited by

Ronald Filiberti Moglia, Ed.D.

Jon Knowles

Three Rivers Press
New York

"Aphrodisiacs and Their Effects" from <u>Our Sexuality</u> by R. Crooks and K. Baur. Copyright © 1993, 1989, 1987, 1983, 1980 The Benjamin Cummings Publishing Co. Copyright © 1995 Brooks/Cole Publishing Company, Pacific Grove, CA 93950, a division of International Thomson Publishing Inc. By permission of the publisher.

"10 Guidelines for Healthy Relationships" Kelly/Byrne, <u>Exploring Human Sexuality</u>, copyright © 1992, p. 274. Adapted by permission of Prentice Hall, Upper Saddle River, New Jersey.

Published by Three Rivers Press, 201 East 50th Street, New York, New York 10022. Member of the Crown Publishing Group.

Random House, Inc. New York, Toronto, London, Sydney, Auckland
http://www.randomhouse.com/

THREE RIVERS PRESS and colophon are trademarks of Crown Publishers, Inc.

Printed in the United States of America

Design by Jerry O'Brien

Library of Congress Cataloging-in-Publication Data is available upon request.

ISBN 0-609-80146-5

10 9 8 7 6 5 4 3 2 1

First Edition

Contents

Acknowledgments

Editors
Ronald Filiberti Moglia, Ed.D., and Jon Knowles

Contributing Authors
Cecily C. Criminale, M.A.
Shauna Croom, B.S.J.
Melinda Gallagher, M.A.
Amy Jo Goddard, M.A.
Jillian Juanita Gonzales, M.A.
Linda L. Hendrixson, Ph.D.
Jon Knowles
    Director of Sexual Health Information
    Planned Parenthood Federation of America
Francesca M. Maresca, M.A.
Pierce Mills, M.A.
    Senior Sexuality Educator
    Planned Parenthood of New York City
Ronald Filiberti Moglia, Ed.D.
    Associate Professor
    Graduate Studies in Human Sexuality
    New York University

Planned Parenthood Federation of America Staff
Gloria Feldt, President
Karla Buitrago, Editorial Associate/Production Coordinator
Michael S. Burnhill, M.D., D.M.Sc., Vice President for Medical Affairs
Roger Evans, Esq., Senior Director, Public Policy Litigation and Law
Jon Knowles, Director of Sexual Health Information
Kim Lafferty, Special Assistant, Office of the President
Wendy Lund, Vice President for Marketing
Mike McGee, Vice President for Education (Acting)
Eve Paul, Esq., General Counsel
Barbara Snow, Vice President for Executive Affairs
Kate Thomsen, M.D., M.P.H., Associate Medical Director

Special Thanks

Jim Beers, Ph.D., New York City

Martin Guggenheim, J.D., Department of Law, New York University

Jan Lunquist, M.A., C.S.E., C.F.L.E., Vice President
   of Education/Professional Development, Planned Parenthood
   Centers of West Michigan

Scott McCann, Ph.D., L.C.S.W., Director of Education, Planned
   Parenthood of Santa Barbara, Ventura, and San Luis Obispo
   Counties, California

Jeffrey Craig Miller, Esq., New York City

**Editorial Coordination and Production
by the People's Medical Society**

Charles B. Inlander, President

Karla Morales, Vice President of Editorial Services

Bill Betts, copy editor

Jerry O'Brien, book design

Marika Hahn, illustrator

Nancy Rutman, proofer

Sally Lutz, indexer

Introduction

The year was 1916, and it was illegal to distribute sexual health information in the United States. A young nurse, Margaret Sanger, challenged state and federal laws by opening America's first family planning clinic in the Brownsville community of Brooklyn, New York. She and her staff offered married women the information they needed to plan their families. In a matter of days, Sanger and her coworkers were arrested and jailed. That is how America's modern birth control movement began and how the organization that became Planned Parenthood Federation of America was founded.

All About Sex reflects the continuing dedication Planned Parenthood devotes to Sanger's belief that access to information about human sexuality improves our lives. *All About Sex* provides important information about sex and sexuality in simple, straightforward language that families can understand and use. It reflects Sanger's belief that sex is a pleasurable and positive aspect of our lives; that positive attitudes toward human sexuality can make the world a better place; and that we must have honest information to make responsible decisions about sex.

The information included in *All About Sex* can help deepen our understanding and comfort with the many aspects of our sexuality. It not only provides important information about the sexual and reproductive anatomy of women and men but also gives special emphasis to the equally important ways in which our sexuality develops, changes, and grows throughout all the stages of our lives.

Human sexuality is wonderfully diverse. *All About Sex* provides positive insights into the ways in which we form our unique preferences, relationships, and values. It also offers perceptions about our sexual traditions and the laws that affect our sex lives. These observations will help stimulate intelligent thinking about the ways in which our society influences our individual sexual identities.

And of course, no book from Planned Parenthood about human sexuality would be complete without useful and comprehensive information about family planning, reproductive health, and safer sex.

No matter what the subject—from the anatomy of sex to the psychology of sex, from sexual science to the physiology of orgasm—*All About Sex* is written in plain, concrete, and commonsense language that offers clear information and reassuring guidance for every member of the family.

We believe *All About Sex* is a comprehensive and comprehensible source of information that can help you and your family maintain sexual health and develop positive, healthy values about sex and sexuality.

For more than 80 years, Planned Parenthood has been America's uncensored source for sexual health information. In *All About Sex,* we provide accurate and complete information about the most common and the less common aspects of sexual experience. In presenting this information, we have taken care to respect the diversity in sexual values that guide our readers' lives. We believe that this uncensored, honest information can enhance our understanding of the individual and social implications of human sexuality.

All About Sex is shaped around four basic facts:

• Sexuality is a healthy, natural, and normal part of being human.
• Sexuality is inherently diverse and complex.
• All people are sexual from birth to death.
• Sexuality serves many important purposes other than reproduction.

The basic value that underlies this presentation of information is that sexually active people have a responsibility to help protect the health and well-being of their partners.

We believe that this encyclopedic guide will also be useful in helping you to make satisfying and responsible decisions about your sexuality throughout your life.

Like Margaret Sanger, Planned Parenthood believes that understanding our human sexuality is the first step toward establishing an enriching and responsible sex life. And we believe that *All About Sex* is a positive approach to understanding ourselves and our world.

One of the heartbreaking stories that Sanger told to persuade the public of the importance of sexual health information was about a young woman named Sadie Sachs. Sadie and her husband, Jake, had three children. Times were hard, they couldn't afford to have a larger family, and Sadie had been told that another pregnancy would kill her.

When Sadie asked her doctor how to avoid any further pregnancies, the only advice he had to offer her was "Tell Jake to sleep on the roof."

As we know, sexual desire is very powerful. Eventually, Jake and Sadie decided to take their chances, and Sadie became pregnant again. In desperation, she tried to give herself an abortion and died from her attempt. Sanger said her life's career was inspired by Sadie's painful and unnecessary death.

Thanks to Sanger, we no longer need to take the chances that Sadie and Jake felt compelled to take.

We live in a time when we can get the sexual health information we need to celebrate and express our sexuality *while* we protect ourselves and our partners against physical and emotional harm. Planned Parenthood offers *All About Sex* to you and your family for positive, sound, and helpful guidance. Enjoy it in good health.

Terms that appear in **boldface** type are defined in the Glossary beginning on page 318.

CHAPTER 1

Our

Sexuality

There may be some things better than sex, and some things worse, but there is nothing exactly like it.
—W. C. Fields (1880–1946)

We live in a very sexual world. There are messages about **sex** all around us—on radio and TV, in movies, magazines, and music. Sexual imagery is used to sell everything from soap to sports cars. Political and religious leaders have a lot to say about sex, too. So do people in locker rooms, in malls, and in our own homes.

But how much of this information is actually useful? Not much. Even with all the sexual messages to which we are exposed, many people still lack accurate and understandable information about their own **sexuality.** That's because sex is often talked about as something bad, disgusting, shameful, sinful, weird, or just plain silly. So instead of learning to be comfortable with the subject of our sexuality, most people feel embarrassed, scared, guilty, or confused about their sexual thoughts and behaviors.

This makes it very difficult, if not impossible, for many people to talk about sex, even with their sex partners. As a result, many kids grow up not understanding their sexuality. As many discover the power of their natural sexual urges, they may engage in high-risk **sex play** before they are prepared to protect themselves from unintended pregnancy and sexually transmitted infections. Others become frightened and may be pressured into sexual **intercourse** before they are ready—physically, emotionally, or financially.

Sex is a big deal. Learning to talk about sex openly and honestly is very important. We all need to be comfortable with our sexuality.

Sexuality is a very important part of life. Not only is it the way in which we can give life to the next generation, it also gives us some of the greatest pleasures and rewards of life, yet it can also cause great sorrow. Sexuality has been used to create **intimacy.** It has been used to avoid intimacy. Individuals have been brutalized and wars have been fought over sexual issues. But human sexuality also inspired many of humanity's greatest achievements—in art, literature, and life. It has a powerful influence on us all.

Learning about our **culture**'s powerful influence on human sexuality can help us better understand our world, ourselves, and our personal **values.** Understanding our sexuality can:

- provide us with a basic key to our own personal happiness
- make us comfortable with our sexual thoughts and feelings
- allow us to take care of ourselves, as well as to respect the rights and decisions of others
- strengthen our families
- give us the ability and confidence to make our own sexual decisions and help protect us from being victims of **sexual abuse**
- help us protect ourselves and our partners against **STIs (sexually transmitted infections)** and unwanted pregnancy
- enhance our relationships with other people
- greatly enhance our sexual pleasure

However, in our culture we often hear about the negative aspects of human sexuality. Dirty jokes and sexual ridicule and put-downs are common. Sexual relationships, whether or not they are based on **love,** can cause pain and sorrow. Some even end in violence and tragedy. Sex is also often used to demonstrate power and to exploit other people. Sexual abuse, **sexual harassment, rape,** and unwanted pregnancy are all too familiar headlines. Many of us have experienced them ourselves.

SEXUALITY IS A HEALTHY, NATURAL, AND NORMAL PART OF BEING HUMAN

If you were to ask other people to think about their *sexuality*, most would define it in terms of their sexual behavior. However, that would more accurately be called sex.

"Sex" usually refers to a physical act involving the **genitals,** or sex organs. Of course, the specific activities can vary tremendously. Thus, what counts as "sex" may be different for everyone. For some, just touching someone else's **penis** or **vagina** counts as sex. For others, it doesn't. For some people, **oral sex** is "sex." For others, it isn't. For some people, anal sex is "sex." For others, it isn't. Some people would only define sex as having **vaginal intercourse** with a penis. Obviously, a simple word like "sex" means different things to different people.

Then, what is "sexuality"? Sexuality is even more complicated, because it is about much more than any sex act.

When you think of your sexuality, what do you think about? What if you were asked to name the sexual parts of your body? What would you say? Most people immediately think of their genitals. But a more correct answer would consider other parts of the body, too.

Every part of the body is capable of receiving pleasure. The biggest sex organ of all is not the penis or vagina, but the brain. Our sexuality has much more to do with how we think and feel than how we behave. Sexuality is a basic part of our physical, mental, emotional, and spiritual lives.

Our sexuality includes our **gender,** both in terms of our physical anatomy and our feelings about what it means to be and act like a woman or man. Another important aspect of our sexuality is our **sexual orientation.** It refers to the gender of the people to whom we are attracted. Sexuality influences how we experience love, compassion, joy, sorrow, and pleasure. It is shaped not only by our bodies and feelings but also by our society and religion. Thus, our sexuality affects our beliefs and values about life, the people our lives touch, and our culture.

So when we think about our sexuality, we do not only think about our genitals or sex acts, our ability to reproduce, or our ability to have an **orgasm.** We think about our entire selves. Our sexuality is not only a part of everything we do, it also influences everything we feel and everything we are.

Try to imagine what life would be like without your sexuality. Try to imagine yourself without the feelings about life your sexuality inspires. Frightening thoughts, aren't they? Our sexuality makes us feel alive. It is one of the most vital elements of our personalities. It is a wonderful, empowering, and liberating part of being human.

Our sexuality is not something to be ashamed of or embarrassed about. It should be enjoyed and celebrated. Believing sexuality is healthy allows us to be open, flexible, and creative as we explore our sexual thoughts and feelings. It lets us recognize that sex can be fun and exciting and can also fulfill many emotional needs. Having a healthy attitude toward sexuality means knowing our values, beliefs, attitudes, limits, and boundaries, and respecting that knowledge by being responsible. It allows us to feel attractive, regardless of our age,

SELF-ASSESSMENT QUIZ
HOW DO YOU FEEL ABOUT YOUR SEXUALITY?

Yes No Not Sure 1. I think my sexuality is normal.
Yes No Not Sure 2. I see my sexuality as a healthy characteristic of myself.
Yes No Not Sure 3. I like my body.
Yes No Not Sure 4. I like my gender.
Yes No Not Sure 5. I like my sexual orientation.
Yes No Not Sure 6. I can talk about my sexual feelings and desires with my partner.
Yes No Not Sure 7. I am able to have sexual experiences without **guilt.**
Yes No Not Sure 8. I am able to give and receive sexual pleasure.
Yes No Not Sure 9. I take responsibility for my sexual behavior.
Yes No Not Sure 10. I am clear about the differences between sex and intimacy.
Yes No Not Sure 11. I see sexuality as a lifelong experience that will always be a part of me and will always be changing.

If you circled a "No" or "Not Sure" for any of these questions, you are quite normal. It's hard for most people to feel good about their sexuality in a world that tells us to be embarrassed about it. Like sexuality itself, sexuality education is a lifelong, ongoing process. If you circled "Yes" for all of these questions, you are doing very well with your sexuality education.

gender, sexual orientation, race, religion, height, weight, or physical or mental ability. It lets us be ourselves.

Knowing as much as possible about our sexual selves, in terms of our beliefs, values, physical needs, and legal rights, will help us create responsible, healthy, and satisfying sexual lives.

HUMAN SEXUALITY IS DIVERSE AND COMPLEX

We go through a lot of changes while we grow up. Between the ages of eight and 20, we grow from being girls or boys into being women or men. During this process, our bodies change, and our feelings change, too—our feelings about ourselves, our family, and other people.

We go through all of these changes whether or not we are ready, whether or not we want to, and whether or not we know what is going on. Sometimes it seems the changes happen too fast. Sometimes we feel they don't happen fast enough. It is often very confusing.

Through all of this personal development, almost everyone has profound fears about being "different" from everyone else. What people want most is to be "normal."

But what most people don't understand as these changes are happening, and what many adults still don't realize, is that *being different is normal.* This is especially true when it comes to our sexuality. No two people are exactly alike in the way they look, think, or feel. Nor should they be. Imagine living in a world where everyone was the same. Think how boring it would be.

Far too often, people fear difference simply out of ignorance. We fear what we don't understand. But once we realize that it is our differences that give our society its excitement, we see that our **diversity** should be celebrated!

Sexuality is inherently diverse and complex. In other words, there is no one right way for women, men, or children to be sexual. Instead, human sexuality varies tremendously. Below is a brief explanation of how people differ in their sexuality in four very important ways: **gender identity,** sexual orientation, sexual tastes, and relationship characteristics. Many of these differences are common, and many of them are less common.

Gender Identity

Gender is a primary difference in human sexuality. Gender can refer to the many physical differences between girls and boys and men and women.

Gender identity means the degree to which someone is considered to act **feminine** or **masculine.**

Feminine traits are ways of behaving that our society associates with being female. Masculine traits are ways of behaving that our society associates with being male. But as in all things related to our sexuality, gender identity really isn't that simple. Everyone is different in the degree to which they live up to society's expectations about femininity and masculinity. Almost all men have some feminine traits, and almost all women have some masculine traits.

So how do someone's ideas about femininity and masculinity develop in the first place, and what causes us to conform or not conform to these ideas?

Our awareness and behavior as boys or girls develop after we are born, mainly from the socialization we all receive from our parents and others while growing up. Socialization refers to the ways in which a society conveys its expectations to someone about her or his behavior. The process that persuades someone to adopt behaviors that are considered socially appropriate for his or her gender is called **gender scripting.**

Through gender scripting, infants are slowly but continuously trained to believe what it means to be a girl or boy by the ways in which they are treated by those who raise them. Parents, caregivers, teachers, and peers treat girls very differently than they do boys. For example, as babies, girls are more likely to be held gently, cuddled, and sung to by parents, while boys are more likely to be bounced around when handled. While most parents buy dolls for girls, they buy footballs and baseball bats for boys.

As children grow, they respond to gender scripting by adopting behaviors that are rewarded by parents and their peers. They stop or hide behaviors that are ridiculed or punished. Thus, by age three, children have usually learned to prefer the toys and clothes that society considers appropriate for their gender. These behaviors and preferences form our **gender roles,** socially defined expectations that people have of either gender.

While gender roles vary greatly from one culture to the next, from one ethnic group to the next, and from one social class to the next, gender roles are universal—that is, all societies have expectations of female and male dress, behavior, and grooming.

Our perceptions of gender roles are greatly affected by **gender stereotypes** that can cause unequal and unfair treatment because of a person's gender. This is called **sexism.**

FOUR BASIC COMPONENTS OF GENDER STEREOTYPES

1. *Personality traits.* For example, women are often expected to be passive and submissive, while men are usually expected to be self-confident and aggressive.
2. *Domestic behaviors.* For example, caring for children is often considered best done by women, while household repairs are often considered best done by men.
3. *Occupations.* For example, until very recently most nurses and secretaries were women, and most doctors and construction workers were men.
4. *Physical appearance.* For example, women are expected to be small and graceful, while men are expected to be tall and broad-shouldered.

Because gender stereotypes are still so strong in our society, sometimes people are verbally, physically, or financially punished if they don't act according to how society expects someone of their gender to behave. For example, women are sometimes not hired for certain jobs simply because of their gender. In a divorce hearing, a judge might automatically award custody of a child to the mother because of the belief that women make better parents. Behavior that is called "aggressive" in a man may be called "bitchy" in a woman. What may be called "emotional" in a woman may be called "wimpy" in a man.

We sometimes find ourselves trapped by our gender roles, and we limit our own behavior. In order to avoid being criticized, men are often reluctant to show their true feelings. Some fathers won't hug their own sons because it is not considered "manly." Women are often passive, giving in to whatever someone else wants. Many women also put limits on their sexual behavior because the slightest sexual suggestion in a woman's behavior may result in an accusation that she is a "slut."

Over the past several decades, however, many people have been learning to reject the stereotypical roles that our society expects each gender to fill. Americans are now free to express their gender identities in more ways than ever before in history. For example, many parents no longer dress their children in either pink or blue, but in a gender-neutral color such as green. Some also allow their children to choose their own toys.

Some schools now have as many athletic programs for girls as they do for boys. More women than ever before in history are entering the workforce in positions equal to those of men. And some men are taking a more active role in parenting by staying home to raise their children. Many men are also taking pride in their emotions, becoming more willing to express their feelings, thereby becoming more sensitive and better friends, lovers, and fathers.

All people—adults and children—are entitled to the same opportunities regardless of gender. All of us should be allowed to make our own choices about what roles are appropriate for ourselves. While we each may have very different characteristics and hopes for our futures, as girls and women, boys and men, we share equal talents, strengths, and dreams.

Diversity in Gender

Most people deal with their gender by accepting the social expectations associated with their biological gender. Others deal with their gender in less common ways. Here are some examples of gender diversity.

Cross-Dressers

Many people enjoy experimenting with their gender roles. People of one gender may like to occasionally wear various articles of clothing identified with the other gender simply to mock or defy society's rules of what is considered "normal." For others, cross-dressing can turn into a career. Many **cross-dressers** become professional entertainers. Men who cross-dress are commonly referred to as female impersonators or drag queens. Women who cross-dress are called male impersonators or drag kings.

Transvestites

Some people dress in the clothes of the other gender because it gives them sexual pleasure. Such people are usually referred to as **transvestites.** Sometimes they cross-dress publicly, sometimes only in private. For example, a transvestite man may enjoy wearing women's panties and stockings under his business suit. Many transvestites are **heterosexuals** who have no interest whatsoever in sexual encounters with people of the same gender.

Transgender

Some people dress in the clothing of the gender other than their biological one because they enjoy being treated as someone of the other gender. This is not done for sexual thrill. These people consider themselves **transgender.** Transgender people typically have two different identities, and even two names for themselves—one female and one male. For them, cross-dressing is like acting, playing a role, trying to see what it's like to walk in a woman's, or a man's, shoes. How often a transgender person plays this role depends on the individual. Many transgender people are also heterosexual and have no desire to actually change their biological anatomy.

Transsexual

A **transsexual** is someone who fully identifies with the gender other than her or his biological one. Most transsexual people remember feeling, from a very early age, that they have been trapped inside the wrong body. Oftentimes transsexual people are unhappy with their female or male anatomy. Most like to live full-time as the other gender. Many use hormone therapy and surgery to change their sexual anatomy so it matches their gender identity.

Sexual Orientation

Sexual orientation refers to the gender to which a person is physically and emotionally attracted. Someone who is sexually attracted to people of the other gender is called heterosexual or **straight.** People who are attracted to others of their own gender are called **homosexual** or **gay.** Gay women are also called **lesbians.** Those who are attracted to people of both genders are called **bisexual.**

Each person's sexual orientation is more complex than these simple labels—humans are all different, and each individual's sexual orientation is unique. Each of us is at a different place somewhere along the range between exclusively heterosexual and exclusively homosexual orientations.

Many people wonder what causes their sexual orientation. While there is strong evidence pointing toward biological factors, this remains a subject of great debate among scientists and politicians alike. Regardless of the cause, whether people are straight, gay, or bisexual is usually established before **puberty** and before they begin having sex. And although sexual orientation may begin to develop before birth, it may shift in the course of a lifetime. But sexual orientation is not something that people can decide for themselves or for others. In other words, being physically and emotionally attracted to people of a certain gender is not a conscious choice.

Homophobia

In our society, there is a tremendous amount of fear and hatred of people who are gay, lesbian, or bisexual. This fear is called **homophobia.** Homophobia is caused by ignorance, or misinformation and lack of understanding about what gay, lesbian, and bisexual people are really like.

Instead of learning about and respecting people of diverse sexual orientations, many people simply believe **myths** that gay people are

For a more complete discussion of the relationship between our bodies and our sexuality, see Chapter 3, "Our Sexual Bodies."

dangerous, sick, evil, sinful, weird, disgusting, and perverted. But these are not truths; they are **stereotypes.** A stereotype is a generalization about an entire group of people based on the actions of a few individual members of that group. Just as it is wrong to draw conclusions about all straight people because of a few examples, making generalizations about all gay people is very harmful. For example, one stereotype of gay men is that they will harm or molest children in sexual ways. As a result, many gay people who tell the truth about their sexual orientation are fired from jobs as teachers and camp counselors. In reality, however, the majority of people who sexually abuse children are heterosexual.

All too often, homophobia prevents people from getting to know gay people as individuals and as friends, so they never learn the truth and rid themselves of these harmful stereotypes.

Homophobia also makes many people worry about their own sexual orientation and the sexual orientation of their children. For example, some people believe that sexual orientation is formed by early childhood experiences. Therefore, many parents worry about sex play between children of the same gender. However, it's very common for young children to look at and touch the sex organs of friends of *both* genders. It is simply one of the ways in which they learn about physical similarities and differences. This kind of sex play does not make a child straight, gay, or bisexual.

Many people also worry that having an occasional sexual **fantasy** about someone of the same gender may mean that they are gay. In reality, people of all ages and sexual orientations may have sexy dreams and fantasies about either gender. Dreams and fantasies don't mean that someone is straight, gay, or bisexual.

Because of homophobia, children who realize that they are strongly attracted to people of the same gender often react with fear, confusion, and self-hatred. They absorb their culture's homophobia at very young ages. That's why most gay, lesbian, and bisexual teenagers spend these years feeling depressed and isolated, thinking they have no one to talk with who will understand and accept their feelings.

Parents and friends can play an especially important role in reassuring gay, lesbian, and bisexual people that their feelings are healthy, normal, and natural. We all have a better chance of being able to enjoy our sexuality if we fight against homophobia.

Sexual Appreciations and Preferences

Humans differ tremendously in their sexual feelings, desires, and behavior. What some people find revolting others might find beautiful. What turns one person on may disgust someone else.

Lovemaps

There may have been times when we've wondered why we are attracted to certain people and not others. Or why certain sexual situations really turn us on or off. These preferences are part of what some sexologists call our **lovemap.** Our personal lovemaps form our ideals for lovers and the ways we prefer to engage in sex. The lovemap determines who and what we fantasize about.

We begin to form our lovemaps even before we are born. Specifically, our genders, and most likely our sexual orientation, are determined by our genetic makeups and prenatal **hormone** levels. But most of our lovemaps develop while we are growing up, due to people and situations we are exposed to as children. Because our experiences while growing up are so vastly different, so are our lovemaps.

This is why some people are physically attracted to people with blond hair, others get turned on by red hair, and still others are attracted only to people who are bald. Likewise, some people are attracted to women with large **breasts,** others to women with small breasts. While some people are attracted to a man with lots of chest hair, others prefer no body hair at all. Because our lovemaps are so diverse, what we find sexually attractive varies tremendously.

Paraphilia

The sexual behavior most common in human lovemaps is sexual intercourse. But sometimes childhood experiences affect a person's lovemap so that she or he becomes turned on by sexual practices that many people would consider bizarre or kinky. For example, some people enjoy **sadomasochism,** or S and M. They may become just as sexually aroused by either giving or receiving pain as they do by having sexual intercourse.

If someone can become sexually aroused only by S and M, or any other sexual practice that society judges as uncommon or unacceptable, he or she is said to have a **paraphilia.**

Paraphilias become problematic if consent is not given by other people who become involved. For example, **voyeurs** are people who become aroused by secretly watching other people undress or engage in sexual behavior. **Exhibitionists** are those who, without asking, expose their genitals to people, usually in public.

Paraphilias are unacceptable if they involve pressuring, forcing, or exploiting another person for sexual pleasure. Mutual consent is needed at all times, for any sexual activity; otherwise the activity is inappropriate and punishable by law.

Common or uncommon, our lovemaps never stop developing. It is possible and normal for our own sexual likes and dislikes to change over the course of our lifetimes. Our shifting lovemaps are a vibrant and fluid part of our lives.

Sexual Relationships

Besides the many differences in our sexual orientation, gender, and lovemaps, there is also a wide variety of sexual relationships that people create. Of course, the form of our relationships is closely related to our unique sexuality. For example, people who identify themselves as gay or lesbian will probably date people of the same gender, while those who consider themselves heterosexual will most likely date only people of the other gender.

The levels of commitment in relationships can vary from one person to the next and from one couple to the next. If both people in a relationship are involved only with one another, they are engaged in a **monogamous relationship.** Some people are more comfortable in an **open relationship,** in which both partners are free to also become involved with other people. There are also those who choose to have no sexual relationships. They may choose to express their sexuality by practicing **celibacy**—having no sex at all.

Whatever form relationships take, the length of time they last may vary tremendously. Depending upon the happiness, satisfaction, and commitment of both partners, romantic or sexual relationships can last for months and years, or for only hours and days. Furthermore, while many people would like to find someone with whom to spend the rest of their lives, others are simply not interested in limiting themselves to one sexual partner.

WHAT PLANNED PARENTHOOD BELIEVES

Here is a brief set of statements that describe the Planned Parenthood point of view.

We believe that:

- Sexuality is a natural, healthy, lifelong part of being human.
- Every individual has a right to pursue sexual health information and services without fear, shame, or exploitation. That right involves access to adequate, accurate, and age-appropriate information about sexuality, including the advantages and disadvantages of sexual expression.
- All people, regardless of gender or sexual orientation, have rights that need to be respected, and responsibilities that need to be exercised.
- It is unacceptable to pressure, force, or exploit another person sexually.
- In a pluralistic society, we must respect diverse sexual attitudes and behaviors, as long as they are based on ethics, responsibility, justice, equality, and nonviolence.
- Information about becoming pregnant and about postponing, preventing, continuing, or terminating pregnancy should be easily available; the choice of whether or not to parent should be free and informed.
- Every child deserves to be wanted, loved, and cared for.
- Abstaining from sexual intercourse is the most effective method of preventing pregnancy and sexually transmitted infections.
- Young people explore their sexuality as part of a process of achieving sexual maturity; adolescents are capable of expressing their sexuality in healthy, responsible ways.
- There are many healthy ways to express sexual feelings, alone or with a partner; sexual intercourse is only one form of sexual expression.
- Uninformed or irresponsible sexual behavior poses risks.
- Women, men, girls, and boys benefit from fairness and flexibility in gender roles.
- Individuals and society benefit when children are able to discuss sexuality with their parents and/or other trusted adults.
- Individuals and society benefit when childbearing is postponed until maturity.

Endorsed by the Planned Parenthood membership on November 17, 1996.

Many people get married and become monogamous. This is one of the most common sexual relationships in the world. Other people never marry. This may be because of personal preference, or it may be involuntary, as in the case of gay and lesbian people, who are not legally allowed to marry. Many people—straight or gay—live together as couples without ever getting married. Sometimes romantic or sexual relationships are broken off and then resumed months or even years later.

SEXUAL RELATIONSHIPS—BASIC GUIDELINES

What people find enjoyable and comfortable in sexual relationships varies tremendously from person to person. However, to help ensure that the interests of both people involved in a relationship are being protected, certain guidelines should be followed.

1. Sexual relationships should be consensual whether or not the partners are married. Each partner should be able to enter and leave the relationship without any physical, financial, or emotional pressure put on them by the other partner. This means that we must make sure we have the other person's full permission before engaging in any sexual behavior.
2. Any behavior that harms someone is unacceptable. All relationships bring with them the risk of becoming emotionally hurt, but such harm should never be intentional.
3. We must be open and honest about our actions with anyone with whom we are sexually involved. For example, both people in a relationship should be aware if either partner is also having sex with someone else.
4. In order to reduce the chance of any physical harm, people who are sexually active with each other need to also practice behaviors that protect both partners against sexually transmitted infections and unintended pregnancies.
5. Sex partners should try to have a clear understanding of each other's feelings and expectations if an unintended pregnancy occurs.

The kinds of sexual activities couples engage in within a relationship can also vary. It depends on what both people are comfortable with, interested in, and enjoy. Their sexual behavior may be limited to mutual masturbation, oral sex, or vaginal or **anal intercourse.** Other couples may enjoy none or all of these forms of sex play.

Sometimes two people will have intercourse on their first date. Other couples wait until they have dated for months. Some wait until they are married. Some never have intercourse. Although monogamous relationships are most common, some couples will agree to switch partners. Such an arrangement is called mate-swapping. Some people engage in group sex, either with other couples or other single people or with both. Even people who are legally married sometimes have open relationships.

Just as our individual sexualities change with time, so can our relationships. What may have started as a monogamous relationship can turn into an open one. Open relationships can also become monogamous. Someone who had sexual relationships only with men may become romantically involved with women.

For a more complete discussion on how we form our ideas about love, attraction, and dating, see Chapter 4, "Our Sexual Journey through Life."

ALL PEOPLE ARE SEXUAL— FROM BIRTH TO DEATH

Everyone is sexual—young or old, woman or man, straight or gay, married or single, rich or poor, abled or disabled. Being a sexual person does not necessarily include having sex. It means that we all have sexual feelings about ourselves and other people, whether we act on those feelings or not.

Sometimes these feelings include **sexual desire.** Sexual desire is a strong physical attraction. We could be attracted to someone we just see on TV or on the street, but whom we never meet. Or perhaps it is someone we talk to every day, at work or at the gym. Sometimes our attractions are just passing flirtations. Sometimes they may be all we can think about. Or sometimes the people we are attracted to are only fantasies we create in our minds.

There are many personal qualities that can attract us. We may be attracted to people because of their intelligence or ambition. We may be attracted to people who have an interest or sense of humor similar to our own. We may be attracted to people who treat us with kindness, sensitivity, and respect. Or we may be attracted to people simply for the way they smile.

Sexual desire and love are not the same thing. Love is a strong caring for someone else. It comes in many forms. There can be love for romantic partners, for close friends, for parents and children, for God, and for humankind. Love can exist without sexual desire, and sexual desire can exist without love. Many people are happiest when both love and sexual desire are shared between both partners.

When Does Sexuality Start?

We begin learning about sexuality as infants and never stop learning. As our bodies, minds, and social environments change during our lifetimes, so do our feelings, beliefs, behaviors, and sexual knowledge. Here is a brief guide to show how sexuality is experienced at different ages and what role parents and other caregivers can play in developing their child's healthy sexuality. But remember, everyone is sexually unique! People can grow and change in very different ways—physically, mentally, and emotionally. So if we or people we know experience this process differently, that is perfectly normal, too.

Birth to Two Years Old

Children learn about sexuality from the day they are born. By constantly observing the people who care for them—what they do and how they act—infants pick up lots of information about themselves. Babies feel secure or insecure by:

- the way they are held and touched
- the way they are fed, washed, and diapered
- the tone of voice of those around them
- being allowed to feel comfortable with their bodies and emotions

Children can develop healthier feelings about themselves and their sexuality if all these things are done in a pleasant, loving, and caring way.

It is normal for babies to explore their bodies. They are quick to learn that touching their sex organs feels good. They should be allowed to enjoy this. If parents yell at them or slap their hands, they may do it, anyway—but they'll feel guilty about it. Such disapproval sends a strong message that children should be ashamed of their bodies and sexuality. It may also prevent kids from turning to their parents later in life when they're looking for guidance about sex.

Three to Five Years Old

By the time they are three, kids are ready to know that women and men have different sex organs. They may have already wondered about it for a while. It is most helpful if parents talk about genitals in the same way they talk about elbows and noses, fingers and toes. Using the right names for sex organs, saying "**vulva**," "penis," and "breasts," instead of family or street words is very helpful. If the genitals are never mentioned by adults, or are identified only by slang terms, kids may get the idea that something is "wrong" with these parts of the body. Their discomfort may lead them to become confused when health care providers discuss these body parts and functions with them.

Toddlers are curious about the bodies of their parents and other children. Nudity within the family is a matter for each family to decide, depending on each family member's level of comfort. Children may "play doctor" to look at each other's sex organs. This is a normal way for kids to find out differences and learn about their sexuality. Parents can choose to allow it or not. But punishing children for such self-discovery will do nothing to foster their comfort and understanding of sexuality.

Three-year-olds may also begin asking, "Where do babies come from?" Parents don't need to describe sexual intercourse at this point. Answers should be simple. Parents might say something like, "Babies grow in a special place inside the mother." As the years pass, other details can slowly be added as the child becomes able to understand them.

It is normal for four-year-olds to become very attached to a parent—even an absent parent. Kids may even be jealous of the other parent or partner. They can become attached to parents or caregivers of both genders. None of these attachments has anything to do with whether a child is gay or straight. Parents should let their kids be comfortable with whatever attachments they form. It's also best not to tease children about having "girlfriends" and "boyfriends."

Four-year-olds may want to snuggle in bed with parents or caregivers. They may also want to see them without clothes on. Parents can set limits that make all family members comfortable. But it may be harmful if children are punished for having such a healthy curiosity and desire for intimacy.

Five to Seven Years Old

At this age, children begin to develop positive or negative feelings about their bodies. They develop attitudes about the bodies of others. They are also beginning to realize their perception of what it means to be and act like girls and boys. And they can get very clubby about it. That's why it is very common for them to say they hate children of the other gender. Again, it's better that parents and other caregivers not tease them about it.

It is common for kids to become less attached to parents and caregivers at this time. Children in primary school may be shy about asking questions. But that doesn't mean they don't have questions. Many of them have heard about such things as **AIDS,** rape, and **child abuse.** And they wonder about these things even if they don't say anything. So parents need to keep talking with them.

Sexual fantasies about family members of both genders are common, too. Kids may find these thoughts upsetting. Parents can reassure them that just dreaming or thinking about things doesn't make them happen.

Most children enjoy touching their genitals and other parts of their bodies. The **clitoris** is designed to give women and girls great pleasure when touched. The penis, especially the tip, gives men and boys great pleasure when touched.

Touching one's own genitals for pleasure is called **masturbation.** Masturbation is not harmful, even though some people believe it is. Children at this age usually do not have sexual fantasies while touching their genitals. They are just enjoying the physical stimulus of the touch. That is why some sexologists call this **autoerotic** activity. The lack of fantasy distinguishes autoerotic activity from the adult form of masturbation. At any age, masturbation is a normal, healthy part of life, and it is common during this time. Parents can reassure kids that it is normal to masturbate—but that it is something to enjoy privately. Masturbation becomes dysfunctional only if it becomes obsessive.

Preteens—Eight to 12 Years Old

Puberty is the stage in a child's development when sexual maturity and reproductive capacity begin. In addition to the physical transformations that occur, puberty brings with it many mental and emotional changes. The first stages of puberty usually start around the age of 10 for girls and

11 for boys, but it can begin earlier or later. Lean children usually develop slightly later, because body fat encourages hormone production.

Parents can make sure that their preteen children have all the facts about **menstruation, wet dreams,** and other signs of maturing so they will be prepared when their bodies start to change. Sometimes children become frightened by the changes they go through. We can ease their concerns with information and reassurance.

Kids are fascinated with the way their bodies change. Boys and girls of this age may have sex play with friends of either gender. But sexual contact at these ages does not predict adult sexual orientation or behavior.

Preteens are very concerned about whether their bodies are developing "normally." Boys worry about their penis size. Girls worry about their breast size. Parents can reassure their children that no two people are the same and that it is normal to be different.

Preteens are also very concerned with their changing relationships with parents and their need to establish independence. They also want to know about social and sexual relationships. Most 12-year-olds are ready to know about sexual behavior and reproduction. They need to know about **abstinence,** sexually transmitted infections, birth control, and the consequences of teen pregnancy. And they need to know how all of this can affect their lives.

Teenagers

Teenagers need to know how to make healthy, appropriate, and responsible decisions about their sexuality, so they will know how to have relationships without getting hurt or without hurting others—either physically or emotionally. This includes knowing how to protect themselves and their sexual partners from unwanted pregnancies and sexually transmitted infections *before* they start having sex. And they must be able to take responsibility for their actions.

Like adults, teenagers will benefit by understanding the differences between "love" and "**lust**." They also need to understand how to have constructive relationships with people of both genders. Parents should allow teenagers to try to fit in with their peers. But teens should also be strongly encouraged to think for themselves so they can avoid peer pressure and bad advice.

Adults

While it's difficult for many parents to admit their children are sexual, it's just as difficult for some adults to admit that they themselves are sexual. This shouldn't be surprising, considering that many people were taught by their parents that sex is too "dirty" for words.

In addition to negative childhood lessons by parents, another social barrier that keeps teenagers and adults from enjoying their sexuality is the media. By using actors and models who are almost always very young, thin, and white, TV commercials and other advertisements constantly promote the idea that there is only one way for a woman or man to look attractive. The message seems to be that anyone who doesn't conform to the look that is portrayed in the media—a "perfect" body and "beautiful" face—won't be attractive to others and won't be able to find a sex partner.

The vast majority of people do not measure up to this narrow physical "ideal." Many grow up disliking the way they look. Women and men often try to change their appearance by using very dangerous or expensive means, such as starving themselves, taking steroids to build up their muscles, and undergoing **cosmetic surgery** to increase the size of their breasts, penises, calves, or buttocks—all in the hope of becoming more attractive to others. Some people who feel that the ideal "look" is beyond possibility for them may "let themselves go," becoming out-of-shape and obese. Other people, those who fear their sexuality, may feel safer by allowing themselves to become less sexually attractive.

In reality, however, beauty is in the eye of the beholder. What people find physically attractive varies tremendously. No matter what we look like, many people will find us physically attractive. Sexual attraction is diverse. No two men or women are exactly alike in the way they look, think, feel, or act, and no two people have exactly the same sexual desires or attractions.

But even if we are comfortable with our appearance, being a sexually healthy adult is not always easy. Adults of all ages continually face many difficult choices related to their sexuality. They need to repeatedly identify and evaluate their beliefs and the values with which they want to live. Adults are also expected to demonstrate respect for people who have different beliefs and values than theirs.

Adults should also be able to communicate effectively and interact with family and peers of both genders in respectful and appropriate ways. Adult relationships must also be consensual, nonexploitive, honest, and pleasurable. Adult partners should protect one another against sexually transmitted infections and unintended pregnancies. Sexually healthy adults will also have regular medical checkups and examine their breasts or **testicles** regularly to identify potential sexual health problems early.

Older Adults

As we age, our bodies, minds, and environments change. These changes affect our sexuality, which also changes throughout our lifetimes. Women commonly experience changes in their sexuality during and after pregnancy, and also after **menopause.** As they age, men experience a natural increase in the time it takes to become aroused and a decline in their ability to get and maintain an **erection.** Certain medications; physical problems, such as strokes or heart attacks; and emotional problems, such as **depression,** may also affect sexual performance. But our sexual feelings and interest are always with us. Despite media images of exclusively youthful sexuality, sex is not only for people in their 20s. Some women and men enjoy healthy, active sex lives well into their 90s.

People with Physical Disabilities

The sexuality of people with physical disabilities is often denied, but people with physical disabilities have the same needs and desires as able-bodied people—whether they are paralyzed, disfigured, blind, or deaf, or suffer from a congenital illness like cerebral palsy or cystic fibrosis. Because we know that sexual pleasure is in our minds and emotions and all parts of our bodies, it is very sensible to assume that women and men with physical disabilities are sexual.

Disabled people should be encouraged to explore their sexuality and enjoy physical pleasure however they are able. In some instances, attendants of severely disabled women and men may be very helpful. They may assist positioning partners for sex play. On the other hand, some people with disabilities may have limitations or neediness that exposes them to the risk of sexual abuse from partners or attendants. Similar risks face able-bodied women whenever their relationships are greatly imbalanced in terms of power. All bodies are special and should be respected, including those that are disabled.

To learn more about how our sexuality and bodies develop and constantly change, see Chapter 3, "Our Sexual Bodies," and Chapter 4, "Our Sexual Journey through Life."

People with Emotional or Developmental Disabilities

People with emotional or developmental disabilities also have an especially difficult time in enjoying their right to be sexual. Far too often, their families and friends mistakenly think that they are not competent enough to make decisions for themselves regarding how, when, and with whom they may enjoy sex play. Paid caregivers, both within the home and in residential facilities, are sometimes under strict orders to stop anyone from engaging in sexual behavior—even masturbation!

Caregivers often fear the consequences of unintended pregnancy in the belief—founded or unfounded—that emotionally or developmentally disabled people in their care may be incapable of caring for children. This fear has often led to forced **sterilization.** It is often difficult to balance what may be in the best interest of the disabled person with what may be in the best interest of the caregiver, institution, or family. The question of sterilization in such cases should be discussed with a trusted health care advisor.

We all have a right to express our sexuality however we want, just as long as our behavior is consensual. Nobody has the right to hurt anyone else, either physically or emotionally—or by depriving him or her of responsible sexual pleasure.

SEX HAS MANY IMPORTANT FUNCTIONS BESIDES REPRODUCTION

Reasons People Have Sex

The belief that reproduction is the only reason for two people to have sexual intercourse has been a major theme in the history of humanity. It became particularly strong during the development of the early Christian church. The idea led to our society's efforts to strictly control the sexual lives of its citizens—especially women. Because women give birth, control focused on their bodies. Eventually, however, all sexual activity was condemned, unless it was performed by married couples for reproductive purposes.

Fortunately, most people have learned to appreciate the fact that reproduction is not the only purpose for our sexuality. There are actually many reasons for two people to enjoy sex play other than to have a baby. Not all of them are good reasons. People have sex to:

- express love, commitment, caring
- feel loved or cared for
- experience physical pleasure
- give someone else physical pleasure
- experiment
- fulfill curiosity
- have fun
- make up with their partners after a fight
- reduce **stress**
- exercise
- prove their masculinity or femininity
- demonstrate power over a partner
- prove maturity
- punish—"get even with"—another person
- get money or drugs

For a more complete discussion on how sexuality is affected by history and culture, see Chapter 2, "Our Sexual Traditions, Beliefs, and History—Some Perspectives."

Some of these reasons can be healthy reasons to have sex; some of them can be unhealthy. Our choices have a lot to do with our circumstances. We all decide to act on our sexual feelings for different reasons. We have different reasons at different times of our lives.

When Should We Have Sex?

Because all people are sexual, we all have to make decisions about what we decide to do with our sexual feelings. We don't always act on our sexual desires. We often don't want to. We may not be able to control whom we are attracted to, but we can decide when, where, and with whom we will be sexually active and what kinds of sex play we will enjoy.

There are important personal motivations and issues to consider as we decide whether or not to engage in a sexual relationship. We need to decide if we are having sex because we want to or because someone else wants us to. We must also consider how having sex will affect us—physically and emotionally. If we ponder having sex with someone important to us, we should also think about how our relationship with that person might change afterward.

SELF-ASSESSMENT QUIZ

DECIDING TO HAVE SEX

Here is a self-assessment quiz to help you think about the reasons you might have sex.

Yes No 1. Am I embarrassed about being sexually inexperienced?

Yes No 2. Does having sex make me feel different about myself?

Yes No 3. Do I ever let myself be pressured into having sex when I don't want to?

Yes No 4. Do I ever have sex to try to keep a relationship together?

Yes No 5. Do I ever have sex to get back at someone?

Yes No 6. Do I know which sexual activities I enjoy and which activities I don't want to engage in?

Yes No 7. Am I able to tell a sex partner about what sexual activities I enjoy and those that I am not willing to engage in?

Yes No 8. Am I able to stand by my personal choices for sexual activity?

Yes No 9. Do I know how to protect myself against pregnancy and infection?

Yes No 10. Am I able to talk about using **contraception** and **condoms** with this person?

Yes No 11. Am I emotionally and financially ready to accept the responsibilities of pregnancy or sexually transmitted infections?

Yes No 12. Do I really care about this person, and does this person really care about me? Does that matter to me?

Yes No 13. Do I respect this person, and does this person respect me? Does that matter to me?

Yes No 14. Do I trust this person, and does this person trust me?

Yes No 15. Does this person want to work on having a committed relationship? Does that matter to me?

There are no right or wrong answers to these questions. We must all decide for ourselves when and with whom we act on our sexual desires. That is our right as sexual persons.

SEXUALLY ACTIVE PEOPLE HAVE A RESPONSIBILITY TO HELP PROTECT THE HEALTH AND WELL-BEING OF THEMSELVES AND THEIR SEXUAL PARTNERS

Being sexually active brings with it many responsibilities. This includes helping to protect ourselves and our romantic partners, both physically and emotionally. Three of the most important ways to attend to each other's health and welfare are to prevent sexual abuse, to prevent sexually transmitted infections, and to prevent unintended pregnancy.

Preventing Sexual Abuse

An important part of being sexually healthy and responsible is never forcing anyone to engage in any sexual activity that she or he doesn't want to do or hasn't consented to. People who do this are sexual abusers. Some people may even try to force themselves on people who are young or on those who find it difficult to defend themselves. Often sexual abusers are well known to the people they hurt. They may be their friends. They may even be members of their families.

Sexual abuse is not limited to forcing someone to have sexual intercourse. It also includes *unwanted* touching, fondling, watching, talking, and giving baths, **douches,** or enemas. And it includes forcing someone to look at one's sex organs. It happens whenever sexual privacy is not respected.

When someone is forced to have sexual intercourse, it is called rape. If someone's husband, friend, or date forces him or her to have sexual intercourse, it is called **acquaintance rape.** If people within the same family have sexual intercourse, it is called **incest.** Sexual abuse, rape, acquaintance rape, and incest are all serious crimes that are punishable under law.

For a more complete discussion of sexual abuse, see Chapter 5, "Our Sexual Feelings— the Psychology of Sex."

Preventing Sexually Transmitted Infection and Unwanted Pregnancy

Not only do we have to be sure that all our sexual activity is consensual, we also need to protect ourselves and our sex partners from sexually transmitted infection and unintended pregnancy. Half of the 31 million women aged 13 to 44 in the United States are at risk of unintended pregnancy.

THE BASICS FOR SEXUALLY HEALTHY RELATIONSHIPS

Sex partners should always:

- have one another's consent
- be honest with one another
- treat one another as equals
- accept responsibility for their actions
- be attentive to one another's pleasure, comfort, and health
- protect one another against emotional and physical harm, including unintended pregnancy and sexually transmitted infection

For more information about family planning, see Chapter 7, "Planning Our Families."

For more information about safer sex and sexually transmitted infections, see Chapter 6, "Our Sexual Health—Taking Care of Our Bodies."

More than half of the 6.3 million pregnancies that occur in the United States every year are unintended. Forty-four percent of these end in **abortion,** 43 percent in birth, 13 percent in miscarriage.

Sexually transmitted infections (STIs) are spread through sexual contact, including vaginal, anal, and oral intercourse. Some can be spread through touching and kissing. Approximately 12 million new cases of STIs are diagnosed each year in the United States. Most of these infections have dangerous consequences and require professional medical treatment. Some can cause sterility. Some increase the risk of getting certain cancers. And others, such as **HBV (hepatitis B virus), syphilis,** and **HIV (human immunodeficiency virus),** can be fatal.

Nobody is immune to sexually transmitted infections. But most people who have one don't know it because they don't notice the symptoms or they don't have any symptoms. Millions of people don't know they're infected until serious and often permanent damage has occurred or they pass the infection to someone else.

Being sexually healthy is more than preventing infections, abuse, and unintended pregnancy. It involves developing fulfilling and responsible relationships, enjoying satisfying sex lives, becoming comfortable with our bodies, planning our families, and understanding our sexuality in relationship to our society. In the following chapters we will look at all of these elements of human sexuality.

CHAPTER 2

Our Sexual

Traditions,

Beliefs, and

History—

Some

Perspectives

*If you know your history, then
you would know where you're
coming from.*
—Bob Marley, "Buffalo Soldier"

HOW WE LEARN
OUR SEXUAL BELIEFS

How each of us expresses our sexuality depends on our understanding of it. We learn about our sexuality from our families, our peers, the media, schools, religion, laws, government, and our personal experiences. This mix is very different for each of us. That is why each of us has an understanding of our sexuality that may be very different from other people's.

What We Learn from Our Families

Every family teaches messages about sexuality. We base our beliefs about sexuality on what we see others do and on the moral, religious, and philosophical values that bind our families together.

Some families never talk about sexuality, but they still send messages about sexuality by *not* talking about it. It may be confusing for members of the family to interpret these silent messages or understand the values that are intended. The silence could mean that sex is considered something private that should not be discussed within the family. It could mean that members of the family are not comfortable discussing it. It could mean that sexuality is not considered important. It could also mean that sex is considered too dangerous to talk about.

Open discussion about sexuality helps family members understand the family's values and what its messages about sexuality really mean. Children and adults in such families are better informed and more likely to share accurate information. They are also more likely to be able to provide guidance and comfort to one another as they learn about themselves on their sexual journey through life.

What We Learn from Our Peers

It is good to be able to talk about our sexuality with friends. They can provide us with comfort, understand-

27

ing, love, and advice. In fact, many of us trust our friends more than we trust other sources of information. Unfortunately, many rumors and myths about sexuality get passed on through word of mouth among peers.

Some of these myths result from wishful thinking and can be dangerous. For example, it is important to know that girls can get pregnant the first time they have sex or if they are raped. Lots of people, adults as well as kids, don't know this because they believed and repeated incorrect information. It is important to know where our friends learn what they tell us. Likewise, we should double-check information before we pass it on to our friends.

What We Learn from the Media

There's a lot of sex in the media, and many people get their sexuality information from the media. The problem is that the media rarely depict sex accurately. They offer us a lot of mixed messages about sexuality as they exploit sex and sexuality to sell products and ideas. Our families may teach us that sex is serious and that sexual responsibility is important. In the media, sex is glamorous! Sex is for the beautiful! Sex is impulsive! Sex has no consequences!

Advertisers use sex as a selling strategy because young people often have a good deal of money at their disposal. Young people are also naturally very curious about sex. Sex is the perfect hook to hold their attention while products are being pitched. The technique works just as well for people who are no longer young. Most of us remain curious about sex throughout our lives.

We may learn valuable information and ideas about sexuality from TV programs, magazine articles, music videos, or movies. There are some very informative programs and publications, but it is important for us to be critical users of the media so we can sort the realities from the fantasies and the healthy messages from the unhealthy ones.

What We Learn at School

We learn about sexuality at school from our teachers and school officials—whether or not there is a formal sexuality education program. While most schools have some kind of program, most "sex ed" is fairly haphazard and too often reflects the personal biases of teachers and administrators. For example, most do not teach methods of contraception or **safer sex** or allow discussions about sexual orientation. Many programs include **abstinence-only curricula** that urge young people to "just say no" until they are married. Other schools have responsible, **reality-based sexuality education** programs that include age-appropriate information about birth control, safer sex, and sexual orientation.

What We Learn through Religion

Most religions have strong teachings about sexuality. These are moral and ethical viewpoints that members of the religion share as matters of faith and conscience. There is a wide range of religious viewpoints on sex and sexuality. Each takes a particular view of the morality of issues such as sex before marriage, sexual orientation, divorce, and sexual **fidelity.** Many people find great comfort and guidance in the religious teachings they receive.

Some religious teachers, however, attempt to reinforce their moral teachings with information that is not scientifically true. For example, stories that masturbation can make you insane or that women can't get pregnant from rape are used as arguments against masturbation, birth control, and abortion.

Although many people have a casual attitude toward their religion's teaching about sex, religious denominations have a powerful influence on the sexual attitudes of our society. We are all affected by the myths as well as the moral teachings that become accepted in our culture, whether or not we share them.

What We Learn from Our Laws and Government

Every society expresses its sexual values through its laws. Human sexuality is often highly regulated by lawmakers. Depending on the political climate of the times, certain viewpoints prevail, and laws are passed that reflect those values. For example, laws governing **sex workers,** the **age of consent,** marriage, **sexual assault,** sexual orientation, and who can use birth control have changed greatly in the last 100 years.

Many laws about sexuality have been created to protect us, such as those about rape and sexual harassment. Many, however, reflect religious and political viewpoints that are not based in scientific or historical fact. For example, more than 30 states have laws against oral sex that are based on religious beliefs that sex is only for procreation. Often laws that are passed on controversial issues about sexuality reflect the **sexual norms** of the most powerful or the most vocal members of the society and restrict the expression of others.

What We Learn through Personal Experience

One of the most important ways we learn about our sexuality is through our own exploration. We learn from our own experiences with our bodies and minds what it is we like, what it is we don't like, how and where we like to be touched, what turns us off, what turns us on, and who turns us on.

We begin to learn as babies through autoerotic play. As children we may learn more by "playing doctor" with other children. Some of us may remember the curiosity that prompted us to say, "I'll show you mine if you show me yours." We all have a natural desire to learn about our bodies and other people's, too.

Masturbation is one of the ways we can get to know our sexual selves. As we get older, we learn more about our sexual selves when we are ready to have sex with other people. Because we are all different sexually, we may explore new areas of our sexuality with each new sexual relationship we have.

We continue to learn about our sexuality throughout our lives. It is a dynamic dimension of our lives that is always changing and evolving.

OUR CULTURE DETERMINES OUR SEXUAL KNOWLEDGE

Although we have a basic human right to express our sexuality, our sexual knowledge, behavior, and attitudes depend largely on the culture within which we live. Our society determines what sexual information and behaviors are permitted.

Social permission for sexual information and behavior is based on:

- the traditions, customs, values, and beliefs of a people
- economic and political conditions
- the history and experience of the culture

Here are four examples. The first is from religious life. The second is from Africa. The third is from around the world. The fourth is from Indonesia.

- A Catholic priest who takes a vow of celibacy and lives in a monastery with other celibate priests accepts certain restrictions on his sexuality. His sexual knowledge and attitudes will be formed by the customs and traditions of the monastery and his church. He will probably experience his sexuality very differently from women and men who live in different settings.

- In some African countries, the labia and clitorises of young girls are removed to make them marriageable. This ancient custom, called **female circumcision,** is based on the belief that female sexuality must be tamed in women who are going to marry. Increasingly, people within those cultures have come to believe that the health of young girls is more important than this cultural tradition. In most places of the world, this practice is seen as very harmful to young girls, and it is called **female genital mutilation (FGM).** But many people in the cultures that practice female circumcision believe it is their cultural right to do so.

- At first, AIDS was mistakenly identified as a homosexual disease. The world's societies reacted in two different ways. Some enforced stricter sanctions, laws, and punishments against gay men. Others mobilized medical and educational efforts to assist the afflicted and deter the spread of the disease. All societies had the same medical knowledge about AIDS. How each reacted was a result of its cultural attitudes toward homosexuality. Societies that first afforded people with AIDS the full protection of their society were those in which homosexuals had equal status—the Netherlands and Sweden, for example. Cultures that initially discriminated against homosexuals and other people with AIDS were those in which homosexuals had lower status—Cuba, Haiti, and the United States.

- The Sambia of New Guinea believe that women mature naturally, but that boys need to participate in certain rituals in order to become men. The boys' initiation into manhood includes being separated from the women and performing oral sex on the older men. The Sambia believe that the ritual enables the boys to become men and have children. They do not consider the behavior homosexual. In fact, homosexuality is condemned in this culture.

Understanding the Sexual Norms of a Culture

Every culture has **cultural norms** about sex and sexuality. To understand the sex life of any culture, including our own, we look at the culture's sexual norms. No two cultures have the same sexual norms.

People often express **ethnocentric** views by thinking that their culture is better than other cultures or that their culture's norms are the "right" ones. Arguing that one culture is better than another is of little value. It is important to understand that there is great cultural diversity in the world and that we can learn a great deal about ourselves and others by understanding that diversity.

There are basic sexual issues around which sexual norms develop in all cultures. To understand a culture's sexual norms, we need to understand how the culture deals with:

- gender roles
- marriage, partnerships, and family
- childhood sexuality
- sex laws and the punishment of unapproved sexual behavior
- **prostitution**
- homosexuality
- birth control
- sexual assault, abuse, and incest
- sexuality education
- sexual **taboos**
- sex customs

We do not have the space in this book to compare the sexual norms of various cultures with ours. But here are the considerations we would include if we were to do so.

Gender Roles

The social roles assigned to women and men are the foundation of any culture. The answers to these and other questions about gender role will reflect a culture's sexual norms:

- What are the roles of the women and men in the society?
- Do women do the domestic work while the men work outside of the home for food or income?
- Do women and men share equally in the duties of the family and the community? Who raises the children? Who gets an education?

- Who assumes leadership and powerful roles in the society? Men or women?
- Is there a sexual **double standard?**
- Do both genders have equal opportunities and access to resources?

Marriage, Partnerships, and Family

Our family relationships have a great impact on our sexuality. The answers to these and other questions about relationships will reflect a culture's sexual norms:

- Do people choose their spouses, or do their parents arrange their marriages for them?
- Are wives and husbands considered equal partners?
- Is divorce common, rare, accepted, or taboo?
- Are same-sex couples allowed to marry?
- Can a man have more than one wife? Can a woman have more than one husband? Can people live together without marrying?
- How do other family members relate to the wife and husband?
- Do grandparents or elders live with the family? What is their role?
- Are unmarried, same-sex, or interracial couples allowed to become parents?

Childhood Sexuality

We can tell a great deal about how a culture feels about sexuality by looking at how it deals with childhood sexuality. The answers to these and other questions about childhood sexuality will reflect a culture's sexual norms:

- Is children's sexual curiosity about their bodies accepted?
- Are children allowed to express their sexuality?
- Are children allowed, forbidden, or encouraged to have sex play with other children?
- Are children allowed to observe adult sexual activity?

Sex Laws and the Punishment of Unapproved Sexual Behavior

Every culture regulates sexuality on some level. The answers to these and other questions about sexual law will reflect a culture's sexual norms:

- Are there laws restricting prostitution, homosexuality, abortion, and sexual abuse?

- What sexual behaviors are considered "normal"?
- What sexual behaviors are considered "deviant"?
- Are the laws in keeping with the ideals, values, and practices of the culture?
- What sexual behaviors does the culture punish?

Prostitution

Prostitution exists in nearly every culture. The answers to these and other questions about prostitution will reflect a culture's sexual norms:

- Is prostitution an acceptable sexual practice, or is it taboo?
- Are prostitutes required to undergo health checks to guard against the transmission of sexually transmitted infections?
- Do laws force prostitutes to work "underground," making their work more dangerous and less healthy?
- Are prostitutes treated like others who work to support themselves?
- Are prostitutes penalized more than their customers?

Homosexuality

Homosexuality occurs in every culture and throughout the animal kingdom. The answers to these and other questions about homosexuality will reflect a culture's sexual norms:

- Is homosexuality respected as a natural way of life for some people?
- Does the culture condemn homosexuality and discriminate against people perceived to be lesbian, gay, bisexual, or transgender?
- Are lesbian, gay, bisexual, and transgender people able to live openly in heterosexual communities?

Birth Control

People have used birth control since the dawn of time. The answers to these and other questions about birth control and abortion will reflect a culture's sexual norms:

- Is birth control legal, illegal, or taboo?
- Is abortion legal, illegal, or taboo?
- Are birth control and abortion easy to obtain?
- Do women have contraceptive choices to find the method best suited for them?
- Are women forced to use contraception, have abortions, or bear children against their will?

Sexual Assault, Abuse, and Incest

Cultures have very different definitions of rape and other forms of sexual abuse. The answers to these and other questions about sexual abuse will reflect a culture's sexual norms:

- How does the culture define sexual abuse?
- Are the victims stigmatized?
- Are there harsh or lenient penalties for sex offenders?
- Are there laws against incest?
- Are there laws that define age of consent?

Sexuality Education

Sexuality education is fundamental to our sexual growth. The answers to these and other questions about sexuality education will reflect a culture's sexual norms:

- Is sexuality education left entirely to the family?
- Are there formal sexuality education programs for adults and children?
- Are fear tactics used to teach about sex in a negative way?
- Are programs designed to be comprehensive and reality-based, or are they restricted to the teaching of one set of values?

Sexual Taboos

All cultures forbid certain behaviors. The strongest prohibitions are called taboos. For example, sex between mother and son is taboo in most cultures. The answers to these and other questions about sexual taboos will reflect a culture's sexual norms:

- Must a woman be a virgin at marriage?
- Is sex outside of marriage forbidden?
- What sexual behaviors and relationships are forbidden?
- Is talking about sex forbidden?

Sex Customs

All societies have sex customs. They include rituals such as marriage, **circumcision,** and initiation; behaviors, such as kissing, courtship, and waiting until marriage to have sex; and rules, beliefs, and attitudes about sex and sexuality. The answers to these and other questions about sex customs will reflect a culture's sexual norms:

- Who benefits from the custom?

- Who is penalized by the custom?
- Is the custom in keeping with the laws and moral teachings of the culture?
- What is the origin of the custom?

We can ask these questions about our own culture as well as others'. The answers can help us understand our culture's effect upon our own sexuality.

SOME EASTERN ATTITUDES ABOUT SEXUALITY

Many teachings in the Eastern world emphasize the naturalness of sexuality and its spiritual potential. Sexual ecstasy is often seen as a way to spiritual awakening, understanding of self, and transcendence. Sexual pleasure and ecstasy are celebrated by both women and men. Human sexuality is regarded as an integrated part of the daily life of the whole person. It is considered a necessary element of good health.

Many women and men are looking for ways to explore the spiritual potential of their sexuality. The ancient East offers us some models for human sexuality that are different from those that have become familiar in the West.

The *Kama Sutra*

In ancient India, the Hindus believed that there were three aims in life: virtue (*dharma*), prosperity (*artha*), and love (*kama*). The *Dharma Shastra* is a compilation of teachings on ethics; the *Artha Shastra* is a treatise on politics and economy; and the *Kama Shastra* is a discourse on love, eroticism, and the other pleasures of life. The *Kama Shastras* were first compiled into a written text, the *Kama Sutra,* nearly 2,700 years ago, when they were already 1,000 years old.

The *Kama Sutra* is an instructional work that describes various ways of obtaining pleasure. It describes the duties of lovers and marriage partners, whether of the same or other gender, and extols the virtues of marriage for love and the advantages of having only one wife. Much of the text describes various lovemaking techniques, but the fundamental message is that "friendship and love must be practiced between equals, neither with superiors nor with inferiors."

The first English version of the *Kama Sutra* was first widely published in 1960. It became a kind of handbook for the sexual revolution of the 1960s. Written and rewritten throughout the long history of India, however, the version that was popularized in the West reflects Moslem attitudes of the tenth century more than the original Hindu views that inspired it. In the popular version, gender roles are much more delineated, women are subordinate to men, marriage and childbirth are the assumed goals of lovemaking, and same-sex love and marriage have been edited from the text.

Taoism

Taoism is an ancient Chinese teaching that offers insight and guidance in the art of living a harmonious life. There are Tao teachings on health, spirituality, and sexuality. The Tao teaches that sex is necessary for the general health of all people. To deny the sexual energy in the body can create health problems. The Tao teaches that to be against sex is to be against life.

The foundation of the Tao teaching is the concept of the energies of the yin and the yang. Yin energy is water and feminine—a receptive, calm, and negatively charged energy. Yang is fire and masculine—active, stimulating, and positively charged. Everyone has yin and yang energies and must keep them in balance. No one is purely female or male.

The Tao of Loving teaches that sexual union is the way women and men share and balance their yin and yang. Various meditation techniques and sexual positions provide healing for the body by stirring and regulating the flow of energy.

The Tao of Loving opposes masturbation in men in the belief that **semen** contains vital energies needed by the body. **Ejaculation** sacrifices a man's spiritual, mental, and physical energy. The Tao teaches men to remain strong and satisfy their sex partners by reserving ejaculation. It suggests that sex will be more enjoyable if ejaculation is not the goal. Many positions and techniques are suggested, including **erotic** deep kissing and oral sex, as well as ways to induce **retrograde ejaculation,** in which semen is ejaculated into the **bladder** instead of out of the penis. Experimentation is encouraged to find out which techniques and positions best suit each couple.

Women have become more subordinate in Taoist teaching in the years since it began, more than 2,300 years ago. They are now regarded as less than equal to men. But great importance is still given to women's pleasure in the Tao of Loving.

Tantrism

Tantric sex is meant to be a divine meditation and a way to connect to God. Tantrism is believed to have originated in India thousands of years ago. It is an aspiration to spiritual enlightenment that is achieved by channeling the life energy, *kundalini,* through the seven energy points of the body that are called *chakras.* Spiritual ecstasy or bliss can be achieved by controlled breathing, energy flow, and assuming certain positions.

As in the Tao, everyone has female and male energies that should be kept in balance. Because the spiritual energy of men is more limited than that of women, the Tantra teaches men to enjoy sex without the loss of semen, which is associated with spiritual energy. Men learn to control ejaculation so that intercourse is prolonged for hours. Sexual arousal is considered an energy that is maintained for its own sake, not for reaching orgasm.

The Rite of the Five Essences is a Tantric love ritual performed using the "five enjoyments"—wine, meat, fish, cereal grain, and sexual intercourse. Music, incense, candlelight, and flowers are also used to enhance this "communion." Meditation is used to awaken the *kundalini.* Centuries ago, a guru would preside over such Tantric rituals. The guru would watch over several couples to ensure they used the correct techniques to aspire to the higher order of the Tantra without becoming self-indulgent. The original meaning of the beliefs and rituals may be lost in the practice of Tantrism in today's Western cultures.

OUR SEXUAL NORMS HAVE CHANGED THROUGHOUT OUR HISTORY

Sexual norms are an important means of social control. As the needs of a society change, so do its sexual norms. These shifts and changes can have a dramatic impact on an individual's personal life. Here are some examples of sexual norms and how they were changed in the history of our culture.

Native Americans

Before the arrival of the Europeans, Native Americans lived in a great many different cultures with diverse cultural and sexual norms. Nevertheless, many viewpoints were commonly held. Sexual attitudes were more Eastern than Western in many ways. In general, sex was considered normal and healthy.

Native Americans exercised a great deal of personal freedom of choice in their sexual expression. With some exceptions, childhood sexual experimentation, same-sex sex play, cross-dressing, **polygamy, premarital sex,** and **extramarital sex** were common aspects of Native American sex lives.

In many tribes, homosexuals were regarded with spiritual respect. There were special ceremonies or initiations to celebrate these members of a tribe. Many tribes believed homosexuals belonged to a third gender. Some tribes referred to homosexuals as two-spirited—female and male. In many tribes, such as the Mohave, two-spirited people were viewed as highly evolved spiritual people who could use their supernatural healing powers to become shamans for their tribes. They were called berdache.

Colonial Americans

Compared to Native Americans, the colonists had much less accepting views of sexuality. Colonists and early settlers were English, Dutch, Spanish, Portuguese, French, Russian, Scandinavian, and German. Although their sexual norms varied, many were shared in common. They were generally Protestant or Catholic. Nearly all were Christian. In the Christian view, sex was for procreation. Sexual pleasure had been considered sinful in early Christian times, and for most Europeans, the taint of sinfulness was still attached to sexual activity outside of marriage and reproduction.

These rigid views clashed with the more accepting views of the indigenous people. Colonists and settlers considered the sexual norms of Native Americans to be "immoral," "impure," or "unnatural." It was largely the difference in sexual norms that led European settlers to depict Native Americans as "savages."

Eventually, missionaries and government agents were sent into native communities to try to teach and enforce Western religion and sexual norms. Territorial and state governments went so far as to kidnap native children and send them to boarding schools, where they were isolated from their native cultures and forbidden to speak their native languages. The assault on native culture was very effective. Native Americans of today face great challenges in their attempts to restore and revive their cultural heritage.

Slavery and Sexuality

One of the ways that the institution of slavery was maintained was to enforce sexual norms for slaves that were different from those of the **dominant culture.** Independent and proud people had been stolen from their homes and sold into slavery. Slave owners had to do something to keep them from becoming defiant and rebellious. The strategy they decided upon was to treat these human beings as though they were animals in order to make them docile.

The sexuality of slaves was systematically violated. They were not allowed to marry or maintain love relationships. They were not allowed to wear underwear. Boys were not allowed to wear trousers until they were fully grown; both genders wore gender neutral "shimmies."

In the effort to dehumanize them, slaves were forced to breed like cattle regardless of affection or pleasure. They were used for sexual pleasure by their owners. They were forced to share loved ones with their masters. They were paraded naked and publicly inspected in slave markets. They were kept from knowing their birthdays. They were kept ignorant of their parentage. Children were forced to eat their meals from troughs and accept sexual abuse from their owners. Slaves who refused to submit to these norms were beaten, killed, or sold.

Damaging sexual myths and stereotypes were developed to absolve "masters" of their roles in degrading the women and men they owned. Black women, whose sex lives were forced upon them, were considered sexually permissive. White women, often ignored by slave owners, were depicted as sexually virtuous, pure, and chaste. After the repeal of slavery, black men were characterized as sexual predators by white property owners who feared reprisals for the centuries of mistreatment black people had experienced.

These **sexual stereotypes** pushed black women into relationships they didn't want, forced many white women to be chaste despite their real desires, and made black men the objects of fear and suspicion.

There were exceptions, of course. Some plantation owners were more humane than others. In general, however, slaves were deprived of their basic human rights, including their sexual rights, for more than 200 years. It is a tribute to them, their descendants, and the valor of the human spirit that African-Americans have come so far from the horrors of that heritage. They, too, face great challenges, as they try to restore and revive their preslavery cultural heritage.

Interracial Sexual Relations

Although common, interracial relationships were taboo during slavery. They still carry a social stigma today. After the Civil War, laws were passed in most states against **miscegenation**—sex, **cohabitation,** or marriage between people of different races. People who had interracial sex were punished by imprisonment and fines. If a couple left their state to avoid laws against interracial marriage and returned to that state after marriage, they could be prosecuted.

Laws against interracial sexual relations also reflected the sexual and racial double standards of the times. White men could have sex with African-American, Spanish-American, or Native American women and escape unpunished. If white women had sexual relationships with black men, however, they would experience scorn and social stigma and could be sent to jail. Their partners were the targets of mob violence and lynching. Interracial love relationships were commonly characterized as rape in order to uphold the myth of the pure white woman as victim of the predatory black man.

It wasn't until 1967 that the U.S. Supreme Court overthrew all miscegenation laws in its decision *Loving v. the Commonwealth of Virginia.*

The Victorians

Named after the reigning Queen of England, the Victorian period extended from about 1840 to 1900. The economic changes of the Industrial Revolution during this time greatly affected the sexual norms of Europe and America. Factory labor required most men to work away from home. Most women were required to stay at home to provide child care and domestic support for their husbands.

Urban industrial life offered increased sexual opportunities for laborers in the cities. In an effort to protect the family from the effects of this potential promiscuity, extreme social pressures were developed to compel women and men to strictly control their sexuality. Once again, sex and sexuality became regarded as dangerous and dirty, and bizarre myths and practices were fostered.

Leading health authorities suggested that married couples should have sex only once every three years, that men were too frail for sex until they reached the age of 30, that women could take no pleasure in sex, and that masturbation caused insanity. The myth that "good girls" and wives were incapable of sexual excitement led men to the habitual use of prostitutes for sexual pleasure. "Virtuous" Victorian families were headed by men whose secret sex lives included regular visits to brothels. As a result, the sexual double standard grew to enormous proportions and sexually transmitted infections became epidemic.

Torturous methods were sometimes employed to preserve the sexual innocence of children and adolescents. **Chastity belts** were devised for girls and boys. Parents applied ointments to the genitals of their children to make them painful to touch. Surgeons inserted rings into the foreskin of the penis so boys could urinate without touching themselves. Carbolic acid was used to burn the clitorises of girls who masturbated. Castration was used to cure boys of "excessive" masturbation.

Birth Control

It wasn't until 1965 that married women and men won the right to use birth control everywhere in the United States. It was another six years before unmarried couples won that right. Since the beginning of the twentieth century, America's family planning movement has been in the forefront of the battle for women's sexual equality. During this time, women firmly established their right to make and carry out their own decisions about when or whether to bear children. This liberty is so fundamental, it is hard to believe that only a short time ago those who fought for reproductive freedom went to jail.

By gaining the right to control their fertility, women also vastly improved their own health conditions and those of their children. Death rates for mothers and infants have plummeted since birth control was legalized. The quality of family life has also improved. When women can limit their family size, they can give more attention, love, patience, and guidance to the children they have. They are happier, and their children are healthier.

The desire for family planning began with the dawn of human history, when women attempted to prevent pregnancy with amulets and incantations. Before the discovery and distribution of modern contraceptives, women and men tried all sorts of remedies to prevent unintended pregnancy.

In colonial America, sexuality was about reproduction. Women and men were expected to enjoy sex, but the primary function of sex was to produce children. Women were expected to marry and bear children. That was their exclusive role for many generations.

Men learned "self-control" as a birth control method. They were to go without, or reserve, ejaculation in order to decrease the chance of pregnancy. This method was called by its Latin name, *coitus reservatus.* Self-control could also mean abstaining from sexual intercourse entirely. These methods were suggested in health books and pamphlets for married couples in the eighteenth, nineteenth, and early twentieth centuries. It is hard to say how many couples actually used them.

Women also used herbal treatments before and after intercourse to prevent pregnancy. They also placed pessaries made of various ingredients in their vaginas to keep sperm from moving into the **uterus.** Recipes for the methods that seemed to be effective were handed down, generation to generation.

Between the 1830s and the 1870s, information about contraceptive methods was widely circulated in the United States. The most commonly used method was probably *coitus interruptus,* which required a man to withdraw his penis from the vagina to ejaculate outside the woman's body. This method is now called **withdrawal.** "Female syringes" were available for women. They were used to douche the vagina with chemicals such as alum or sulfates of zinc or iron.

Cervical caps and condoms made of animal membranes were also available, but they were expensive. The first **diaphragm,** "the Wife's Protector," was patented in 1846. It was made of wood, sponge, and cotton.

Diaphragms and condoms could be made more cheaply after the invention of the vulcanization of rubber in 1844. By 1870, the prices of contraceptives had dropped, and most people could afford them. Contraceptives had become so popular that various groups of people, including many doctors, began to protest their use.

Many feared that the use of contraception would make women promiscuous and "lower" them to the status of prostitutes. Many also feared that birth control would lower the rate of population growth among white people and lead to social domination by people of color.

In 1873, anti-family planning crusaders won a major victory when the U.S. Congress passed the first **Comstock Act,** named after Anthony Comstock, the man who wrote it. This law prohibited the distribution of contraceptive information or devices through the U.S. mail.

The Reproductive Rights Movement

In 1915, Mary Ware Dennett founded the National Birth Control League. It was the first birth control organization in the country. The league worked to repeal the Comstock laws. Dennett believed that information about sexuality and contraception was crucial to the health and happiness of the American family.

Dennett wrote *The Sex Side of Life,* a sexuality information guide for young people. She was charged with **obscenity** under the Comstock laws in 1929 and was found guilty and jailed. When the verdict was reversed in 1930, Dennett won one of the first victories against Anthony Comstock. Despite her efforts, however, the National Birth Control League was short-lived.

Margaret Sanger and America's First Birth Control Clinic

The reproductive rights movement was firmly established on October 16, 1916, in the Brownsville community of Brooklyn, New York, when Margaret Sanger, her sister, Ethel Byrne, and an associate, Fania Mindell, opened the first birth control clinic in America. They provided contraceptive advice to desperately poor, immigrant women who lined up hours before the clinic doors opened.

Less than a month later, all three women were charged with violating New York's antiobscenity statutes. They were arrested, indicted, and sent to prison for discussing and distributing contraceptives. The resulting publicity caused great widespread anger against the injustice of forcing women to bear children they could not afford and did not want.

In 1923, Sanger founded the Birth Control Clinical Research Bureau. The bureau treated patients and kept comprehensive records that would demonstrate the need to broaden the interpretation of federal and state Comstock laws and allow women to contracept for health reasons.

In 1936, the birth control movement achieved one of its greatest victories. Judge Augustus Hand, writing for the U.S. Circuit Court of Appeals in the case of *U.S. v. One Package of Japanese Pessaries,* ordered a sweeping liberalization of federal Comstock laws as applied to the importing of contraceptive devices.

Federal agents, acting under the Comstock laws, had seized a shipment of contraband diaphragms—Japanese pessaries—that was addressed to Sanger's Birth Control Clinical Research Bureau. Judge Hand decided that birth control could no longer be classified as obscene in his jurisdiction—New York, Connecticut, and Vermont. He cited contemporary data on the health consequences of unplanned pregnancy and the benefits of contraception.

In the years following *One Package,* the ideas that had made Sanger controversial ceased to be shocking and gradually became entrenched in American public life. In 1939, the two organizations Sanger had founded—the American Birth Control League and the Birth Control Clinical Research Bureau—merged to become the Birth Control Federation of America, which was later renamed the Planned Parenthood Federation of America.

Advances in Contraceptive Research

Sanger avidly supported the development of a "magic pellet"—an inexpensive, medically safe, completely reliable contraceptive that could be taken orally or by injection. Years of scientific and advocacy efforts were rewarded in the early 1950s, when Dr. Gregory Pincus demonstrated that injections of the steroid **progesterone** could stop ovulation in laboratory animals. In 1960, the U.S. Food and Drug Administration approved the sale of oral steroid pills—"the Pill"—for contraceptive use.

Shortly thereafter, the first **IUDs (intrauterine devices)** became available. While later findings revealed that neither the Pill nor the IUD was problem-free for all users, they heralded major advances both in science and in attitudes about sexual and reproductive freedom. The advent of safe, effective, and inexpensive contraception helped propel the contemporary women's liberation movement.

Legalization of Family Planning

Legalization of family planning and reproductive rights for women took a great step forward in 1965, when the U.S. Supreme Court, in *Griswold v. Connecticut,* struck down state laws prohibiting the use of contraceptives by married couples. The decision paved the way for the nearly unanimous acceptance of contraception that now exists in this country. Two years later, the United Nations Declaration on Population proclaimed family planning a basic human right and established the United Nations Fund for Population Activities.

Legalization of Abortion

The most dramatic advance in reproductive rights during the 1970s took place in the midst of a reawakened civil rights movement, the winding down of the war in Vietnam, and the drive for the Equal

Rights Amendment. On January 22, 1973, the U.S. Supreme Court handed down its decision in *Roe v. Wade,* which struck down restrictive abortion laws throughout the nation. It declared that the U.S. Constitution protects a woman's right, in consultation with her physician, to choose to have an abortion.

The Anti-Abortion Backlash

Not surprisingly, the more the family planning movement was absorbed into the mainstream, the more vigorously reactionary, religious opposition marshaled its forces. The first anti-family planning organizations were launched in several U.S. communities in the 1960s, with strong support from the Catholic church. In 1973, the National Right to Life Committee was organized by the U.S. Catholic Conference's Family Life Division. Its express purpose was to overturn *Roe v. Wade* and the new state statutes that had made abortion safe and legal.

Many supporters of these **anti-choice** organizations oppose contraception as well as abortion. They have proposed statutes and constitutional amendments that would outlaw the IUD and some forms of the Pill and severely restrict access to federally funded family planning services. Opposition to contraception within the anti-abortion movement continues to this day.

In the mid-1970s, the impact of anti-abortion organizing began to be felt in public policy. Congress passed the first version of the Hyde Amendment in 1976, barring any government support for abortions for poor women. Anti-abortion restrictions were added to numerous bills in subsequent years, continuously reducing the number of women eligible to receive federal assistance for abortions.

Anti-Abortion Terrorism

Many religious-political extremists turned to terrorism in the 1980s and 1990s as a result of their continuing failure to decisively overturn *Roe v. Wade* through the courts or by a constitutional amendment. Efforts to barricade clinics and the harassment of patients and reproductive health care workers have become commonplace. In the past two decades, there have been hundreds of bombings, acts of arson, and bombing or arson attempts launched against family planning and abortion clinics. Death threats and kidnapping have also become terrorizing weapons of the anti-choice arsenal.

In the early 1990s, clinic doctors and workers were shot and killed by anti-abortion protesters in Florida and Massachusetts. Five people were murdered at the women's health centers where they worked.

Not since Margaret Sanger opened the Brownsville clinic have family planning activists had to fight such opposition and harassment from the anti-choice minority and from the government. Nevertheless, the overwhelming majority of Americans continue to believe that individuals should be able to make their own reproductive decisions without government interference.

Sexually Transmitted Infections

Throughout history, sexually transmitted infections were often seen as physical evidence of moral decay rather than health problems. There has been a great tension between those who wanted to improve public morals at the expense of public health and those who wanted to improve public health regardless of public morals. The tension between those two viewpoints has had an enormous impact on our sexual norms.

Gonorrhea and Syphilis

There were overlapping epidemics of syphilis and **gonorrhea** in Europe and the United States from the sixteenth to the early nineteenth centuries. The common hiring of prostitutes by men before and during marriage spread the infections throughout entire families and communities. It was assumed that gonorrhea and syphilis were the same until 1837, when a French **venereologist** proved that they were two different infections.

Each caused many serious health problems and illnesses. Gonorrhea caused sterility and blindness in newborns. Syphilis caused birth defects and could lead to madness and death. Many of the available treatments were painful and not very effective. Some, such as large doses of mercury, had serious side effects. Others were brutal. For instance, one doctor recommended placing the penis on a table and hitting it with a book to cure the curvature that resulted from gonorrhea!

Progressivism

The Progressive Movement was formed at the end of the nineteenth century to seek more government and state intervention in social and economic issues. "Venereal disease" was a major concern within Progressive reform.

Progressive physicians tried to address the problem of venereal disease within the changing social context of American life. They were the first to promote sexuality education as a way to protect women and men from sexually transmitted infections. They also sought to break the American man's habit of using prostitutes. They saw prostitution as the vice that caused infection and the breakdown of families. Many doctors saw themselves as protectors of families and guardians of women's role as mothers.

The Social Hygiene Movement

A New York physician named Prince Morrow believed that as long as there was shame attached to sexually transmitted infections, people would not seek treatment. In 1905, he formed the Society of Sanitary and Moral Prophylaxis to break the silence. The social hygiene movement called for frank discussion of sexuality and for sexuality education in schools.

Like many conservatives of today, social hygienists were motivated by what they observed as "moral decay." Social hygienists, however, advocated the use of comprehensive sexuality education. They wanted to teach people how to avoid temptation. They supported state-mandated blood tests before marriage and compulsory reporting of diagnosed sexually transmitted infections. They also became the loudest voices in the movement against prostitution.

World War I

Soldiers, away from home, want sex. That's why sex workers flock to military camps. During World War I, sexually transmitted infections among soldiers were viewed as undermining the efficiency of the military. At home and abroad, soldiers lost nearly 7 million days of work as sick days because of sexually transmitted infections. Infection was also seen as a moral issue.

The Committee on Training Camp Activities was formed a few days after Congress declared war in 1917. It provided recreation to keep off-duty soldiers busy so that they would not succumb to sexual temptations. The committee also provided sex education for the soldiers. The teachers used fear tactics and advocated abstinence. Condoms were not discussed. Of all the soldiers in Europe during

World War I, Americans had the highest rates of infection. They were the only ones who were forbidden the use of condoms.

Social hygienists volunteered to aid the committee's moral reform effort. They urged soldiers to avoid infection for the good of their country and to protect the virtuous women at home from infection.

A law enforcement division of the committee was also formed to clear prostitutes out of cities near military camps. Most cities in America had "red-light districts" of brothels in which sex workers entertained customers. The committee closed these districts all across the country. Despite the shutdown, rates of infection remained unchanged. Sex workers simply moved to other neighborhoods. As brothels were closed, working the streets became common, and the risk of violence against prostitutes increased.

Although prostitutes were working-class women with few other employment options, many were stigmatized and blamed for the spread of infection and moral decay. Men who hired them, however, were neither arrested nor blamed.

As brothels near military bases closed, soldiers turned to young women who were hanging around looking for excitement, adventure, and love. Soon these young women were being called promiscuous and blamed for infection rates among the soldiers. Public health campaigns were mounted that suggested it was women's responsibility not to arouse the passions of men. Health messages suggested that "easy" women were usually infected and were not trustworthy.

Treatment centers, called prophylaxis stations, were set up in the camps to kill any infection a soldier might pick up before it got into his bloodstream. The social hygienists disapproved. They thought prophylaxis encouraged soldiers to have "illicit" sexual contacts.

Soldiers were supposed to be treated within three hours of sexual intercourse. Unsanitary conditions, long waiting lines, and embarrassment discouraged many of them. A man had to urinate, then wash his genitals and have them inspected by an attendant. The attendant injected a liquid solution into the penis that the man had to hold in his **urethra** for five minutes. He wasn't to urinate for four or five hours after expelling it.

To encourage prophylaxis, men were threatened with court-martial if they became infected. Their pay was docked as well.

Between the World Wars

The events of war created a new openness about sexuality. American soldiers overseas became acquainted with the sexual norms of other cultures. As brothels in the United States were closed, men were more likely to establish sexual relationships with women who were not sex workers, especially unmarried women. Despite the increase in sexual activity during the 1920s, federal funding was cut for programs to fight sexually transmitted infections.

During the Great Depression, rates of infection increased because so few people could afford treatment. People with sexually transmitted infections were stigmatized. Hospitals refused to treat them. As a result, infections increased and the stigma against people with them became stronger.

In the 1930s, social hygienists came under fire. President Franklin D. Roosevelt appointed Thomas Parran as U.S. Surgeon General in 1936. Parran was determined to deal with sexually transmitted infections as a health problem, not a moral dilemma. He had a five-point plan to control syphilis:

1. Identify women and men with syphilis.
2. Treat them.
3. Contact and screen their sex partners.
4. Mandate blood tests before marriage and early in pregnancy.
5. Educate the public about syphilis.

Parran rejected the moral stigmas that prevented the development of effective public health programs. In 1938, his National Venereal Disease Control Act was passed by Congress. It provided funding for treatment and prevention programs.

Moral stigma and the fear of syphilis—syphilophobia—undermined Parran's program, however. Myths emerged that associated syphilis with certain ethnic groups and social classes. Twenty-six states prohibited marriage of infected people.

In 1932, the Public Health Service began a tragic experiment that would last for 40 years. This unethical experiment was known as the Tuskegee Syphilis Study. Public health officials wanted to find out what would happen if syphilis went untreated. Four hundred African-American sharecroppers in Alabama were selected for this study. For 40 years, they believed they were receiving treatment for syphilis when they were not. About 100 men died as a result. It wasn't until the public found out about the experiment in 1972 that it ended. The doctors who designed the study made the racist assumptions that all blacks were infected and that the subjects would not have sought treatment, anyway.

Although the condom was known to protect against sexually transmitted infections, the American Social Hygiene Association opposed its use, despite the commonsense arguments of the Birth Control Federation of America. Discovered in 1928, penicillin wasn't found to be an effective treatment for syphilis or gonorrhea until the 1940s.

World War II and Condoms

As many as 50 million condoms were distributed to American soldiers each month during World War II. The army also provided fear-based sexuality education classes and medical prophylaxis. The law that docked the pay of infected soldiers was repealed.

Prostitution was suppressed once again, although a number of health officials saw "benefits" to prostitution. They suggested that prostitution reduced the incidence of rape and homosexuality. They advocated segregating prostitutes in areas near the bases and providing them with regular medical exams. Despite this advice, more than 700 cities and towns closed their red-light districts.

From Herpes to AIDS

Many people had many partners during the "sexual liberation" of the "swinging" 1960s and 1970s. One result was an epidemic of herpes. Many infected women and men felt great shame and guilt, even though herpes is not a serious health condition. The stigma once attached to syphilis and gonorrhea was transferred to people with herpes. For some time, they were seen as sexually promiscuous, perhaps even immoral. In time, hot lines and support groups were formed to help restore a sense of normalcy to the lives of people with herpes.

In the early 1980s, the stigma associated with herpes was overshadowed by the stigma associated with AIDS. First known as gay-related immune disease, AIDS was first identified among gay men and later among intravenous drug users—groups that were already severely stigmatized. People with AIDS were commonly discriminated against or refused medical and social services in the first years of the epidemic.

As the epidemic progressed, other groups became targets for discrimination. Even children fell into the line of fire. Many people thought that children with HIV should not be allowed to go to school. Some parents kept their children at home when students with

HIV were allowed in school. Women were viewed as transmitters of the infection, and only pregnant women were included in most studies. It was more than 10 years into the epidemic before the definition of AIDS was changed to include conditions specific to women.

It is now very clear that all IV (intravenous) drug users and sexually active women and men, all over the world, are at risk for AIDS. Despite public education campaigns and media attention, however, ignorance about AIDS still exists, and arguments continue about the morality of the use of condoms by people at risk of HIV. Today, teenagers and women have the fastest-growing rates of HIV infection.

There is now widespread research being done on AIDS. Although there are improved treatments for many conditions associated with HIV disease, there is still no cure. We have to rely on preventive techniques, including sexual health education. Early in the epidemic, the gay community buckled down to educate itself about HIV and safer sex. Its efforts paid off, and the infection rate in the gay community has fallen. Although the IV drug community was more difficult to mobilize than the gay community, needle-exchange programs have been effective in urban areas.

Despite the evident effectiveness of educational campaigns, the majority of high school students in the United States are still deprived of responsible sexuality education that includes information about contraception, sexual orientation, and safer sex. The old stigmas about sexually transmitted infections still haunt us.

The AIDS epidemic, however, is forcing our society to deal more openly with sex and sexuality. Educators, the media, public health officials, medical professionals, parents, young people, and children are all much more likely to speak frankly and directly about sex than our great-great-grandparents did at the beginning of the century.

"Sexual Revolutions" That Have Affected Our Sexual Norms

Sexual norms and gender equality have been crucial concerns of various social and political movements throughout our history. These include the civil rights and antiwar movements as well as the movements for women's equality and gay liberation. They all have had a major impact on our attitudes toward sex and sexuality today. Here are some of the highlights:

First-Wave Feminists: The Women's Movement— Suffragists and Abolitionists

Women began fighting for the right to vote—suffrage—20 years before the Civil War. The suffrage movement was born out of the abolitionist movement that fought to outlaw slavery. Elizabeth Cady Stanton and Lucretia Mott held the first women's rights conference in Stanton's home in Seneca Falls, New York, in 1848.

The suffrage movement split from the abolitionist movement before the Civil War began. Some women found it unacceptable that men in the movement wanted to postpone the suffrage effort until after slaves were emancipated. Many women remained with the abolitionists under the leadership of Lucy Stone. Others formed their own movement under Stanton, Mott, and Susan B. Anthony. They widened the suffrage agenda to include issues such as divorce reform, sexism in the church, and assistance for workingwomen.

Temperance and Moral Reform

In 1874, the Women's Christian Temperance Union was established to work for moral reform. The union worked toward eliminating prostitution, improving public education, and enacting universal suffrage. Its chief goal, however, was temperance—abolishing the sale of alcohol. Union members believed that drinking was a threat to the American home—that drunken husbands wasted money on liquor and were abusive to their wives and children.

The social purity campaign against prostitution grew out of the temperance movement at the end of the nineteenth century. Its members worked to create a single standard of sexual conduct in the belief that prostitutes were the victims of male vice.

The Sexual Revolution of the 1920s

The soldiers who experienced the sexual norms of Europe during World War I changed the sexual norms of the United States when they returned home. They became much more likely to have intercourse with women for whom they cared than with prostitutes or casual sex partners. Young women and men began to develop equality in romantic relationships and sexual behaviors. The number of women who had sexual intercourse before marriage increased from 25 percent at the turn of the century to 50 percent by the 1920s.

The Sexual Revolution of the 1960s

The 1960s were marked by enormous political and social upheavals. President John F. Kennedy and civil rights activist Dr. Martin Luther King, Jr., were assassinated. The Civil Rights Act was passed, the anti-war movement led to mass protests across the country, and the Equal Rights Amendment for women was debated in statehouses across the nation. The increasing availability of contraception allowed women and men to seek sexual pleasure with decreased fear of unintended pregnancy. A new "singles" culture developed among young people, and marriage was no longer seen as the only option in women's lives.

Second-Wave Feminists: The Women's Movement of the 1960s and 1970s

Since the beginning of the century, women had gained the right to vote, they were more competitive in the workplace, and they had made many strides in gender equality. But American culture remained dominated by men. Women's share in positions of political and economic power was still small. In 1966, Betty Friedan founded the National Organization for Women to support the Equal Rights Amendment, end sexist discrimination in the workplace, and make abortion safe and legal.

Women began to meet in consciousness-raising groups to talk about sexism, gender roles, and the oppression of women. Out of this work came the understanding that "the personal is political"—that the sexual double standard, motherhood, and marriage had become elements in a system of gender roles that made women subordinate to men.

Women of the 1960s demanded the right to control their own bodies and broke the silence that concealed the crimes of rape, sexual abuse, and domestic violence. Hundreds of women's groups and organizations were formed focusing on issues from **pornography** to prostitution, from lesbian rights to sexual pleasure, from child support to domestic violence.

Black Feminism

African-American feminists found unacceptable levels of sexism in the often male-centered civil rights, Black Nationalist, and Black Panther movements. Many also felt excluded from the mainstream women's movement. In 1973, Audre Lorde and other black feminists formed the National Black Feminist Organization to address the combined effects of oppression related to race, gender, class, and sexual orientation. In recent years, the black feminist movement has generated a variety of organizations that address specific concerns of the African-American community.

Third-Wave Feminists

For many young women, the term "feminist" has become suspect. Many, however, still speak out for increased gender equality and for the recognition of the many other problems women yet face in our culture. The 1990s ushered in a new era of young feminists. Rebecca Walker founded an organization for young feminists called Third Wave. Diversity is the hallmark of this chapter in the history of the women's movement. It addresses the dynamics of ethnic, racial, class, and sexual diversity.

Gay Liberation

On a Friday night in the summer of 1969, a group of police officers raided a gay bar in Greenwich Village in New York City in order to arrest women and men who they thought were gay. Such raids were common, but on this night the patrons of the Stonewall Inn decided they had had enough of this legalized form of harassment. Lesbian, gay, bisexual, and transgender people resisted arrest, overcame the police, and launched a demonstration that lasted several days.

Within weeks, the Gay Liberation Front was formed to seek justice and equal protection under the law for all members of the gay community. Lesbians, gay men, bisexuals, and transgender people began making themselves visible at political rallies and antiwar demonstrations. Gay activists challenged the socially approved **heterosexism** that oppressed them, and they began to "come out"—to publicly acknowledge their gayness. Finally, in 1974, the American Psychiatric Association removed homosexuality from its list of mental disorders.

The **gay liberation movement** continues to seek changes that will make it illegal to deprive women or men of their civil rights because of their sexual orientation.

The Struggle for Responsible Sexuality Education

Most American parents want their children to receive comprehensive, age-appropriate, reality-based sexuality education. Public schools, however, have become major battlefields in the struggle to provide young people with the information they need to develop sexual health and well-being.

Many of the same people who oppose legal abortion, safer sex education, birth control, and civil rights for lesbian, gay, bisexual, and transgender people also oppose responsible sexuality education. Few in number, but well organized and often belligerent, opponents include political extremists affiliated with the religious right. They belong to organizations such as the American Family Association, Citizens for Excellence in Education, the Christian Coalition, the Eagle Forum, the National Association for Abstinence Education, Concerned Women of America, and Focus on the Family. These advocates of abstinence-only, fear-based programs continue to infiltrate school boards by mounting "stealth candidates" whose political ties and agendas are disguised until after election ballots are counted.

In contrast, Planned Parenthood, the Society for the Scientific Study of Sexuality, the American Association of Sex Educators, Counselors and Therapists, the Sexuality Information and Education Council for the United States, and more than 90 other organizations are committed to exposing and opposing these political maneuvers. The outcome of this struggle remains to be seen.

SEXOLOGY—THE STUDY OF SEX AND SEXUALITY

The study of sex and sexuality is called **sexology,** or sexual science. We learn a great deal about sexuality by comparative studies of sex in animals, insects, and humans. Sex research helps us sort reality from myth. It helps us learn how to maintain sexual health and understand the physical, medical, and emotional problems related to sex and sexuality. For example, in the 1940s, men who admitted they masturbated could be rejected from serving in the armed forces because masturbation was thought to form dependent, weak, and irrational personalities. Careful scientific research proved this assumption to be untrue. Masturbating, privately or with a partner, is now understood to be a normal and healthy part of human sexuality.

Some Pioneers of Sexual Science

Sexual science is a comparatively young research area. The community of sexologists continues to grow. Sexologists come from many different scientific disciplines. They provide perspectives on the social, medical, psychological, biological, historical, and physiological aspects of sexuality. An increasing number of community activists is also at work to advance the general public's knowledge of sexual issues.

Many people have contributed to our knowledge about sexuality. Their work has had a major impact on changing the sexual norms of our culture. Here are brief descriptions of some of the key pioneers in the development of sexual science:

Havelock Ellis (1859–1939)

Ellis was an early English sexologist who promoted tolerance for sexual diversity. He worked to reform repressive sex laws. He tried to convince society that sexual exploration by infants and adolescents, masturbation, and homosexuality were all natural behaviors. He believed birth control was the key to sexual liberation. He believed sex to be natural and good, and asked, "Why...should people be afraid of rousing passions which, after all, are the great driving forces of human life?"

Sigmund Freud (1856–1939)

Freud was a very influential psychoanalyst who believed that we must understand human sexuality if we are to understand human nature. He understood that children have strong sexual feelings, and believed that everyone is naturally bisexual. He developed a theory—the **Oedipal conflict**—which maintains that children have natural sexual impulses toward their parents. He also theorized that girls have "penis envy" and want to have penises just as boys have.

Freud's ideas were not always based on scientific facts. Many of them have since been refuted or disproved. His work is enormously important, however, because it established the wide discussion of sexuality that continues to this day.

Clelia D. Mosher (1863–1940)

Mosher began surveying her women patients about their sexual histories in the late nineteenth century. She wanted to find out more about what married women knew and felt about sex so that she could counsel women with better sexual advice before they married. She found that women had little accurate information about sex and often entered marriage in complete ignorance about sex and reproduction.

Mosher could be called a closet researcher, because she never published the results of her survey. The research she began in 1892 was not published until 1974, long after her death.

Katharine Bement Davis (1860–1945)

Davis completed the first major study on women's sexuality. In 1929, she published her study "Factors in the Sex Lives of Twenty Two Hundred Women." She gathered data for more than 10 years about the sex lives of middle-class women. She also worked extensively with prostitutes in prisons. She examined such topics as sexual desire, masturbation, frequency of intercourse, use of birth control, marriage, sources of sexual instruction and information, and same-sex intimate relationships.

Her study challenged the narrow reproductive view of women's sexuality common at the beginning of the twentieth century. It was our first real glimpse into the sex lives of real women.

Magnus Hirschfeld (1868–1935)

Hirschfeld was a German sexologist who founded the Institute of Sexual Science in Berlin in 1919. He studied human sexuality in order to provide counseling for sexual problems. He published one of the world's first sexological journals to encourage open debate about sexual issues. He also believed masturbation and homosexual behavior were normal and healthy. He challenged many of the repressive ideas about sexuality of his time. The institute's and most of Hirschfeld's research were destroyed by the Nazis in 1935.

Alfred Kinsey (1894–1956)

Kinsey has been the most influential American sex researcher of the twentieth century. His research was unique and groundbreaking. In extensive live interviews, he and his team of researchers took thousands of case histories of the lives of women and men. No one else, before or since, has questioned such a huge **sample** of people so thoroughly about their sexuality. Although his sample did not precisely reflect the full range of diversity of the American people, he and his team provided us with important data from which we have learned a great deal.

William Masters (1915–) and Virginia Johnson (1925–)

Masters and Johnson are responsible for our understanding of the human **sexual response cycle.** They used minicameras and other electronic devices to observe what was going on inside and outside the body during the various phases of sexual arousal.

They noticed and measured functions in the bodies of women and men that no one else had been able to observe. They first developed the concept of **sex therapy** by working with couples to help them overcome sexual problems, including **sexual dysfunction.**

Michel Foucault (1926–1984)

Foucault was a French philosopher who wrote three volumes on the history of sexuality. He challenged Freud's view that women and men are sexually repressed by their cultures. He theorized about the role of power in sexual relationships. He suggested that power does not always come from the top down, but from the bottom up as well. He believed that people have sexual power as individuals, despite sexual law or cultural norms.

Although his ideas were not always based in scientific or historical fact, Foucault's work enabled many people who belonged to oppressed sexual minorities to view themselves as powerful individuals, capable of resisting dominant sexual norms.

Foucault died of AIDS in 1984.

The rich and changing traditions, history, and beliefs described in this chapter have shaped our society with extremely diverse messages and values about sex and sexuality. The differences between the various messages and values may often seem confusing and conflicting. In the following chapters, we will look at the ways in which people develop their own **sexual identities** within this world of sexual diversity.

CHAPTER 3

Our Sexual Bodies

How beautiful are thy feet with shoes, O prince's daughter! The joints of thy thighs are like jewels, the work of the hands of a cunning workman. Thy navel is like a round goblet, which wanteth not liquor. Thy belly is like a heap of wheat set about with lilies. Thy two breasts are like two young roes that are twins.

—Song of Solomon 7:1–3 (The Bible)

Whenever a child is born, family and friends always want to know the child's gender because most people treat girls and boys differently from the day they are born. Actually, the human bodies of girls and women and boys and men are not that different. All have hearts, brains, stomachs, bones, muscles, blood, and many other commonalities.

The one very important difference between female and male is in the nature of their sex and reproductive structures and functions. The sexual anatomies of women and men are different inside and outside their bodies.

Everyone's body is made up of many parts. Some of these parts, such as fingernails, **scrotum,** eyebrows, and vulva, are structures. Some body parts have more complicated functions and are called organs. A leaf is an organ of a tree; an ear is an organ of an animal. Our hearts, **ovaries,** brains, penises, and lungs are organs.

We have special structures and organs that are a part of our sex and reproductive systems. The parts *outside* the body are the external sex structures and organs—commonly called genitals. The structures and organs *inside* the body are the **internal sex and reproductive organs** and structures. These are linked to the **external sex and reproductive organs** and structures.

Our sex and reproductive organs identify us as girls and boys or women and men. They are also the source of sexual pleasure in our lives. But they are not the only sexually sensitive parts of our bodies.

Different people find the skin in many different areas of the body sexually stimulating. These areas include the nape of the neck, ears, throat, underarms, thighs, soles of the feet, hands, lips, eyelids, buttocks, toes, fingers, and knees. Touching hair or being touched by hair can also be very sexy. That goes for the hair on our bodies as well as our heads.

The breasts are also sources of sexual pleasure. Many women and men like to have their breasts and **nipples**

60

caressed during sex play. Many also receive pleasure when the **anus** is touched.

Almost any part of the body may be sexually sensitive—to someone. Each of us is different, and each of our bodies is different. Each of us will find different parts of our bodies to be sexually sensitive. One of the pleasures in life is the exploration of our bodies to discover what parts we find sexually sensitive. Babies begin this exploration at birth.

SEXUAL ANATOMY OF MEN

Men's External Sex Structures and Organs

The two most obvious external sex organs and structures of men are the penis and the scrotum.

Penis

The penis gets a great deal of attention for several reasons:

- It is the most obvious sex organ because it extends out from the body.
- It gets handled often. Every time a boy or man urinates, he handles his penis. The penis is the organ through which urine passes out of the bodies of boys and men.
- The penis is the most sexually sensitive organ in boys and men. From the first moments of sexual excitement, the penis begins to enlarge and stiffen—become erect.

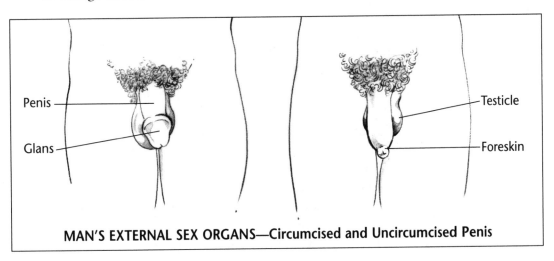

MAN'S EXTERNAL SEX ORGANS—Circumcised and Uncircumcised Penis

At the height of sexual excitement in adolescent and adult men, a fluid called semen spurts out of the penis.

The penis has two parts: the **shaft** and the **glans.**

The shaft is the largest part of the penis. It is shaped like a tube. At one end, it is connected to the body; at the other end is the glans—sometimes called the head or tip of the penis. The glans is made up of softer, fleshier tissue than the shaft. It is highly sensitive and can be a source of sexual pleasure. It is equivalent to the clitoris of a woman. There is a small opening at the tip of the glans called the urethral opening. Urine and semen pass out of the man's body through this opening. The sensitive area of skin that attaches the underside of the glans to the foreskin is called the frenulum.

At birth, all penises have a loose tube of skin called the **foreskin** that covers the glans. The foreskin protects the glans. Shortly after birth, the foreskin is removed from the penises of some boys. The operation to remove the foreskin is called circumcision. A penis that has no foreskin is called a circumcised penis, and one that has not had the foreskin removed is called **uncircumcised.**

Circumcision was popularized in the United States during the early part of this century in a misguided effort to decrease masturbation among boys. Religious and cultural beliefs and hygienic concerns are the reasons that parents now have their sons circumcised. The other common reason for circumcision today is that fathers want their sons to look like them.

The foreskin can easily be pulled back to allow a boy or man to urinate or clean himself. It is important to clean under the foreskin; otherwise, **smegma** forms. Smegma is a sticky, white substance that often has an unpleasant smell. It is formed by oils produced by the body and bacteria that feed on the oil. Proper cleaning of the glans and shaft of the penis is important.

The inside of the penis is made up of the urethra and two tissues called the **corpus spongiosum** and the **corpus cavernosa.**

The urethra is a very versatile structure within the penis. It is involved with both functions of the penis—urination and ejaculation. It is a long tube that passes from the bladder, through the center of the penis, to the urethral opening. Urine flows from the bladder through the urethra during urination. The male urethra is also connected to the reproductive system. It carries semen through the penis. The spurting of semen from the urethra is called ejaculation.

The shaft of the penis is formed of tissue called the corpus spongiosum and corpus cavernosa. These tissues form caverns and spongy areas. Normally, blood passes through these tissues and around the caverns and spongy areas, which remain empty. During sexual excitement, however, tiny muscles in the tissue relax and open, allowing the caverns and spongy areas to fill up with blood. As these tissues fill with blood, the penis becomes "tumescent." It gets longer and thicker and becomes less flexible and more stiff. This is called an erection.

When sexual stimulation ends, the muscles close off the emptied caverns from the bloodstream, the erection ends, and the penis softens into its normal flaccid state.

Boys and men are often concerned about the size and shape of their penises. There is no standard penis size, shape, or length. Some are fat and short. Others are long and thin. There is no truth to the idea that a bigger penis is a better penis.

Size has little to do with any reproductive or sexual function. It is true that some people prefer that their partners have a certain size penis. Preferences for penis size can be compared to preferences about height—there are just about as many people who want tall lovers as want short lovers.

Scrotum

The other external sex organ is called the scrotum—the sac that hangs directly under the penis. The scrotum contains some internal reproductive organs. In the scrotum are two ball-shaped glands. These are called **testes,** and they produce **sperm.** Part of the function of the scrotum is to protect the testes. Another word for the testes is testicles.

The scrotum changes in appearance. Sometimes the scrotum is loose so that the testes hang far from the body. At other times the scrotum is small, and the testes are tight against the body.

Changes in the shape of the scrotum are necessary for the production of sperm. The testes produce sperm only if they are at temperatures a few degrees below the temperature of the body. The scrotum holds the testes away from the body to maintain this cooler temperature. On hot days, the scrotum becomes larger, and the testes hang far from the hot body. On cold days, or after a cold shower or swim, the scrotum draws the testes closer to the body to share its heat.

A muscle named the cremaster muscle is attached to the scrotum.

It is responsible for adjusting the distance that the testes hang from the body. The cremaster muscle also tightens or relaxes the scrotum when the inside of a man's thigh is touched. The cremaster muscle operates involuntarily. Men and boys have no control over it. The muscle's response to temperature and touch is called the **cremaster reflex.**

Some men notice that their testicles are lopsided. It is normal for one side of the scrotal sac to hang lower than the other side. It is also normal for both sides to hang at the same level.

Self-examination of the external sex organs and structures once a month is an important part of good health care. Men should ask for medical advice if they notice any sores, swellings, or bumps on the penis or scrotum.

Men's Internal Sex and Reproductive Organs and Sperm Production

The penis and scrotum are connected to the internal reproductive organs and structures. The internal organs and structures are responsible for making and moving sperm. Sperm are the **reproductive cells** in men. It takes two reproductive cells, or **gametes,** to unite and begin the long, complex process of making a new individual. One cell has to come from the male and one from the female. When a sperm meets a female reproductive cell, the **egg,** or ovum, they can unite. This is called **fertilization.**

Testes

The testes are the ball-shaped glands inside the scrotum. Within each testis is a network of thin tubes, 750 feet long. These tubes are tightly coiled. They are called the **seminiferous tubules.** Sperm are formed inside these tubes. The name for the process of making sperm is **spermatogenesis.** Men's bodies make sperm all their lives, from puberty on. New sperm develop every minute. The supply never ends.

In between the seminiferous tubules are cells that produce male sex hormones. Hormones are chemicals that influence the changes in our bodies. Hormones also direct the work of glands and organs. If a hormone is found in greater quantities and has greater importance to the reproductive process in the male body than in the female body, it is categorized as a male sex hormone. Another name for male sex hormone is **androgen. Testosterone** is the major androgen that stimulates the production of sperm.

Epididymis

On top of each testis is another highly coiled tube. This tube is called the **epididymis.** When sperm are nearly mature, they move into each epididymis. Here, the sperm mature and gain the ability to swim. Mature sperm are stored in the epididymis until they are forced out of the body at the peak moment of sexual excitement. This is called ejaculation. This process is also called emission. At this point, boys and men usually have an orgasm, which is a very pleasurable feeling that may involve the whole body.

An orgasm is an uncontrollable release of tension that has built up in the body during sexual activity. This can happen during sex play, such as masturbation or intercourse, or during erotic fantasy. Orgasm does not always occur with ejaculation, and ejaculation does not always occur with orgasm.

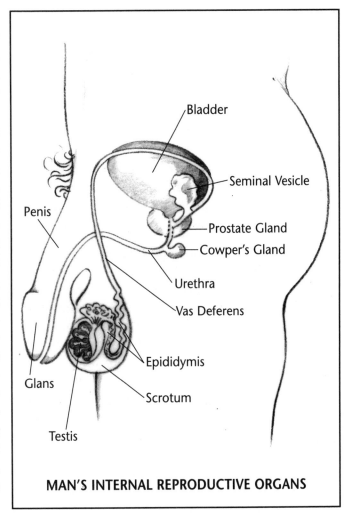

MAN'S INTERNAL REPRODUCTIVE ORGANS

Bladder
Seminal Vesicle
Penis
Prostate Gland
Cowper's Gland
Urethra
Vas Deferens
Epididymis
Glans
Scrotum
Testis

Vas Deferens

Mature sperm are pushed out of each epididymis into a long, thin tube called the **vas deferens.** The vas deferens connects the epididymis to the **seminal vesicle.** It moves sperm to the seminal vesicle by contracting and pushing them on their way.

Seminal Vesicles

The seminal vesicles are two small organs that are located beneath the bladder. It is here that the sperm are combined with a fluid called the **seminal fluid.** This fluid gives the sperm more room to move and also provides nourishment.

Prostate

The **prostate** is the next important place on the sperm's journey. The prostate gland is located below the bladder and is very sensitive. Some men like to have it stimulated during sex play. When sperm, combined with the seminal fluid, reach the prostate, another substance is added to the mixture. The prostate produces a thin, milky fluid that is secreted into the urethra at the time of emission of semen. The substance helps give the sperm an environment in which it can swim easily.

A muscle at the bottom of the prostate gland keeps the sperm out of the urethra until ejaculation begins. Then the sperm move through the urethra in the penis and out of the body.

Cowper's Glands

While the sperm are waiting, something else is happening to make the voyage easier. Located below the prostate are two **Cowper's glands,** which are attached to the urethra. The Cowper's glands deposit a fluid into the urethra before ejaculation. This fluid acts as a lubricant for the sperm and coats the urethra while flowing out the penis.

If there are sperm in the urethra from a previous ejaculation, they will mix with the Cowper's fluid. This means that sperm can slide out of the penis before ejaculation. The lubricant is often called **pre-ejaculate.**

Ejaculation happens when the prostate muscle opens and the prostate gland pumps the seminal fluid into the urethra. It then gets pumped out of the body through the urethral opening. When the final mixture leaves the body, it is called semen.

Some men worry that they may urinate instead of ejaculating. This is impossible. When the penis is erect, a muscle closes off the bladder so no urine can pass through the urethra. It is also not possible for semen to mix into urine during urination because the prostate closes when urine moves into the urethra.

If these muscles are not working correctly, semen can be ejaculated into the bladder instead of out of the body. This is called retrograde ejaculation. This does not happen often. It is most likely to happen to men who have had prostate surgery or who have diabetes or multiple sclerosis. Men who have retrograde ejaculation are still able to have fulfilling sexual relationships and orgasms.

SEXUAL ANATOMY OF WOMEN

Women's External Sex Structures and Organs

Vulva and Mons Pubis

The external sex organs of girls and women are nearly hidden from view. A girl will see only some of her external structures—an indentation with two folds of tissue on each side. Her external sex and reproductive organs and structures are inside this area, which is called the vulva. A mature or adolescent woman looking in a mirror will also see her vulva, but it will be covered with **pubic hair.** Above a woman's vulva is an area of fatty tissue that helps protect the sex and reproductive organs inside her body. This is called the mons pubis.

The best way for women and girls to see the parts of their vulvas is to use a mirror and move and separate the folds of the vulva. The parts inside the vulva are:

- the outer lips (**labia majora**)
- the inner lips (**labia minora**)
- the clitoris
- the opening to the vagina
- two **Bartholin's glands**

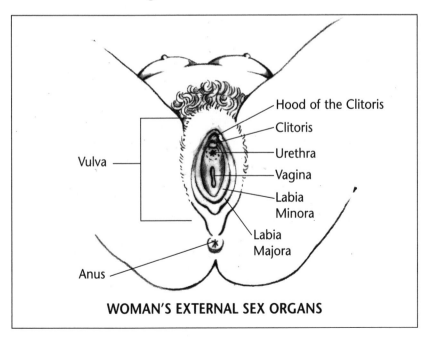

WOMAN'S EXTERNAL SEX ORGANS

Labia Majora and Labia Minora

The labia majora and labia minora are two folds of fleshy tissue on the outermost part of the vulva. The labia majora—the outer lips—are on the outermost part of the vulva, closer to the legs. Pubic hair often grows on the labia majora of adolescents and adults. The labia majora contains fatty tissue, so it is thicker than the labia minora. The fatty tissue helps protect the rest of the vulva.

If you hold back the labia majora, you will have a clear view of the labia minora lying inside.

The labia minora surround and protect the rest of the inner vulva. They do not have pubic hair. The inner and outer lips meet at the top and bottom of the vulva. The size and shape of women's labia may vary greatly.

Clitoris and Clitoral Hood

Located toward the top of the vulva, in the soft folds where both labia meet, is a very important organ. It is called the clitoris. The only purpose of the clitoris is to give girls and women sexual pleasure.

The tip of the clitoris is called the glans. The size of the clitoris varies from woman to woman, but it is often about the size of a pea.

FEMALE CIRCUMCISION

Female circumcision is performed in some African, Middle Eastern, and Southeast Asian countries—and in the United States among immigrants from these countries who still follow customs of their original cultures. Female circumcision is an operation that removes the clitoral hood, the clitoris, and, often, the labia. Female circumcision is practiced for cultural reasons. It is often done in unsanitary conditions, can lead to severe health problems, and reduces sexual sensitivity. For these reasons, there is a growing international movement to ban the practice. Female circumcision is often called clitoridectomy or FGM (female genital mutilation). There are no health or medical reasons to perform FGM. Although they can still lead a sexual life, women who have been circumcised will not enjoy the same clitoral sensations during sex play.

The shaft that supports the glans of the clitoris separates into two "legs" that straddle each side of the vagina inside the woman's body. The shaft and glans of the clitoris are covered by a **clitoral hood.** The glans of the clitoris is extremely sensitive to the touch. The clitoris contains corpus cavernosa tissue that causes it to swell with blood during sexual activity.

Opening of the Urethra

In girls and women, the urethral opening is located below the clitoris and above the vaginal opening. The urethral opening is not easy to see because it is in the vulva area. Because it is somewhat hidden, some young girls mistakenly believe urine comes out of their vaginal openings.

Young people may become confused about the functions of the urethra. The urethra in girls and women is not a part of the reproductive system. Its sole function is to provide a passageway for urine to flow from the bladder to the outside of the body.

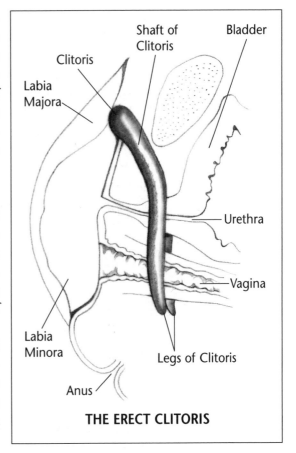

THE ERECT CLITORIS

Vaginal Opening

Directly under the urethral opening is the vaginal opening. The tissue surrounding it is called the **introitus.** The vaginal opening has three important functions:

- It is the opening that allows **menstrual flow** to pass from the body.
- It is where the penis is inserted during vaginal intercourse.
- It is the opening through which a **fetus** passes out of the body during birth.

Bartholin's Glands

The two internal glands on each side of the vaginal opening in the labia minora are called Bartholin's glands. They secrete fluids that act as lubrication when a woman is sexually excited.

Breasts

Women's breasts are important physical and psychological sources of pleasure. In most cultures, they are a major element of female attractiveness. Stimulation of the breasts during sex play can give women sexual pleasure. A woman's breasts can also support and nurture human life by producing milk for a baby after a woman has given birth. Many mothers also experience erotic pleasure during breast-feeding.

On the exterior of the breast is the nipple. The nipple has openings from which milk flows from the breasts. The area around the nipple is the **areola.** The nipple and areola are made of tissue and muscles that contract when it is cold or when sexually aroused—this happens in both males and females.

Milk is produced in special cells in the **alveoli** sacs inside of the breasts. These sacs are grouped together in areas called **lobes.** These cells, sacs, and lobes begin to produce milk only when a woman is pregnant. At that time, the body produces a hormone that stimulates milk production. When the fetus passes out of the womb and the woman is no longer pregnant, the milk passes into **milk ducts.** These are tubelike structures that connect to the nipple. When the baby sucks on the woman's nipple, milk is drawn from the ducts to the nipple.

Women's Internal Sex and Reproductive Organs

These include the following:

- vagina
- **cervix**
- uterus
- **fallopian tubes**
- ovaries

All these organs are supported by a bone and muscle structure called the **pelvic girdle.** Both men and women have a pelvic girdle. It is more developed and wider in women because it has to support a fetus during pregnancy. This is why girls' and women's hips are often wider than the hips of boys or men.

Vagina

The vagina is the structure that connects a woman's external sex organs to her internal sex and reproductive system. The opening of

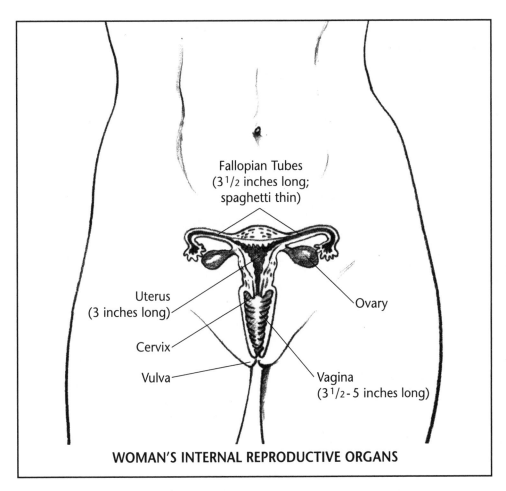

Fallopian Tubes
(3 1/2 inches long;
spaghetti thin)

Uterus
(3 inches long)

Ovary

Cervix

Vulva

Vagina
(3 1/2 - 5 inches long)

WOMAN'S INTERNAL REPRODUCTIVE ORGANS

the vagina is in the middle of the vulva, beneath the opening of the urethra. The vagina is a flexible passage that is four to five inches long. In its relaxed state, the soft, moist walls of this tunnel-like structure touch against each other like the walls of a collapsed balloon. Like a balloon, the vagina has the ability to enlarge a great deal.

The flexible vagina can accommodate the penis during intercourse and the fetus during childbirth—the vagina is also the birth canal. During birth, the fetus passes from the cervix of the uterus through the vaginal canal to the outside of the woman's body. During menstruation, blood and tissue flow along the same path.

Hymen

A thin membrane of skin may stretch across part of the vaginal opening. It is called the **hymen.** An opening in the hymen allows men-

VIRGINITY AND THE HYMEN

The hymen is very important to some people as a sign of **virginity.** They believe that a woman whose hymen is stretched open has let a boy or man put his penis in her vagina. But that isn't always true, because some women are born without a hymen. Others stretch and break theirs open during normal physical activities. Some bleeding may result when a hymen is torn. Something as simple as playing sports, horseback riding, or riding a bicycle can break the hymen.

A bride's virginity is highly prized in cultures that demand that women's only sex partners be their husbands. Bleeding during intercourse is believed to be a sign of virginity. In these cultures, bed sheets are examined for signs of blood after a wedding night. If blood is found, the female is considered to have been a virgin. However, a woman may be a virgin and still not bleed during her first intercourse.

strual flow to pass out of the body. Most girls are born with a hymen. Some are born without it. The condition of the hymen is not a good indicator of sexual virginity for one or more of three reasons:

• A girl may have been without a hymen.
• The hymen can easily be ruptured during normal physical activity and sports.
• The hymen can be stretched open by the use of tampons.

G-Spot

There is a small area called the Grafenberg Spot, or G–Spot, inside the vaginas of some women. It is located about an inch or two inside the vaginal opening in the vaginal wall that is closest to the navel. The G-Spot is sexually sensitive and swells slightly during sex play.

Urethra

Urine from the bladder passes through the urethra and leaves the body through the urethral opening. The urethra of girls and women is much shorter than the urethra of boys and men because it does not extend outside the body, as it does in the penis.

Skene's Glands

The Skene's glands are inside the body—one on each side of the urethra. They open into the urethra. Stimulation of the G–Spot and expulsion of fluid from the Skene's glands may constitute female ejaculation.

Uterus

The uterus is the pear-shaped reproductive organ commonly called the womb. It is formed of powerful, muscular walls and is about the size of the woman's fist.

The cervix is the lower, narrower portion, or neck, of the uterus. Nearly one-half of the cervix is inside the vagina. An opening in the cervix, called the os, is like a canal that connects the inside of the uterus to the vagina. At its narrowest point, the opening of the cervix is about as wide as the lead in a pencil.

Menstrual flow passes out of the uterus through the cervix. The cervix can also stretch to allow a fetus to pass through it. During intercourse, the penis does not enter the cervix. It may tap against the cervix, which may provide sexual pleasure to some women. Others may find this uncomfortable.

The inside of the uterus is a triangle-shaped area. It is lined with thick, plush walls of tissue and blood. The lining is called the **endometrium.** It is like a nest for the fertilized egg if pregnancy happens.

The endometrium stays particularly plush for part of each month. If one of the woman's eggs is fertilized during this time, it may move to the uterus and attach itself to the endometrium. If it does, pregnancy will begin as the endometrium begins to nourish the fertilized egg, or **pre-embryo.** If fertilization does not take place or the pre-embryo does not attach, the endometrium will break down and pass out of the vagina. This is called menstruation.

If pregnancy develops and continues, the pre-embryo will develop into a fetus. When it is time for the fetus to move out of the woman's body, the muscles of the uterus contract in a process called labor to deliver the fetus from the uterus, through the stretched, or "dilated," cervical os, down the vagina, through the vaginal opening, and out of the body.

THE G-SPOT AND FEMALE EJACULATION

The G-Spot is thought to contribute to female orgasm and female ejaculation. It was once believed that only urine passed through the female urethra. However, researchers have recently studied female e jaculation. In some women, a clear fluid spurts out of the urethra during intense sexual excitement and during orgasm. In some women, this fluid is urine and not a true ejaculation. In other women, the fluid is similar to the fluid produced by the prostate in men. It is estimated that about 10 percent of women experience this kind of ejaculation.

Ovaries

The two ovaries are where a woman's eggs are stored and where they mature. They are located in the lower part of the abdomen. If you want to get a sense of where your ovaries are located, put your finger on your navel and move it in a direct line to the top of your leg. When you have moved your finger one-half of the way there, your finger is over your ovary. There is one ovary on each side—one on the left and one on the right. Each ovary is about the size of an almond.

A baby girl has 1 million immature eggs in her ovaries when she is born.

Fallopian Tubes

A fallopian tube opens into each side of the uterus to allow an egg to pass from the ovary to the uterus. One end of each tube opens into the uterus; the other end opens very close to an ovary. When an egg is released, it can easily enter the open end of a fallopian tube. Each tube has fine hairlike fringes (cilia) that sweep a mature egg from the ovary into the tube. The contractions of the fallopian tube and the movements of the cilia move the egg toward the uterus.

Usually, the fallopian tubes are where the sperm and egg join. Sperm that are deposited in the vagina can swim through the cervix, through the uterus, and into the fallopian tube. If the egg meets sperm and joins with a sperm, this is called fertilization.

The egg is the largest human cell. It is about the size of the dot of this "i." The eggs are stored in areas of the ovary called follicles. Each follicle holds one immature egg. A number of follicles grows each month. Only one or, rarely, two, will reach maturity and release an egg each month. This happens during the years a woman can get pregnant. This process is called **ovulation,** and it begins at puberty.

Ovaries also make hormones that are needed for ovulation and a girl's growth during puberty. The hormones made in the ovaries are **estrogen** and progesterone. These and other hormones influence the process of ovulation, the passage of the egg to the uterus, and the eventual elimination of the lining through menstruation every month. This pattern is called the **menstrual cycle.** It does not occur during pregnancy but will continue throughout a woman's reproductive years.

Some women can feel their ovaries become tender during ovulation. The medical name for this is Mittelschmerz. All women are aware of the elimination of the unfertilized egg and the lining of the uterus. This monthly event is called menstruation.

Menstruation

The menstrual cycle is the name given to the process of fluctuations of hormones in a woman's body that cause the building and shedding of the endometrium. The part of the cycle when a woman has the

greatest chance to become pregnant is called the fertile period. It usually begins about six days before ovulation. At other times of the
cycle, her chances of pregnancy are diminished and she is less fertile
or infertile.

Menarche is the name given to the time when menstruation first
occurs, and menopause is the term given to the time when the last
menstruation occurs and the menstrual cycles end. Each woman's
body is different, and these events do not happen at the same age in
all women. Generally, girls enter menarche between the ages of nine
and 14. Menopause occurs when they are 45 to 55 years old.

Knowing how a woman's menstrual cycle works can help her
understand how fertilization and pregnancy take place and how to
plan or avoid pregnancy. The time from the first day of one menstruation to the first day of the next is one menstrual cycle. The length of
the cycle is different for each woman and also may change from
month to month. A typical menstrual cycle can last from 21 to 35 days.

The menstrual cycle is based on what happens to one egg that is
released from the ovary. It has two stages: before ovulation and after
ovulation. The whole wonderful process is controlled by a small gland
in the base of the brain, called the pituitary gland. The pituitary gland
produces chemicals called hormones that stimulate the ovaries and
uterus through the process of a woman's menstrual cycle. The four
hormones that regulate the menstrual cycle are:

- progesterone
- estrogen
- LH (luteinizing hormone)
- FSH (follicle-stimulating hormone)

The first day of the menstrual cycle—Day 1—is marked as blood
and tissue begin to flow out of the vagina. Day 1 results from what
happens after ovulation in the previous month. If the released egg was
not fertilized, the endometrium that was prepared to accept a fertilized egg has to be shed. Once this is done, a new plush tissue lining
will be made for a new egg.

The shedding of the old lining is known as menstruation or having a **period.** This may last from two to seven days. The tissue that is
shed is called menses or menstrual flow because it flows out of the
body. The menses flow through the cervical opening, down the vagina, and out of the body through the vaginal opening.

The menstrual flow includes fluid, tissue, and three to four table-spoons of blood. When girls first begin their menstrual cycle, they may be alarmed at the sight of this flow. That is because all their earlier associations with blood have been with injuries or sicknesses. Some people believe this flow is dirty, unclean, and unhealthy. This is not true. The process of menstruation is a healthy sign.

Sometimes the menses appear brown, causing concern for some women. Brown flow can be perfectly normal. It occurs when the flow of blood is light, usually at the beginning or end of the period. It has turned brown because the blood was sloughed off and was not drawn out swiftly by a brisk flow. When the menses flow slowly, they may turn brown before leaving the vagina.

Women use **sanitary pads** that attach to the underwear or **tampons** that fit inside the vagina to absorb the flow as it leaves the body. These items are made of materials that absorb the flow and prevent damage to clothing.

Shortly after her period, a woman's body begins to prepare a new egg to leave the ovary. The pituitary gland in her brain releases FSH (follicle-stimulating hormone), which stimulates the follicles in the ovaries. Usually, one follicle develops more fully, and the egg within that follicle then begins to ripen and mature.

During maturation, the follicle produces a hormone called estrogen. Estrogen sends a message that makes the endometrium thicken with blood and tissue. It is difficult to know the exact day when the egg is released because it can vary. But sometime between Day 13 and Day 16 after menstruation in a 28-day cycle, a new egg will be released.

The release of the new egg from the ovary is called ovulation. It is caused by a surge of luteinizing hormone (LH) that is triggered by the pituitary gland. Although it is difficult to predict on what day the egg will be released, we know that *after* the egg is released it will be 14 days until Day 1 of the next cycle. This is true for all women's cycles, whether their cycles are 21 or 35 days long.

MENSTRUATION IN BRIEF

A 28-Day Cycle

Day 1: First signs of blood and tissue flowing from vagina. Menstruation begins.

Day 2 to Day 5: Menstrual flow continues.

Day 7 to Day 13: An egg begins to ripen. The lining of the uterus begins to thicken.

Day 14 to Day 16: An egg is released from an ovary—ovulation.

Day 16 to Day 18: The unfertilized egg breaks apart.

Day 25: Hormone levels drop. The lining of the uterus begins to break down.

As soon as the egg is released by the follicle in the ovary, it is swept into a fallopian tube and pushed toward the uterus. The follicle that released the egg remains in the ovary. It is called a corpus luteum. It continues to produce estrogen and begins to produce progesterone to help develop the lining of the uterus.

The egg travels down the fallopian tube toward the uterus. Along the way, it may meet and unite with a sperm and become fertilized. If fertilization occurs, the fertilized cell may implant in the uterus. If fertilization does not occur, the lining of the uterus will begin to break down. The lining of the uterus is shed. It passes out of the uterus, through the cervix and vagina, and out of the vaginal opening. This is the first day of another menstrual cycle and is marked by menstrual flow. Then the whole process starts all over again.

Menstrual cycles will likely go on until a women is 45 to 55 years old and enters menopause. After menopause, eggs no longer mature, and follicles stop making hormones. Therefore, the cycle of hormonal changes is interrupted. This makes a woman's body change. The change can happen slowly or very quickly.

SEXUAL ANATOMY OF CHILDREN: GIRLS AND BOYS

Our sex organs develop before we are born. At first, the sex and reproductive organs of all human **embryos** are alike. They all appear to be female. Unless the fetus has a male genetic code, the fetus will continue to develop as a female. Otherwise, the genetic code signals hormonal changes that cause the sex and reproductive organs to develop into male organs. Tissue that would otherwise become a clitoris becomes the glans of a penis. Tissue that would otherwise form the labia forms the scrotum.

Here is a diagram that compares the placement of these tissues in female and male fetuses during the 12th week of development.

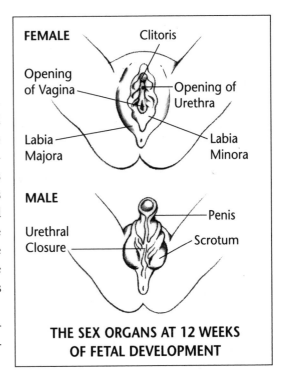

FEMALE — Clitoris — Opening of Vagina — Opening of Urethra — Labia Majora — Labia Minora

MALE — Urethral Closure — Penis — Scrotum

THE SEX ORGANS AT 12 WEEKS OF FETAL DEVELOPMENT

Primary Sex Characteristics

From the first day of our lives, as newborn babies, we have all the major sex organs and structures that we have as adults.

A baby has the same internal and external sex and reproductive organs that an adult does. These characteristics are called **primary sex characteristics.** We will have the primary sex characteristics with which we are born for the rest of our lives.

Secondary Sex Characteristics

As our bodies grow, our sex organs grow, too. As girls and boys grow, changes will happen to their bodies that make girls look more like women and boys look more like men. These changes happen during puberty and affect our **secondary sex characteristics.**

Changes That Occur in Puberty

Puberty is a time when hormones stimulate change in all parts of the body. The changes affect what happens to the body on the inside—girls begin to menstruate, and boys begin to produce sperm and ejaculate. The changes affect our bodies on the outside as well. Girls develop breasts, and boys develop facial hair. Every person goes through puberty, but when and "how quickly" puberty and secondary sex characteristics develop are different for every person. Puberty generally lasts for a couple of years.

Puberty doesn't happen at the same time for girls and boys. Very often, girls begin puberty between the ages of eight and 14. Boys usually begin puberty about two years later, between the ages of 10 and 15.

During puberty, young people of the same age may look very different. In a group of three friends, all age 13, the first may be almost done with puberty, the second may just be starting puberty, and the third may not yet have started. These three people have very different secondary sex characteristics, and they will all be normal (see page 82). The time puberty begins does not indicate whether children will be bigger or smaller than anyone else when they are adults.

Puberty may be embarrassing for young women and men. The numerous changes our bodies go through may feel awkward. Erections or periods may happen at unwanted times. Breasts may make one feel self-conscious. Sweat may be produced in large amounts. Body odor becomes stronger than it was in childhood. Acne—pimples on the face caused by bacteria and trapped oil—may make one feel unattractive.

How Pubescent Changes Affect Girls and Boys

Menarche and Thelarche

Menarche is occurring at younger and younger ages. In 1840, the average age for menarche was between 17 and 18. Today, the average age that girls have their first period is 12.5! It is no longer unusual for girls to enter menarche at the age of 10. Physiologists believe that earlier menarche is related to better nutrition, which leads to increased amounts of body fat in modern girls. The hormones responsible for the menstrual cycle are stored in body fat.

On the other hand, many young women today are very athletic and maintain a naturally lean body. Menarche may be much later for them. Even after menarche, their menstruation may be very irregular and light.

The range of years during which menarche may happen is very wide. It is difficult to predict when it will happen. Family members, educators, and **clinicians** may not anticipate it in time to counsel young women about the changes that are happening in their bodies. This is one of the reasons menarche may come as a complete surprise to many young women—especially if it is early.

Girls who have early menarche are likely to start having erotic dreams earlier than other girls. They are more likely to have sexual intercourse at younger ages. They need earlier counseling about sexuality, safer sex, and birth control.

Girls may experience anxiety about breast development. The beginning of breast development is called **thelarche.** For some, breast development seems to happen too soon and is embarrassing. Others are frustrated that it isn't happening soon enough. Many worry that their breasts won't be the size they want or expect. Many wonder when it is appropriate for them to wear a bra for the first time.

Menarche, thelarche, and other events during puberty are likely to be accompanied by many uncertainties. Girls have a lot to adjust to,

CHANGES THAT OCCUR IN PUBERTY

Girls

Girls have all their sex and reproductive organs when they are born. Girls also have all their **sex cells**—eggs—already formed by the time they are born. At puberty, these eggs mature, usually one a month.

The pituitary gland in the brain stimulates body changes by triggering hormone production in the ovaries. The ovaries begin producing the hormones estrogen and progesterone. Estrogen and progesterone affect the other cells in a girl's body. Secondary sex characteristics begin to appear. Some changes girls can expect during puberty:

- They will grow taller.
- The voice will become deeper.
- Underarm hair will appear.
- Pubic hair will grow on the mons pubis and the labia majora.
- Sweat glands will produce greater amounts of sweat.
- Acne may appear.
- The uterus will enlarge.
- Breasts will develop.
- Hips will widen.
- Menstruation will start.
- Thinking about sex will become more common.
- Mood swings may happen abruptly.

whether puberty is early or late. Menstruation may occur very irregularly. Early periods may be quite uncomfortable or even painful. Often in puberty, girls have a white, sticky vaginal discharge called **leukorrhea.** It may upset girls who do not know it is normal.

It is also normal for one breast to develop faster than another. But the experience may be unsettling. Likewise, the onset of sexual desires and dreams may be very confusing for girls who don't know what to expect. Some girls may become unnerved by the experience and may need counseling. Girls who have been prepared with helpful information may have a much more positive experience with menarche, thelarche, and the other events of puberty.

Boys

Boys have all their sex and reproductive organs at birth, but the testicles do not make sperm until puberty.

The brain stimulates body changes by triggering hormone production in the testes. The testes produce very large amounts of the hormone testosterone. Testosterone affects the other cells in a boy's body. Secondary sex characteristics begin to appear. Some changes boys can expect during puberty:

- They will become taller very quickly.
- Facial hair will begin to grow.
- The voice will become deeper—it may "crack" during the change.
- Underarm hair will appear.
- Pubic hair will begin to grow above the penis and on the scrotum.
- Sweat glands will produce greater amounts of sweat.
- Acne may appear.
- Penis and testicles will become larger.
- Seminal vesicles, the prostate, and the Cowper's glands will begin the adult function of producing semen.
- Erections will be more common and may happen spontaneously without stimulation.
- Thinking about sex will become more common.
- Wet dreams may occur.
- Mood swings may happen abruptly.

Spermarche, Erections, and Wet Dreams

Boys have erections all their lives, starting from the moment they are born. But at puberty, erections occur more often. Many young men think that the occurrence of an erection means that their bodies are ready for sexual activity. This is not true. For example, when a boy or man wakes up from sleep, he may have an erection. This is because his bladder is full. A full bladder may stimulate nerves inside the body near the base of the penis and cause an erection.

Erections normally occur throughout the night during sleep. Erotic dreams cause young men to become aroused in their sleep. Young men undergoing puberty may notice that when they wake up,

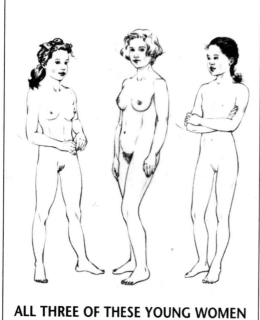

ALL THREE OF THESE YOUNG WOMEN WILL BE 13 IN THREE MONTHS— THEIR BODIES ARE DEVELOPING AT DIFFERENT RATES.

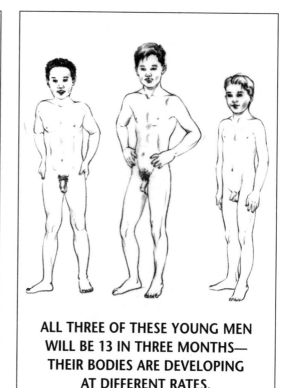

ALL THREE OF THESE YOUNG MEN WILL BE 13 IN THREE MONTHS— THEIR BODIES ARE DEVELOPING AT DIFFERENT RATES.

their bellies, clothing, or sheets are sticky and wet around their penis. This is because young men may ejaculate in their sleep. The ejaculate, or semen, is the sticky substance found when a young man awakens. Ejaculating in one's sleep is often called a wet dream. The clinical name is nocturnal emission. Almost all young men will have wet dreams. Boys and men who ejaculate during masturbation or other forms of sex play are less likely to have wet dreams.

The first time a young man ejaculates is called **spermarche.** Ejaculation can occur during nocturnal emission, masturbation, or sexual intercourse.

Sexual Thoughts and Fantasies

A young woman's body will begin to respond to sexual thoughts and stimulation during puberty. Before puberty, children and babies touch the vulva only because it feels good. Their autoerotic play is usually not a sexual type of pleasure because it doesn't involve sexual thinking or fantasy. At puberty, young women may begin to touch the clitoris and vulva for *sexual* pleasure. They can also be aroused by sexual thoughts or touch. Sexually stimulating dreams may mean that a girl wakes up with her vulva moistened with lubrication.

Sexual arousal—an erection or lubrication of the vulva—may happen without sexual activity. All the sensitive nerve endings that give us sexual pleasure are present from birth in girls and boys. At puberty, young women and men begin to have more sexual thoughts. When they touch themselves in the same way they have done all their lives, but with sexual fantasies while they are doing it, it is more correctly considered sexual activity.

Breast Size Changes in Boys—Gynecomastia

The change in hormones during puberty may cause surplus estrogen to be produced in a young man's body. This usually happens only for a short period of time. It can mean that his breasts become slightly larger. This condition is called **gynecomastia.** It happens in 40 to 60 percent of adolescent boys. Young men feel very self-conscious and embarrassed about having enlarged breasts. During puberty, gynecomastia is usually temporary—it goes away within one to two years. If it happens before a boy goes through puberty, or continues after puberty, a health care provider should be consulted.

TALKING ABOUT OUR BODIES

The Names We Use: Slang or Scientific

As we grow and explore our body parts, we need words to describe them. It is important to learn the proper, scientific names of the parts of the body.

The proper names for body parts are the same names used by scientists and health care workers. The proper names, such as "testes" and "vagina," are technical terms just like "liver," "lung," "leg," and so on.

However, we often learn the slang terms instead. Slang names are words that people use instead of the proper scientific names. Slang names may also be real words that are used incorrectly. Certain slang words are made by using a word we know in place of one we don't know.

For example, when people speak of the testes, they may use the slang term "balls." Another slang word for testes is *"huevos,"* which means "eggs" in Spanish. Because the testes are round, they may remind us of balls or eggs. Balls or *huevos* may seem more familiar, easier to remember, and easier to pronounce than "testes." Another example is that of the slang words "tits" or "titties"—for women's breasts. An animal's nipples are properly called "teats." "Teats" was changed to "tits" and "titties." Other slang words seem to make no sense. For example, a penis is sometimes called a "Johnson." We do not know who or what a Johnson is. Or having vaginal intercourse for the first time is often called "losing one's cherry"—for both women and men. Obviously, there is no cherry or any other fruit inside our sex and reproductive structures. Yet "cherry" has become slang for "hymen."

Slang is handed down from generation to generation. New slang terms are also created by the pop culture or media in each generation. Slang in one family or community is often different from the slang used in another family or community.

Some women and men agree to use slang during sex play to express and increase their excitement. Otherwise, the slang names of the sex and reproductive organs can create communication problems between men and women, people of different ages, cultures, and economic classes, and people of different professions. There are more slang terms for the sex organs and the sex acts than for any other body part or function. For example, it's difficult to think of slang terms for "finger," "toe," or "elbow."

Imagine being a doctor or nurse. To understand your patients, you may need to understand all of the slang terms that your patients use. Imagine being a patient who doesn't understand the words the health care worker is using. A confusing situation for both people! Slang can be a real communication problem.

Respect is another reason to use the correct scientific names of our sex and reproductive organs. The person using a slang term may feel that the word is the right one to use, but the person hearing the term may be offended or hurt. For example, one person may think that "balls" is the right word to use for the testes. Another person may feel that "balls" is a very rude word. Slang names often cause strong negative emotions because many people find them rude, impolite, hurtful, or disrespectful of our own and each others' bodies.

If using slang creates difficulty in communicating and risks the disrespect of others, why do people still use it?

Slang begins at home when parents and relatives teach a child that a "pee-pee" is a penis, "boobies" are breasts, and a "vaginy" is a vagina. These slang terms may seem harmless at the time. The terms may even seem easier for a young child to say. But learning and using slang continue as a child grows. Soon the child becomes an adult who is using a whole vocabulary of slang expressions that she or he passes on to another generation.

It is important for parents to know that children can easily learn the proper names at an early age. When they grow up, they will hand down to their children the correct names of the sex and reproductive organs. Using proper language can help people better understand their sexuality.

If everyone used the proper names for body parts, there would be fewer problems communicating with each other. No matter what family or community, age, sex, or culture, each person would be using the same terms. More important, when we use the proper names, we are showing respect for our bodies, others' bodies, and both genders—male and female. Of course, when we use the correct names, we should use them correctly. Many well-educated people, for example, use the word "vagina" when they really mean "vulva."

Positive Talk and Proud Bodies

The many reasons we have slang tell us something about ourselves. It shows that many of us are not comfortable talking about our bodies—especially our sex and reproductive parts. Slang shows that we may not even know much about our bodies. We create slang to hide our embarrassment. But embarrassment keeps us ignorant. Ignorance keeps us from becoming comfortable with our bodies.

A body is an incredible, fascinating structure. It is normal to want to learn about it. It is normal to ask questions about it. It is normal to be proud of it. Parents, relatives, and friends can help promote greater self-esteem among young children and teens by using the proper names of the sex and reproductive organs.

Talking to children positively about their bodies, puberty, and sexuality helps them develop a positive sexuality. Positive talk replaces embarrassment with pride. It replaces ignorance with knowledge and gives us comfort instead of discomfort. Positive talk also helps children learn to respect the sexuality of others.

OUR BODIES AND
OUR SEXUAL RESPONSE

Sexual Stimulus

Our bodies respond to the world around us. Anything that makes our bodies respond is called a stimulus. We sense **stimuli** by our five senses: touch, sight, smell, hearing, and taste. We may see our bodies' response to a stimulus, such as sweating when it's hot or getting goose bumps when we're scared. Or we may not see the response—it may be inside our bodies, such as digestion of food when we eat, increase in heartbeat when we're scared. These responses happen involuntarily—we don't even have to think about them.

All of our senses pick up sexual stimuli just as they do other stimuli. Sexual arousal can be caused by what we see, hear, taste, smell, and touch. Our bodies become sexually aroused in predictable ways.

Often we think of touch as the main sexual stimulus when we think of sexual activity. Touching our own skin or someone else's can be very sexually arousing. Areas of our body where the skin is very sensitive to sexual stimulation are called **erogenous zones.** Our external sex organs are highly sensitive to touch—such as the glans of the clitoris or penis. However, other parts of our skin can be touched and also produce sexual arousal: arms, legs, back, neck, nipples, buttocks, ears, fingers, feet. In fact, any part of our skin can be an erogenous zone. People have different likes and dislikes about where they like to be touched. Our erogenous zones are unique to each of us.

Touch is not the only sexual stimulus. As we grow, we learn to associate certain sounds, such as music or voices, and sights—parts of the body, for example—with sexually stimulating experiences or thoughts. This is also true of smells and tastes. In each society and culture, there are characteristics, personalities, and behaviors that are thought to be attractive and sexually stimulating. For example, long hair, dancing, a certain physical stature, or shyness may be very attractive and sexually stimulating for someone. Tight clothing or certain kinds of underwear may be stimulating for someone else.

When and how we learn about these characteristics, behaviors, and personalities will affect what we find attractive and sexually stimulating. Later on in life when we see or hear those things again, our bodies respond. What each of us learns and experiences is different from any other person. This learning and experiencing continues throughout the rest of our lives. We are never too old to find new stimuli and new sources of sexual stimulation. Nor do we forget those that aroused us during our younger years.

Imagination can produce stimuli that can be seen, heard, tasted, touched, and smelled in our minds. Sometimes our sexual experiences begin and end in our imaginations. We can also heighten our sexual responses with imagination. The use of our imaginations for sexual arousal is called fantasy. It can be the most stimulating aspect of our sexual experience.

Adult Sexual Response

Sexual stimulation begins with sexual arousal and may continue just after orgasm. The pattern of our response to sexual stimulation is called our sexual response cycle. There are five steps in the cycle: **desire, excitement, plateau,** orgasm, and **resolution.** Some or all of the steps are reached each time one has a sexual experience. However, one can stop at any step before orgasm. Completing the cycle is not necessary for sexual fulfillment.

In order to make the sexual response cycle easier to understand, let's take a look at two people who have just met. For the purposes of showing the responses that are similar and different between men and women, the couple in this example will be a man and a woman.

Desire Phase

The man and woman begin to feel sensations. They are attracted to each other. Their interest grows. This is caused by stimuli—such as seeing one another, hearing one another's voice, smelling one another's cologne or perfume, or holding one another's gaze. Neither the woman nor the man knows why or how this attraction happens. At this point, the woman and man begin to want or "desire" sexual intimacy with one another.

The desire phase can go on for a long time—weeks, months, or years. Or the change from desire to the next phase, excitement, may happen very quickly—within a few minutes.

Excitement Phase

Excitement is the phase during which the body responds to desire. The body reacts automatically to the stimuli of desire. It may be very easy for the woman or man to feel these reactions in her or his own body. If they are wearing clothes, however, it may be difficult for each to know that the other is sexually excited. Communication about their sexual excitement may begin. Communication happens through talking and body gestures. It may be that our bodies produce special chemical substances that attract us through our sense of smell. These substances are called **pheromones.**

Sometimes women and men are embarrassed by their sexual excitement and try to hide it. Sometimes we are attracted to people who are not available to us because of social restrictions. You may be sexually attracted to the spouse of a friend, but your mind tells you that a sexual relationship with that person is not allowed. Sometimes we are very surprised by sexual stimuli. In any case, sexual stimulation

CHANGES IN OUR BODIES DURING EXCITEMENT PHASE

Woman's Body

- Heart rate increases.
- Blood pressure increases.
- Body muscles tense—voluntarily and involuntarily.
- Sex flush—reddening of the skin, especially around chest and neck—may begin in some lighter-skinned women.
- Nipples become erect, and breasts increase in size.
- Clitoris swells and enlarges slightly.
- Labia majora flatten and separate if the woman has never had a baby. They swell and separate if she has had a child.
- Labia minora swell.
- Vagina lubricates and turns darker color.
- Uterus rises a little.

Man's Body

- Heart rate increases.
- Blood pressure increases.
- Body muscles tense—voluntarily and involuntarily.
- Sex flush—reddening of the skin, especially around chest and neck—may begin in some lighter-skinned men.
- Nipples become erect.
- Penis becomes erect.
- Scrotum thickens, and testes rise closer to the body.

is often difficult to talk about. Shy people may wait a long time for a sign of interest from other people before they communicate their sexual excitement.

Excitement prepares our bodies for sexual intercourse or for **outercourse,** which is sex play without insertion of the penis into the vagina or anus. Excitement can lead to sexual intimacy, but the woman and man can experience excitement in their own bodies and not be sexually or physically intimate with each other.

Once a person enters the excitement phase, she or he can leave it at any time. Desire, excitement, and wanting to be sexually intimate are normal, but it is important to remember that it is never "necessary" to be sexually intimate. Whenever women or men do not want to be sexually intimate, their choices must be respected.

For the purposes of our example, this couple is feeling sexually excited. They have been flirting. They have also talked about their sexual excitement. This woman and man agree to continue their excitement through intimacy, **foreplay,** and intercourse. The excitement phase for this couple lasts from the time of their discussion through foreplay. During the excitement phase, the following changes happen inside and outside of the woman's and man's bodies.

Plateau Phase

Excitement continues to rise through many kinds of stimulation. At the highest point of excitement, a certain state of feelings and body changes is reached. This state is the plateau phase. Stimulation continues during the plateau phase. Stimulation during the plateau phase is usually physical. It may include stroking or rubbing of an erogenous zone—face, breast, clitoris, or penis. This can occur during masturbation, intercourse, or outercourse.

Sexual intercourse usually means that the penis is inserted into a part of the body and moved in and out for sexual stimulation. Sexual intercourse occurs between women and men, men and men, and women and women. Trying different types of intercourse depends greatly on how comfortable you are with your own and your partner's bodies. It also depends on your personal, religious, and cultural values.

TYPES OF OUTERCOURSE (FOREPLAY AND ALTERNATIVES TO INTERCOURSE)

- *Masturbation.* Masturbation is the most common way we enjoy sex. Partners can enjoy it together while hugging and kissing or watching one another. Masturbating together can deepen a couple's intimacy.
- *Erotic massage.* Many couples enjoy arousing one another with body massage. They stimulate each other's sex organs with their hands, bodies, or mouths. They take turns bringing each other to orgasm.
- *Body rubbing ("frottage").* Many couples rub their bodies together, especially their sex organs, for intense sexual pleasure. Many are stimulated to orgasm by this "dry humping."
- *Erotic fantasy,* **role play,** *masks.* Reading, watching, or telling erotic fantasies with a sex partner can be very exciting. Acting out fantasies can be exciting, too. Masks and costumes may intensify this kind of sex play.
- *Sex toys.* Sex toys, including vibrators and dildos, can heighten sexual pleasure. They are used to stroke, stimulate, probe, and caress the body.

TYPES OF SEXUAL INTERCOURSE

- *vaginal intercourse (coitus)*—inserting the penis into the vagina
- *anal intercourse*—inserting the penis into the anus
- *axillary intercourse*—inserting the penis under the armpit
- *interfemoral intercourse*—inserting the penis between the thighs
- *mammary intercourse*—inserting the penis between the breasts
- *oral intercourse*—inserting the penis into the mouth. Sex play that involves putting the tongue into the vulva is also often called oral intercourse.

In our example, the woman and man began foreplay during the excitement phase. They are now having vaginal intercourse during the plateau phase. Some of the changes that take place inside and outside the body during the plateau phase are shown in the following table.

CHANGES IN OUR BODIES DURING PLATEAU PHASE

Woman's Body

- Breathing becomes more rapid.
- Heart rate continues to increase.
- Blood pressure continues to increase.
- Sex flush may continue.
- Muscle tension continues—small spasms occur.
- Bartholin's glands secrete lubrication.
- Glans of clitoris withdraws.
- Areolas around nipples become larger.
- Labia majora continue to swell with blood.
- Labia minora become deeper in color.
- "Orgasmic platform" develops: Lower part of vagina swells so it is more narrow and tight; uterus tips so it is now standing higher in the abdomen.

Man's Body

- Breathing becomes more rapid.
- Heart rate continues to increase.
- Blood pressure continues to increase.
- Sex flush may continue.
- Muscle tension continues—small spasms occur.
- Cowper's glands secrete pre-ejaculate.
- Glans of penis becomes larger.
- Testes enlarge and continue to rise closer to the body.

Orgasm

A high peak occurs during the plateau phase. This peak is called orgasm. Orgasm is defined as the phase where sexual tension is released. This is the shortest of all the phases and lasts less than a minute. However, when an orgasm occurs, more than just muscles are relaxed. During orgasm, the body releases chemicals—called endorphins—that produce good feelings. These are chemicals that reduce pain. Endorphins are produced in both men and women.

Ejaculations and orgasms in men often occur at the same time. Orgasms are not the same as ejaculations. The stimulation of the shaft and glans of the penis helps create sexual and muscle tension. The release of this tension is an orgasm. An ejaculation is the pushing and contractions of the prostate and seminal vesicles to move semen out of the penis. A man can ejaculate and not have an orgasm. A man can

TYPES OF ORGASM IN WOMEN

Type	Stimulus That Causes Orgasm
clitoral/**tenting** orgasm	stimulation of the clitoris alone
vaginal/A-frame/uterine orgasm	stimulation of the vagina alone (includes stimulation of the G-Spot alone)
blended orgasm	stimulation of the vagina and clitoris

also have an orgasm and not ejaculate, as in retrograde ejaculation. Orgasm in men is usually limited to the genital area.

What is an orgasm in a woman? This question has caused many arguments, discussions, and much research, because it was once believed that women did not have orgasms. However, women's bodies do create and maintain sexual and muscle tension. The release of this tension, combined with the muscular contraction felt in the pelvic organs, and the release of endorphins create orgasms in women. Women, like men, can be stimulated to orgasm. Unlike men, however, women seem to have more than one way in which they experience orgasm, and they are more likely to have orgasms that involve more than the genital area.

Clitoral and vaginal orgasms may produce different effects inside the body. Stimulation of the clitoris causes the vagina to become longer. It also causes a pocket to be formed beneath the uterus. The indentation it creates looks much like a tent or a balloon. Stimulation of the vagina or G-Spot makes the uterus drop lower. This shortens the vagina.

Some researchers believe that there is only one type of female orgasm. They believe that there is no such thing as a vaginal orgasm. Instead, they believe that a clitoris is necessary in stimulating a vaginal orgasm. Other researchers disagree. In fact, women's diverse experiences with orgasm make it difficult to define the female orgasm in one way. Some women may not feel contractions of their uterus during a uterine orgasm. Some women can reach orgasm with imagination as the only source of stimulation.

It is important for women to understand what feels good and what orgasm is for them as individuals. Ideally, women can ask their partners for the kind of satisfying physical contact that they need. This may be more important than striving to create an orgasm defined in terms that may have no relevance for a particular woman.

CHANGES IN OUR BODIES DURING ORGASM PHASE

Woman's Body

- Heart rate, breathing, and blood pressure reach highest peak.
- Sex flush spreads.
- Loss of muscle control—spasms occur.
- No change in clitoris.
- Vagina and/or uterus, anus, and muscles of pelvic floor contract five to 12 times, with 0.8 second between each contraction.

Man's Body

- Heart rate, breathing, and blood pressure reach highest peak.
- Sex flush spreads.
- Loss of muscle control—spasms occur.
- Ejaculation becomes unstoppable. **Ejaculatory inevitability** is reached as the vas deferens, seminal vesicles, and prostate begin contractions.
- Urethra, anus, and muscles of pelvic floor contract three to six times, with 0.8 second between each contraction.
- Ejaculation occurs.

Women and a few men can have **multiple orgasms.** This means that a person can have more than one orgasm while staying inside the high state of the plateau phase. Multiple orgasms are more common in women. Most men enter the next phase—the resolution phase—before they are able to have another orgasm or ejaculation.

In the box above are the changes that take place during orgasm in women and men.

Resolution

Resolution is the last phase of the sexual response cycle. This is the time after orgasm when the body returns to the way it was before sexual excitement. Both women and men enter this state. While a man's body is returning to a nonaroused state, he loses his erection and experiences a **refractory period.** During this time, men cannot get another erection. The length of the refractory period for young men is normally very short. The length of the refractory period increases with age. It will take an older man longer to be able to get another erection after he has ejaculated.

Women do not have a refractory period. They can be sexually aroused immediately after orgasm. The box on the next page shows what happens to our couple during the resolution phase.

CHANGES IN OUR BODIES DURING RESOLUTION PHASE

Woman's Body

- Heart rate and blood pressure dip below normal and soon return to normal.
- The whole body sweats, including hands and soles of feet.
- Breasts and areolas decrease in size. Nipples are no longer erect.
- Clitoris moves out from under the clitoral hood and shrinks slightly.
- Labia return to normal size and position and become a lighter color.
- Orgasmic platform disappears, and color of vagina lightens.
- Opening of cervix remains open to help semen travel up into uterus. After 20 to 30 minutes, the opening closes. Uterus lowers into upper vagina.

Man's Body

- Heart rate and blood pressure dip below normal and soon return to normal.
- The whole body sweats, ncluding hands and soles of feet.
- Nipples are no longer erect.
- Penis becomes soft and smaller.
- Scrotum relaxes and testes drop farther away from the body.

Children and Sexual Response Cycle

It may be hard for us to imagine children as sexual creatures. Boys and girls may say that they think that the other sex is "yucky." Therefore, we think of sexual attraction as something we grow into at puberty and in adulthood. Or we may think that we *learn* sexual attraction. We mistakenly think that without sexual attraction there is no physical response of the sexual systems.

Erotic response is not a learned behavior or a process that happens only in adult life. Children respond to stimulation and touch from the moment they are born. Baby girls are capable of lubricating. Their clitorises swell. Baby boys get erections. The sexual response system is a reflex that we are born with. It is associated with sexual desire, attraction, and fantasy as we grow older.

Aphrodisiacs

Drugs, foods, drinks, and odors that are supposed to create or increase sexual desire are called **aphrodisiacs.** "Aphrodisiac" comes from the name of the mythical Greek goddess of love and beauty, Aphrodite. Some well-known examples of so-called aphrodisiacs are rhinoceros horn, oysters, perfume, and vitamin E. Most aphrodisiacs don't work. In fact, some of them may be harmful to your health. There are chemicals that are known to affect sexual desire. However, these chemicals are often illegal and dangerous, and in some people, they may produce a *lack* of sexual desire. All aphrodisiacs may pose health risks during pregnancy—for the woman and her fetus. They may also interfere with our intentions to practice safer sex.

Here is a list of aphrodisiacs, their rumored effect, and the real results.

APHRODISIACS AND THEIR EFFECTS

Name	Street Name	Rumored Effect	Real Effect
alcohol	booze	Increases arousal.	Can reduce inhibitions and stress about sex. In moderate amounts, it can weaken an erection and create problems with arousal and orgasm.
amphetamines	uppers, crystal, crank	Heighten sexual sensation and performance.	If used for a long time, they can impair sexual function. They also reduce lubrication in women.
amyl nitrite/ butyl nitrite	poppers, snappers	Make orgasm and arousal more intense.	The pelvic area may become warm. Time becomes distorted. May cause headaches, dizziness, and fainting.
barbiturates	downers, barbs	Increase arousal.	Much like alcohol in reducing fears to stimulate sexual activity.
cantharis	Spanish fly	Stimulates the genitals to make a person want sexual activity.	Made from ground-up *Cantharides* beetle. This is a powerful irritant that can cause inflammation of the urethra and bladder. The labia may become engorged, and the penis may become erect. This is usually painful. May cause permanent damage to the urethra, bladder, and genitals. In large amounts, Spanish fly can be fatal.

(continued)

APHRODISIACS AND THEIR EFFECTS—*CONTINUED*

Name	Street Name	Rumored Effect	Real Effect
cocaine	coke, crack, blow	Produces more orgasms and more intense orgasms.	Reduces fear of risks and boosts sense of well-being. Regular use can cause depression and anxiety. Sniffing can cause damage, scarring, and holes in the nasal passage.
damiana leaf			Heightens sexual stimulation but standardized product is difficult to find.
ginseng		Increases sexual performance.	A root from China, often used in teas and vitamins.
levodopa	L-dopa	Makes older men more sexually active and able to perform.	In a small percentage of men, hypersexuality was reported. More frequently, it has no effect or causes a painful, constant, unwanted erection. Has no effect on women.
LSD	acid, fry	Makes sexual response "real."	This is a hallucinogen. It has no sexual effects.
marijuana	pot, dope, weed, joint	Heightens mood and arousal.	Similar to alcohol in reducing sexual inhibitions. It stimulates sexual activity and may change perception of time—resulting in an illusion that arousal and the length of orgasm have been increased. Often has no effect.
psilocybin/ mescaline	mushrooms	Heightens sexual response.	These are hallucinogens. They may temporarily alter how one views sexual activity. A "bad trip" results in a very bad experience—sexual or not.
testosterone		Creates sexual arousal and enhances sexual performance.	Can raise sexual desire in men and women. May be prescribed for women after menopause. Side effects include acne and, in women, unwanted facial hair.
yohimbine		Creates sexual arousal and enhances sexual performance.	Made from the bark of an African yohimbe tree. May have aphrodisiac effects in humans in correct dosage form.

BODY VARIATIONS AND OUR SEXUALITY

Most of us know someone—a friend, a family member, or a class-mate—who has a disability. We may be disabled ourselves. People with disabilities are challenged in their everyday lives by activities that may be easy for others. For example, crossing a street, reading a book, or even having a conversation may require extra skills and courage. Disabled people may be physically or mentally challenged. They have emotions, needs, and wants just like people who are not disabled. They are also sexual. They have sexual desires, attractions, imaginations, and sexual response cycles. Sexuality is a major part of their lives, too. Because of their physical or mental challenges, developing their sexuality may require different methods of learning and experiencing.

It is very important to remember that a child who is physically or mentally challenged has the right to be educated about sexuality. It may be awkward for many parents to talk about sexuality to a child who is disabled. The first step in overcoming the fear of talking and educating is to recognize and accept that all people have a sexual birthright.

We must also recognize and deal with the many challenges that people with disabilities may meet while trying to exercise their sexual birthrights. Disabled people may deny their own sexual feelings. They may also fear the sexual advances of others. Some of their fears stem from real feelings of vulnerability. Their other fears reflect the misguided social belief that disabled people are not supposed to be sexual.

Among the many challenges faced by people with disabilities is the development of positive body images and positive attitudes toward sex and sexuality. Family and friends of physically and mentally challenged children and adults need to be especially caring and attentive to these needs.

Just as it is normal for disabled people to become sexually attracted to other people, it is also normal for anyone to be sexually attracted to them. We may fear becoming clumsy if we decide to explore these sexual attractions. We may be embarrassed that we won't know how to deal with disability in a sexual way. We need only remember that relationships and sexual fulfillment do not rely on only one kind of sex play. Sexual relationships and fulfillment come from sharing intimacy and a wide range of physical sensations.

All people are capable of being intimate and of receiving, giving, and sharing sexual pleasure, whether or not they are disabled. Sexuality can be a great challenge for people with disabilities, their abled or disabled sex partners, and their caregivers. If we acknowledge and address their sexual needs, however, disabled women and men can discover, establish, and maintain the fulfilling sexual relationships to which they are entitled.

Blindness

Humans use sight more than any other sense. People who are blind cannot see with their eyes. Instead, they develop their other senses: touch, hearing, smell, and sound. These other senses help them "see." Blind people can read a language by moving their fingers over a code of bumps—this language is called braille. They write, move around in society, play sports, hold jobs, create art, or make music. They have sexual relationships. They are parents and grandparents.

People who are blind from birth are likely to begin puberty at an earlier age than sighted people. Women and men who have early menarche and spermarche are also likely to begin having sexual intercourse at an early age. Blind women may also experience more irregular menstrual cycles than sighted women.

Books about sexuality that are designed for sighted people may not be as useful for blind people. Instead, discussions, models that can be touched, and books in braille can help provide sexuality education for the blind. Being an open and approachable parent will help provide sexuality education for a blind child. Growing up and discovering sexuality as a blind person means discovering what is arousing without sight. It may be a voice, a personality, a certain odor, or a certain touch. Blind people develop sexual preferences just like everyone else.

People who become blind as adults may have already gained a sexuality education. However, adjusting to their loss of sight may be challenged by depression, lower **self-esteem,** and confusion about their sexuality. It is important for friends and family members who become blind to recognize that they are still sexually attractive and capable of enjoying and having sex. In fact, they may even be able to heighten their sexual sensations. Nevertheless, the transition period can be hard for adults and their sex partners. Patience, effort, and education can help both partners through this time.

Deafness

Deaf people are those whose hearing is impaired, as well as those who cannot hear. People who are deaf from an early age do not learn to speak as hearing people do. They "listen" by watching a language of hand signals called sign language. Some deaf and hearing-impaired people may become very good at lipreading—but this is less usual. Some may learn to use their vocal cords to produce words and speak as hearing persons do.

It is difficult for deaf people to learn to read because so much of our vocabulary is learned by hearing. The vocabulary of the deaf may be more limited than that of the hearing. Lack of vocabulary makes learning parts of the body more difficult. It may take special efforts to overcome the problems of communication and meaning when the deaf are learning about their sexuality.

These communication problems can also create great challenges as deaf people learn to socialize. Hearing people are usually illiterate in sign language. They may also be embarrassed and not know any other way to "talk." This can make it difficult and frustrating to establish a relationship. The lack of social interaction that deaf children experience may affect their sexual development. Deaf people may mature more slowly socially. They may have their first sexual encounters at later ages.

Loss of Limb

People may be born without one or more of their limbs—hands, feet, arms, or legs. They may also lose limbs through accident or disease. These people are challenged by activities such as putting on clothes, opening doors, walking, using computers, and playing sports. They may become very good at functioning in society by using special devices—wheelchairs or prosthetic arms, legs, hands, and feet—to get around. For some, the function of the missing limb is replaced by another part of the body—typing with the feet or writing with the other hand, for example.

People who have lost a limb face the challenge of poor body image. Sexuality is deeply affected for anyone who has a poor body image—whether or not she or he has lost a limb. People feel unattractive. They may feel sexually inadequate. They may feel that they are unable to give or share sexual pleasure with a partner. They may

have **performance anxiety.** They may also feel that their coordination and sexual performance will be affected by not having all
their limbs. Certain sexual positions or arrangements may be easier,
more comfortable, and pleasing for someone who has lost a limb. An
attentive partner will understand and help meet these needs. Both
partners can help one another by listening and communicating their
needs and wants.

Spinal Cord Injuries

The spinal cord is the long bundle of nerves in the middle of our
backbones where all of the nerves in our bodies meet before connecting to the brain. The spinal cord stretches from the base of the
neck to the tailbone just above the anus. When we are touched, the
nerves in our skin stimulate nerves in the spinal cord. The spinal cord
stimulates receptors in the brain. The brain translates the stimulation
as pleasure, pain, or discomfort. The head is the only part of the body
that does not depend on the spinal cord for responses to sensation.
Sensations experienced by the head—sight, smell, taste, hearing, and
touch of the face—are experienced directly by the brain.

Different injuries of the spinal cord will affect how different parts
of our bodies experience touch, pressure, and movement. An injury
of the spinal cord damages the nerves that let us know we are being
touched. A serious injury to the spinal cord often results in paralysis—
a part or parts of the body become unable to feel sensation and cannot be moved.

The location of the injury determines which nerves are damaged
and where paralysis will occur. If the injury occurs at the base of the
neck, most of the nerves will be damaged, and most of the body will
be paralyzed. If the injury occurs lower on the spinal cord, the nerves
that are damaged may be only those for the genitals and legs, and
paralysis will occur from the waist down to the toes. People with
spinal cord injuries may have areas of skin that are still sensitive to
touch, even if the areas are limited to the face.

Often, areas of the skin that were not very sensitive before an
injury become erogenous zones after an injury. For example, breasts,
neck, shoulders, or the face and lips may become more sensitive to
sexual stimulation. Imagination may also become a more developed
tool for sexual fulfillment.

Spinal cord injury in women often means that the genitals lose the ability to feel sexual pleasure. Women may experience diminished lubrication. Unless lubricants are used, vaginal tissue may be torn and infection may occur. Orgasms are also affected. Sexual positions are also limited for women with spinal cord injuries. Fertility, however, is usually preserved.

Many men with spinal cord injuries are still able to have erections. However, many may not be able to feel their erections. Or their erections may not last for very long. Furthermore, the sexual positions that partners are able to take may be limited without the use of legs or arms. Ejaculation is possible for some men, but not for others. Orgasm may take more of an emotional form than a physical one. Fertility may also be affected.

For men, injections and special devices are available to help keep an erection for a longer period of time. Men who lose sensitivity in the genital area learn to find sexual pleasure from the touch of another erogenous zone.

Current research is looking at why some people with spinal cord injuries are still able to have orgasms. Our understanding of spinal cord injuries and sexuality is growing. New information about the anatomy of the spinal cord and our sexual nervous systems may provide more insight into the sex lives of people with spinal cord injuries as well as their partners. It is important for women and men with spinal cord injuries to know that they may be able to experience a great deal of pleasure during sexual activity.

Mental Challenges

Mental retardation is a condition of lower-than-average intelligence. Mental retardation has many causes and results in many different IQs. It happens when the development of the brain is slowed or stopped. The cause is often genetic. Trauma, lack of oxygen during birth, or infection during pregnancy are other causes. The retardation can be so severe that people are unable to care for themselves. In other situations, retardation may be so mild that people may be able to learn skills, hold jobs, and live independently.

Regardless of how severe their mental challenge may be, all people are born with the ability to feel sexual pleasure. They also have body images that affect their everyday lives as well as their sexuality.

Positive body images can be reinforced by parents, teachers, and caregivers who make the effort to educate these women and men about their sexuality.

Family and health care workers who deal with the mentally retarded may be afraid of or embarrassed by the sexuality of the mentally challenged. They may fear that challenged people will masturbate in public. They may fear that they will engage in sexual intercourse without using contraception.

Developmentally disabled women, men, and children need to know that sex play in public is not socially acceptable. They also need to know about safer sex and birth control. Many will be able to effectively use a reversible method such as the condom, **vaginal pouch,** or the Pill. Some, however, may not be able to protect themselves from unplanned pregnancy.

It may be appropriate to provide some high-risk individuals with long-term reversible contraceptives such as **Norplant®** and **Depo-Provera®** or permanent methods such as **vasectomy** and **tubal sterilization.** Whenever contraceptive choices need to be made for the developmentally disabled, they must always be made in the best interests of the disabled person.

For more information about these and other dysfunctions, see Chapter 5, "Our Sexual Feelings— the Psychology of Sex," and Chapter 6, "Our Sexual Health—Taking Care of Our Bodies."

Sexual Dysfunctions

Dysfunction means to not work well. A sexual dysfunction can be either physical or mental. Or it can be both. It means that a sexual process or response is not functioning normally. For example, if a man is not able to get an erection for some time, his penis is not functioning normally. This is commonly called impotence. It can be caused by physical problems—the penile tissue may be damaged, for example. It can also be caused by mental problems such as anxiety, fear, stress, and depression. For example, a man who is very fearful of impregnating a woman may not be able to get an erection. The correct term for impotence is **inhibited arousal.** In women, inhibited arousal results in a lack of lubrication. Inhibited arousal can also be caused by certain drugs and medications.

There are numerous sexual dysfunctions that affect our sexual abilities. Dysfunction can happen at any point during the first three phases of the sexual response cycle—desire, excitement, or plateau.

Health Conditions and Our Sexual Function

All illnesses and diseases can affect our sexuality. An illness can make us too exhausted to join in or enjoy sexual intimacy. It can also cause physical problems that affect our sexual response cycle and our ability to perform. Disease and illness also affect how we view our bodies. We can develop a poor body image if we feel our bodies are unhealthy, unattractive, or unresponsive.

Our sexuality is also affected by medications that are prescribed to treat illness and disease. Medications can affect us physically and psychologically. They can also affect how we view ourselves sexually and

HEALTH CONDITIONS AND OUR SEXUALITY

Health Condition	Possible Sexual Problems—Women	Possible Sexual Problems—Men
arthritis	Pain in joints and restricted movement can make it difficult to masturbate or to have sexual activity in certain positions.	Same.
cancer breast cervix or uterus prostate testicles ovaries	Radiation treatment causes hair loss, fatigue, and nausea, which greatly reduces sexual desire. Radical surgery may cause changes in self-image, reduce the function of sexual organs, or halt the production of hormones. Women who have a hysterectomy will no longer experience uterine contractions during orgasm.	Same. Prostate surgery may affect ability to ejaculate or have an erection.
cardiovascular (heart) disease	Fear that sexual activity will lead to a heart attack. Depression and lack of interest in sex because of fears. Physical effects such as shortness of breath and chest pains will limit sexual activities.	Same.
diabetes	Greater likelihood of painful chronic infections, reduced lubrication.	Impotence, retrograde ejaculation.
mood disorders (either depression or euphoria)	Depressed persons often experience a reduction in desire for sexual activity. Certain antidepressant medications can decrease sexual desire and performance.	Same.
spinal cord injury	Effects will depend on where the injury has occurred in the spinal cord. It could result in different forms of paralysis. Paralysis may limit the positions sex partners can take. Decreased sensation may affect sexual pleasure. Could cause loss of lubrication.	Same. Could result in loss of erection.

how we perform. Some medications have side effects that can decrease our sexual desire or performance. They may also be used, however, to treat illnesses such as depression that affect our moods and sense of ourselves. They may help us feel better about ourselves and positively affect our sex lives.

It is important for people who take medications to talk with their health care professionals about the effects any medication may have on their sex lives. Very often health care professionals fail to consider their patients' sex lives. If they do not begin the conversation, make sure that you do.

In the table on the previous page, a few health conditions are listed with the effects these conditions may have on sexual health. If you need more information about these or other health concerns, contact a health care professional or visit your local library.

Our sexuality and our sexual bodies go through many changes during our lives. In the next chapter, we will look at some of those changes as they occur over the life span.

CHAPTER 4

Our Sexual

Journey

through Life

*'Tis better to have loved and lost
Than never to have loved at all.*
—Alfred, Lord Tennyson (1809–92)

We begin our sexual journey through life in childhood. It continues through our **adolescence,** our young adulthood, and our senior years. Our journey is shaped by gender, sexual orientation, disability, special needs, or lifestyles such as the religious life or the military, and physical, emotional, and social changes we experience.

The meanings of love, friendship, and life partnership may also change for us along the way. Although all of us are on this voyage, none of our adventures will be exactly the same.

OUR SEXUAL JOURNEY AS CHILDREN

As children, we may not think of ourselves as being on the beginning of a sexual journey, but we are. We may start our trip by just being curious about our bodies, asking our parents where we came from, or noticing that girls and boys are different from one another. Eventually, we notice the physical changes that our bodies are going through. The timing of the changes is different for each of us, but we all go through them.

Traditionally, childhood sexuality was seen incorrectly as either dangerous or nonexistent. Many still become uncomfortable with a child's normal sexual behavior or interest. They may be concerned for various reasons:

- They worry that their children's sexuality is not normal or is bad.
- They are uncertain or worried about how to deal with their children's sexuality.
- They might be dealing with their own sexual conflicts.
- They fear their own normal curiosity about their children's sexuality.

Rest assured that sexuality in childhood is normal and is also healthy and natural. Our sexual reflexes are already at work when we are babies. We experience and enjoy physical closeness with our parents through hugging, clinging, and cuddling. We are really too young to be aware of the connections that are being made to our sexuality. But we do learn that physical closeness and expressions of affection feel good.

Physical Changes during Childhood

As we grow, the physical changes in our bodies become quite obvious. We lose our baby fat and develop quite distinctive physical features. We learn to walk, talk, dress ourselves, and feed ourselves. We grow taller and stronger month by month. It happens to each of us at different rates. That's why everyone in our fourth-grade class pictures seems to be of different heights.

These changes in growth are not the same as the changes that happen later during adolescence. They do, however, affect our sense of ourselves and our sense of our sexuality. Are we bigger than girls should be? Are we smaller than boys should be? The answers we learn can deeply affect our sense of our femininity or masculinity.

Emotional Changes during Childhood

We develop our basic attitudes about sexuality during childhood. As infants, we form attachments with our parents or other caregivers. How they bond with us is very important to the way we shape our future relationships. Whether they are warm, secure, and loving or cold, insecure, and indifferent affects how we develop our emotional lives into adulthood. Many of our earliest experiences with love and attachment directly reflect our bonds with our parents and caregivers.

Our parents are under a lot of social pressure to try to raise us to be sexually responsible individuals. Some parents try to stop any kind of sexual experimentation by children. They may become upset if they notice their child touching his or her genitals and might say things like "That's not nice" or "Don't touch yourself down there." They may give nonverbal negative messages by slapping or pushing a child's hand away from her or his genitals.

We may become confused if our parents encourage us to be proud of our growing bodies but discourage us from taking satisfaction in our genitals. Such disapproving messages may cause children to develop negative feelings about their bodies and themselves. The message they receive is that sexuality is bad and so are they.

On the other hand, parents can foster positive feelings about sexuality by acknowledging their children's autoerotic pleasure. They can smile to their infants and coo, "That feels good, doesn't it?" To older children, they can say, "I know that feels good, but that's a private pleasure. We do that when we're alone—in private." These approving messages can help children develop positive feelings about their bodies and themselves. The message they receive is that sexuality is good and so are they.

Educational Needs and Responsibilities during Childhood

The sexual curiosity of a child may be surprising to us. It is a good idea to act calmly no matter how surprised we may be. We must be prepared to answer questions. If they are old enough to ask, then they are old enough to receive an answer. When parents don't know the answer, it helps to be honest and admit it. We can invite our children to help us look up the answer, or we can find it by ourselves.

The bottom line is to give the child an accurate and simple answer as soon as possible. In all our conversations with our children, we should try to use proper terminology for all body parts, including the vagina, penis, anus, and breasts. Using slang terms gives the impression that we think there is something shameful about these parts of the body.

By the time we are six years old, sex play between our friends and ourselves is a common way of being curious and learning about the differences in our bodies. "Playing doctor" is just one way that we learn about the physical differences between boys and girls while we satisfy our curiosity. We are also aware of the many social restrictions on our sexual expression, so we probably try to hide our activities from our parents and other adults.

One of the greatest responsibilities that our parents have during our childhood is to make sure we know what is socially appropriate behavior and what is not. Parents can integrate discussions about sexuality into family life in a balanced, frank, matter-of-fact way that allows them to deal with sexual topics openly, whenever appropriate. They can set reasonable limits on our sexual behavior as children just as they set rules for other behaviors. They can also present sexuality as a healthy and positive part of life as they present information about sexual risks and responsibilities.

A balanced view of sexual pleasure and responsibility will help children learn to develop positive decision-making skills.

Sexual Diversity during Childhood

Most children are not aware of their sexual orientation until they become teenagers. Most assume that they are straight. They strive to be what they think is considered feminine or masculine in their culture. They expect to have partners of the other gender when they grow up. They base their expectations on what they observe in their families, their communities, and the images that are presented in the media.

Some children, however, find that they feel somehow different from other children. They may not be able to express how or why they feel different. Later in life, when they are older, they may come to understand what made them feel different. They may have sensed that they didn't quite fit the gender roles and sexual identities they felt were assigned to them. This insight often happens when young people discover that they are lesbian, gay, bisexual, or transgender.

Parents cannot predict if a child will conform to cultural and sexual norms regarding gender identity. They have no way of knowing which, if any, of their children will grow up to be lesbian, gay, bisexual, or transgender. Neither do their children. That's why it is especially important for parents to allow their children to begin their sexual journey through life without feeling pressured to be feminine or masculine or gay or straight.

Children who experience their sexuality differently from cultural norms may have the impression that their families will not accept their true sexual identities and can have a very hard time growing up. They are much more susceptible than other children to depression. They make more suicide attempts and are at higher risk for using alcohol and other drugs. They are also more likely to leave their homes at early ages and to engage in high risk sex practices in order to survive on the streets.

Parents can let their children know, from the very earliest ages, that they will be loved and supported, no matter what their sexual identities and orientations prove to be.

It's a very important responsibility to prepare children for their sex lives, but it's really important to do so before their next stop on their sexual journey—adolescence.

HOW TO TALK WITH YOUR CHILD ABOUT SEX AND SEXUALITY

Here are some tips:

- Try to talk about sexuality often and in a matter-of-fact way—the way you'd talk about anything else.
- Try not to "lecture" about sex or rush through a discussion in 15 minutes. Children need time to digest information and ask questions.
- Include more than **biology**—children need to learn about values, emotions, and making decisions.
- Don't be concerned about providing too much information. Children will filter out what they do not understand.
- If your child is using inappropriate language, calmly explain what these words mean and why you don't want them used. Laughing or joking about their use may encourage continued use.
- Use correct terminology for all body parts.
- Preschool children need to know how to protect themselves from sexual abuse. Let them know that it is okay to say no to an adult and to unwanted touch.
- Don't wait until a child is a teenager to discuss puberty. Physical changes start happening before the age of 10 and vary widely from person to person.
- Educate boys as well as girls about menstruation and erections.
- Be sure to include topics such as sexual orientation, sexual abuse, and prostitution. Most children will hear about these issues on television or from peers.
- Be direct when talking about AIDS and sexually transmitted infections. But don't try to frighten children with facts about death from AIDS as a way to keep them from being curious about sex—it is not a method that works.
- Create a safe environment for your child to come to you with questions. Don't embarrass a child or say, "You're too young." Children who ask need to know.
- If you don't know the answer, admit it and then find it out.
- After you've answered a question, ask if they understand your answer and provide them with the opportunity to ask you further questions.

OUR SEXUAL JOURNEY AS ADOLESCENTS

Adolescence is the transition from childhood to adulthood that includes dramatic developments in mental, physical, and social growth. It extends from the time we are about nine or 10 years old to our late teens. For some people, adolescence may last into their early 20s. Adolescence is a time of change, of pride, self-consciousness, and uncertainty. We do not feel like children or adults, and we are often treated as neither. We wonder about what is going on with our bodies and feelings, and we worry that these changes are noticed by our peers. We also wonder about just how normal we are.

Physical and Emotional Changes during Adolescence

The physical changes of adolescence are probably the most startling and obvious part of growing up. The rapid changes of our bodies, the growing importance of peers, and the sexual development of our lives can all contribute to confusion and stress. The physical changes associated with early or late onset of puberty can be particularly embarrassing. As adolescents, some of us experience weight problems or have severe acne. Whether short or tall, fat or thin, we have an increased self-consciousness about our bodies. We are very aware of our peers and are constantly comparing our stages of development with theirs.

We become very concerned with our appearance. Wearing the right or wrong clothes to school can determine whether we have a good or bad day. Not looking "right" can put barriers in the way of being accepted by our peers. Worrying about being cool or popular is a serious concern for us. We may need a lot of help to bridge the gap of feeling unwanted or disliked.

Feeling unwanted or disliked is quite common. As adolescents, we often have doubts about ourselves. We often don't like ourselves very much. We need a lot of love, affection, and reassurance from our parents. It is really vital. But at the same time that we want our parents to share in what we are feeling from our peers and our own emotional turmoil, our parents become faced with the fact that their children have become sexual people! It can be hard to handle. We all have to be very patient with one another.

As sexual people, we have become more concerned, or even anxious, about masturbation and our erotic desires, dreams, and thoughts. Many of us may hear about sexual intercourse for the first time, and we may not be too happy about what we hear. We might be shocked or unbelieving that sex really happens like that! We may feel safer in the company of people of our own gender. That's one of the reasons that adolescents often split into **homosocial** groups, in which girls make friends only with girls and boys make friends only with boys.

As adolescents, we have important emotional and educational needs. We want to know everything we can about relationships. Communication skills are critical. We need to talk about our feelings of confusion. We need our questions answered. We need open lines of communication. We need to learn these skills in order to make decisions and resolve conflicts. Decision making becomes increasingly complicated as we mature. Should I have sex? Should I drink alcohol? What kind of birth control should I use?

As adolescents, we also need information about pregnancy, contraception, sexually transmitted infections, and sexual abuse, before we are sexually active. We want our parents to give us the facts we need to stay healthy. We also want them to share the underlying values they have used to make their own decisions about sexuality.

Social Pressures and Responsibilities during Adolescence

As children, we learn a lot about what is sexually appropriate. We learn not to touch ourselves except in private. We also learn not to touch others in inappropriate places. As adolescents, the messages become more urgent. "Don't have sex until you are married!" "Only bad teenagers have sex!" "Don't even think about sex!" At the same time, our sexual bodies and feelings are urgently demanding our attention!

It's hard to figure out what we should listen to and what we should ignore. Parents, politicians, educators, and religious organizations might prefer that we ignore the sexual part of our lives. And it may be difficult for our parents to think about us as sexual beings because they remember what it may have been like for them—confusing, exciting, daring, and dangerous. So they try to protect us from unwanted pregnancies and sexually transmitted infections. They often suggest that we just say "No!"

Meanwhile, our friends and peers may be starting to date, going to make-out parties, and, as we get a little older, starting to think about having sex. First dating may start around 12 or 13. Group dating and coed parties are common. Kissing games are popular at these parties. A date may include going to the movies, bowling, or just hanging out. Going steady is still popular and is marked with symbolic gifts like bracelets, rings, caps, and jackets. Early in adolescence, however, we remain rather sexually conservative, usually believing that we should have sex only if we are married.

As we become older teenagers, however, our attitudes may change. Our peers may push us to become sexually active. This is known as **peer pressure.** Peer pressure can often move us to do positive things for ourselves—develop athletic skills, for example. It can also lead us to high-risk activities such as smoking, drinking, and drug taking.

It's hard to resist peer pressure when the need to be accepted by our friends is so great. Being different—especially about sex—isn't something our friends may consider "cool." Our parents, on the other hand, often want us to put off sexual activity.

For many of us, the message is mixed. A son may be pushed to become sexually active by his father or older brother. A daughter may be encouraged by both parents to resist sexual activities. This is a double standard in which one set of rules applies to one person, and a different set applies to another person in the same situation.

There are other conflicting messages about sexuality in our society. Just as we may have strong desires not to disappoint our friends, we may have equally strong desires to please our parents. On the other hand, some of us may feel the normal desire to break away from our parents and set our own rules. We may feel we are ready for sexual activity, or we may want to have sex as a way of rebelling against our parents.

On one hand, we are told about all the bad things that happen to sexually active teenagers, such as unintended pregnancies and sexually transmitted infections. But on the other hand, sexual attractiveness—being sexy—is highly valued. We learn both these lessons from TV, magazines, movies, and music videos.

As adolescents, we also learn a lot of gender stereotypes—what supposedly is right or wrong for girls and boys to do. We feel a lot of pressure about our gender. We try to conform to our society's gender stereotypes. On the next page is a list of positively valued stereotypes that are supposed to be true of women and men.

Of course, these are all characteristics that women and men both possess, but there is a lot of pressure on us as teenagers to fulfill one or the other of these stereotyped roles. We are expected to look feminine or masculine, and we are expected to act that way as well.

As adolescents, we tend to form instant judgments about people's femininity or masculinity on obvious or subtle characteristics, like the way they dress, their hairstyle, or their body language. We develop a lot of our expectations about female and male behavior at home as we observe who does what chores, who takes care of the children, who makes decisions, who brings home the paycheck, and who decides what's done with it.

Dating is one of the crucial gender pressures we experience as teens. We live in a predominantly heterosexual world, and when we reach our teen years, we are expected to be attracted to, pursue, and date the other gender.

Sexual decision making may become a part of dating for older teens. Not only are we pressured to date, we are also pressured to have sex. Sometimes saying no to sex can be really difficult. We worry what it means about us. Does it mean that we do not love our partners? Does it mean we are not feminine or masculine enough? Does it mean we are not sexually desirable? There are probably few experiences in our lives, whether we are adults or teenagers, that can be as exciting and anxiety-ridden as making decisions about when to have our first sexual intercourse.

These are very real questions for us as teenagers. Many of us also believe sexual myths like the ones listed below.

- Having sex makes one become adult.
- Having sex proves love is real.
- "No" really means "yes."
- People can't enjoy sex if they use condoms.
- HIV can't happen to me.

POSITIVELY VALUED STEREOTYPES OF FEMININITY

According to the stereotypes of femininity, women are always supposed to be:

  emotional
  warm
  able to devote themselves to others
  gentle
  helpful
  kind
  understanding
  aware of others' feelings

POSITIVELY VALUED STEREOTYPES OF MASCULINITY

According to stereotypes of masculinity, men are always supposed to be:

  able to perform under pressure
  independent
  dominant
  active
  competitive
  decisive
  self-confident
  determined

DANGEROUS MYTHS ABOUT BIRTH CONTROL AND PREGNANCY

Although nearly 75 percent of all teens have sexual intercourse before they graduate from high school, many believe myths that may lead to unintended pregnancy or sexually transmitted infection. To offset these misconceptions about birth control and pregnancy, young adolescents need to know the following:

- A woman *can* get pregnant even if:
  - she is having vaginal bleeding
  - she doesn't have an orgasm
  - she doesn't have vaginal intercourse often
  - she has vaginal intercourse standing up
  - she urinates right after having vaginal intercourse
  - she douches with Coke®, Sprite®, Fresca®, or anything else
  - the man pulls his penis out of her vagina before he ejaculates
  - she jumps up and down after vaginal intercourse
  - she hasn't had her first period yet
  - she's under 12 years old
  - it's her first time
- Plastic wrap wrapped around the penis is not an effective contraceptive.
- The Pill does not prevent sexually transmitted infections.

Adults also have myths about teenagers and sex. Many believe that if teenagers are given information about their sexuality, they are more likely to have sex earlier than other teens. Actually, the opposite is true. Teenagers who receive information about their sexuality are more likely to delay their first intercourse.

On the next page are some worthwhile questions to ask about ourselves, our partners, our families, and our friends before we decide to have sex with someone else.

Being a sexual person during our adolescent and teen years carries with it a certain amount of responsibility. We are not only accountable for ourselves but are also accountable for anyone with whom we may be sexually intimate. We must be knowledgeable about contraception and sexually transmitted infections. We must come to understand what it means to make emotional commitments

AM I READY TO HAVE SEX?

Questions about Myself

1. Have I thought enough about myself and my sexuality to know that I am ready to have sex?
2. Am I prepared to protect myself or my partner against unintended pregnancy?
3. Am I prepared to deal with an unintended pregnancy if it happens?
4. Am I prepared to protect myself and my partner against sexually transmitted infections?

Questions about My Relationship

1. Do we feel comfortable talking with one another about sex?
2. Do we both agree that we are ready and want to have sex?
3. Are we committed to protecting one another physically and emotionally?
4. Are we using sex to hold our relationship together?

Questions about My Parents

1. Do I ever talk about sex with my parents?
2. Do I understand my parents' values about sex, and do I share them?
3. Will I be able to talk with my parents about my decision? If I can't, how would it feel if I lied to them?
4. Am I planning to have sex to hurt, anger, or spite my parents?

Questions about My Friends

1. Are my friends pressuring me to have sex?
2. Would I be considered "not cool" if my decision about sex isn't the same as theirs?
3. Do I become tempted to have sex when I get drunk or high with my friends?
4. How much does it matter what my friends think?

to another person. Being able to communicate and make decisions together can make these experiences more rewarding and much healthier for both partners.

Sexual Diversity during Adolescence

Many teenagers struggle to understand their sexual identities. We wonder if certain things about us mean that we are women or men, straight, gay, lesbian, bisexual, or transgender. We may not want to have sex with anyone, or we may like hanging out only with people of the same sex. We may have crushes on or fall in love with people of the same sex.

Exploring our sexual identities and orientation during our teen years can be a scary experience. Our society pressures us to be heterosexual—to be feminine women and masculine men. As young people, we are well aware of society's negative attitudes toward homosexuality. We learn to use words like "fag," "fem," and "queer" on the playground to hurt other kids. We hear negative things about lesbian, gay, and bisexual people in many of our families. We may be reprimanded for dressing too feminine or masculine.

Some of us are called "tomboys." Others are called "sissies." Some people are aware of their sexual identities and orientation from childhood. Others become aware of it later in life. As they come to know their sexual identities and orientation, each youth has to make his or her own decision about **coming out** to family and friends. Coming out is the process of acknowledging, first to ourselves and then to others, that we are lesbian or gay, bisexual, or transgender. There may be great risks involved. We may alienate parents upon whom we are dependent for our daily needs. Coming out at school can be frightening when the approval of our peers and school officials is so very important.

Accepting ourselves as different from society's sexual norms can be very difficult in American culture. Our society fears homosexuality and people whose identities are not clearly feminine or masculine. We are very likely to internalize our society's negative views, and that can make us feel guilty and afraid of our sexual feelings.

These fears and uncertainties can lead to depression and confusion. Feeling isolated, alone, and hated might make us think about suicide. Nearly 30 percent of all teen suicides are committed by lesbian and gay youth. Lesbian and gay youth and those who are perceived to be are two to three times more likely to commit suicide than straight teens and six times more likely to think about suicide.

OUR SEXUAL JOURNEY AS YOUNG ADULTS

Our biggest challenge during adolescence was to develop identities that were uniquely our own. We had to navigate a difficult path from childhood through puberty, accept our changing bodies, and resolve our many emotional issues. As young adults, the changes of puberty are nearly complete, our bodies long for sexual expression, and our struggle for sexual identities may continue. We may have experienced our first sexual relationship, and we may now be beginning to learn more about our sexual likes and dislikes. We are also developing more complex intimate relationships with others and learning more about relationships and commitment.

For more information about coming out and the emotional needs of lesbian and gay and bisexual teens, see Chapter 5, "Our Sexual Feelings—the Psychology of Sex."

Physical Changes during Young Adulthood

Our physical journey is at a slower pace now. The rapid changes of puberty are just about over. Young women have probably stopped growing taller. Young men may have a few more inches to grow. But we are now more accustomed to our adult bodies and their rhythms. Our hormones have reached more balanced levels. Most young women have established a menstrual cycle that is more predictable. Young men are probably experiencing fewer spontaneous erections and nocturnal emissions. Physical changes are more subtle as our bodies and faces slowly change into their adult forms.

Emotional Changes during Young Adulthood

The emotional and mental changes that take place in young adulthood are probably going to be more noticeable than the physical ones. Decisions about careers, living arrangements, and relationships become important. Our educational needs will also change.

One of the biggest concerns we have as young adults is our living arrangements. We usually remain living at home with our parents until we are financially able to have our own apartment or house.

Being a sexual adult while still living at home can have some draw-backs. When we enter adulthood and begin having intimate relationships with others, it may be difficult to express our sexuality when we know our parents are in the house!

Families have to get together and establish ground rules about privacy at home. Every member of the family can express what will allow her or him to be comfortable. Families may want to consider the risks young people take to have sex outside the home.

Sex in parked cars and other public places can lead to dangerous or humiliating situations. If being sexual at home is against the rules, then other solutions can be found. The partner's home may be more appropriate. If neither home is an option, finding our own place might become necessary.

Living alone may offer great potential for personal fulfillment. We may have greater opportunities to travel, entertain, relax, pursue hobbies, and explore our own individualities. Maintaining independence and learning how to be a responsible person are additional benefits. The privacy of living alone enables us to be sexually active, if we choose, without the concerns of being in our parents' home. But living alone—whether by choice or necessity—can also be difficult and lonely.

If living alone is not appealing or practical, sharing a home with a roommate may be the solution. People of the same or other gender can share housing. Roommates can provide companionship and share the costs of the home. They should establish ground rules regarding privacy and houseguests from the start.

As infants, children, and adolescents, we have emotional needs that must be met. We need affection, caring, and education. As adults, we still have these needs. These emotional needs are met through various people in our lives. We still receive and need love and affection from family. Our friends are also very important to us. But as adults, we find ourselves making new friends and forming new relationships that are unconnected to our families or the friendships of our childhood.

Not all of us make new friends when we become adults. Some young adults choose to avoid intimate relationships. They may fear taking risks with their emotions because of some past hurt, or they may be concerned with other changing parts of their lives, such as their careers or their changing relationship with their families.

Forming relationships, however, usually becomes a central part of our lives. Developing relationships, especially intimate ones, can be a challenge. It happens when we become comfortable enough to risk revealing our true identities and our most personal thoughts and feelings to someone else. In order for us to become intimate with someone else, we need to understand our own identities.

Intimacy is a closeness between two people. Intimacy can be an emotional, spiritual, social, or intellectual closeness. It usually involves both sharing and caring. Being free to communicate is essential in an intimate relationship. We can be intimate with family, friends, or sex partners, but sex does not have to play a role in intimacy.

Intimate friendships can be extremely rewarding. Yet forming them can be sometimes difficult. On the one hand, it seems so simple: The major reason we make new friends is that they are similar to us in some way, and they like us. We feel emotionally rewarded when we are with them, so we *want* to be with them. We also want them to feel as good as we do, so we return the emotional reward to them—we "reciprocate," then they reciprocate, then we reciprocate, and so on.

On the other hand, reciprocity can have its downside. Even when both people want to reciprocate, they may fall short of one another's expectations. One of them may be ill. Times may be hard. One person may not be as mature as the other. There are lots of reasons.

We also learn from experience that our judgment isn't always good about the people with whom we choose to reciprocate. We can make mistakes about how much we think someone else cares for us. We can also overlook what it may cost us to reciprocate to the "wrong" person—especially if we have low self-esteem. In other words, we can get hurt.

As we learn more about relationships, we become more careful. Sometimes we become too careful. The better we understand ourselves, however, the more likely it is that we can have safe and secure reciprocal relationships. It can be the work of a lifetime to learn enough about ourselves to be able to manage rewarding intimate relationships with other people. Many women and men have found that the investment is worthwhile.

We have a strong desire to be liked and held in good esteem by others. This is a powerful and motivating force that has been with us

ELEMENTS OF SIMILARITY IN RECIPROCAL RELATIONSHIPS

The women and men with whom we are likely to have reciprocal relationships are often similar to us in:

age
outlook on life
moral values
appearance
mental health
physical health
intelligence
competence
geographic location

(Of course, not everyone we like is going to be just like us. That would be rather boring!)

since childhood and adolescence. Social approval is very important to us in adulthood as well. Having our worth reaffirmed by others really matters to us. We depend on others to help satisfy our needs. Their approval helps us feel confident that these needs will be met. It builds our self-esteem.

Not everyone has his or her sense of worth affirmed. The unaffirmed will find it difficult to feel good about themselves or think that others feel good about them. They are likely to have low self-esteem. People with low self-esteem do not *expect* others to like them, and they have a hard time accepting affection when it is offered. They are also likely to make poor judgments about forming reciprocal relationships.

Sex and Love

Sometimes in our sexually intimate relationships, we care for our partners as much as we care about ourselves. This is called **mutuality.** It means that we are willing to make sacrifices and compromises. Sometimes we may feel as though we are making sacrifices and compromises that are not appreciated by our partners. This can greatly affect the sex play and intimacy in a relationship.

It is always important to open communication about these issues—to discuss what we appreciate as well as what we expect. It helps to carefully evaluate the compromises and sacrifices we make and try to figure out what purpose they serve and what they may mean to the relationship over time.

Intimacy in a relationship can fluctuate. Each one of us has our ups and downs. The nature and quality of the intimacy in our relationships change with each up and each down. It is this emotional intimacy that makes our relationships in adulthood different from the ones we had as adolescents. It also makes possible a mutual sharing of sexual pleasure.

Mutuality is one of the aspects of **romantic love.** Romantic love is a combination of liking, sexual attraction, and intense emotional interaction between two people. There are two kinds of romantic love. **Passionate love** is a strong combination of feelings. It can sometimes be confusing because it can include tenderness, sexual desire, elation, pain, anxiety, relief, altruism, and **jealousy** all at once.

Passionate love often occurs at the beginning of a romantic relationship. As time passes, it usually quiets into companionate love. **Companionate love** is less emotionally intense than passionate love. It remains sexual but is moderated by friendly affection and a deeply emotional committed attachment.

As individuals, we are capable of feeling all kinds of love toward others. Sometimes love grows out of friendship. Other times love is found with a new person in our lives. Some people even fall in love at first sight!

There may be times when we think we are in love but we are not. We may be infatuated with someone. **Infatuation** is a strong sexual attraction to someone, based mainly on her or his resemblance to the ideal in our lovemap. Infatuation is common and healthy. It doesn't take long for us to realize that we are infatuated and not in love. Infatuation often passes when we get to know the person and realize that we were attracted to surface qualities, not the substance of a person. An infatuation so strong that we can't get it out of our heads is called **limerance.**

Jealousy is another emotion that is sometimes a part of our romantic relationships. Jealousy occurs when we believe that there is someone else who is receiving our partner's affection. We all fear the loss of love at some time in our lives. The thought that a loved one might be looking for a new love interest can cause us to feel anxiety and anger. It can lower our self-esteem. Communication and honesty are the best cures for jealousy. We may also find it important to remember that we are all capable of caring for many different people during our lives.

A good, healthy, lasting relationship requires work from both partners. We can't just sit back and think it will happen of its own accord. Communication and honesty are just two ingredients of healthy relationships, but they can go a long way. On the next page are some helpful hints that can strengthen relationships. They may seem simple, but it is often the easy things that we forget!

We are constantly making decisions when we are in relationships.

10 GUIDELINES FOR HEALTHY RELATIONSHIPS

1. Share good news.
2. Respect privacy.
3. Show support and caring.
4. Don't criticize.
5. Offer to help when needed.
6. Keep one another's secrets.
7. Repay favors.
8. Avoid jealousy.
9. Trust one another.
10. Confide in each other.

Kelley/Byrne, *Exploring Human Sexuality,* © 1992, p. 274. Adapted by permission of Prentice Hall, Upper Saddle River, New Jersey

These decisions include such issues as contraception, commitment, and living arrangements. As adults, we become more responsible for continuing to educate ourselves about our sexuality and sexual health. We can no longer depend on family and friends to do it for us.

We should know what contraceptive methods are best suited for our individual needs. We should know about sexually transmitted infections, including HIV/AIDS, and how to get tested. Young women should receive an annual pelvic exam, and young men should receive an annual physical. We should also try to understand what makes relationships healthy so that we can avoid abusive relationships. We should try to develop the communication and negotiation skills that are vital to maintaining healthy relationships.

Sexual Diversity during Young Adulthood

Women and men who have gender identities and sexual orientations that differ from social norms have long-term and committed relationships despite the social constraints against them. The accomplishments, problems, and decisions that these people make within relationships are similar to the ones made by straight women and men who fit the social norms.

Gay and straight couples experience the same frequency of sex, talk about who initiates sex, and decide whether or not to have children. They are equally satisfied with their relationships.

Many gay people live their sexual orientation in a hidden way. The common expression is "in the closet." They keep their sexual orientation a secret out of fear of losing loved ones, housing, or a job. Increasing numbers of gay people and those perceived to be are more overt about their sexual orientation. They live their lives out in the open and are "out" to others. Some people feel safe being out to only some of the people in their lives—to coworkers, but not family, for example. Others feel safe being out to all the people in their lives.

Coming out is a personal decision. It is a decision that gay people have to make over and over again, each time new people are introduced into their lives.

In response to the homophobia and antigay prejudice of our society, gay people have formed communities of their own in which they can feel safe. There is now a growing gay culture. In some cities, such as New York and San Francisco, being gay is becoming socially acceptable. Gay communities have bars, restaurants, dance clubs, community centers, and magazines. Since gay liberation in the late 1960s, lesbian and gay and bisexual women and men have been fighting for the same rights that are afforded to straight people. This includes the legal and civil rights afforded to straight married couples.

Social Pressures and Responsibilities during Young Adulthood

Cohabitation

Some people in relationships do not get married before they live together. Living together unmarried while in a sexual relationship is sometimes called cohabitation. Some people do this because they are not ready to commit to legal marriage. Others may never want to marry. Some people may have been married before and do not want to get married again.

Lesbian women and gay men cannot get married legally. They often share the same desires and reasons all women and men have to live with someone—to gain intimacy, companionship, and security and to live more economically.

Our views of cohabitation are shaped by our moral values and our religious and cultural beliefs. Not everyone approves of couples living together outside of marriage. Many religions do not allow for sexual intercourse before marriage, which may make cohabitation unacceptable. Deciding to live together is a decision that we make with our partners for ourselves based upon our own values and priorities.

Living together is an important commitment that couples make to one another. Like marriage, it requires good communication skills and a commitment to negotiate and compromise. It is important for both people to be clear about the goals and expectations they bring to the relationship.

Marriage

Americans like to get married, even though there is less social pressure to get married today than there was in our grandparents' generation. One reason for this is that there is less of a social stigma on single motherhood. Many women are choosing to have children without being married. Another reason is that many women no longer have to depend on marriage for financial security and can be self-sufficient.

Marriage is public recognition of the commitment that two people make to one another. It is also a legal contract. It is important to be very careful about whom we marry, when we marry, or if we marry. Marriage is not for everyone. Some people may not be socially or emotionally mature enough to get married.

How do we know when we are ready for marriage? Thinking about the following issues might help us to make a good decision:

Age. How old we are when we marry can be a good indicator of how successful the marriage will be. Usually, the older we are, the better. Three out of four teenage marriages fail.

Autonomy. Being economically independent and capable of managing one's own life is also important for successful marriage. Both partners should be able to set their own goals and be able to achieve them.

Emotional maturity. Being able to satisfy our own emotional needs without exploiting anyone else increases the chances of having a good marriage.

Social maturity. Being socially experienced through interactions such as dating, leading an independent single life before marriage, and managing financial affairs are essential to establishing equality between married partners.

Flexibility. Successful marriages require compromise. We must try to meet our partners halfway because no two people are exactly alike in tastes, needs, and desires, and we have to acknowledge and celebrate our differences.

Personality traits. It is helpful if both personalities are similar and if basic moral and religious values are held in common.

Mutuality. It is important that a marriage fulfill the needs of both partners. If it is one-sided, it will cause tension and frustrations.

Power balance. How power is used and shared may determine the long-term outcome of a relationship.

Communication. It is essential that we be able to talk about *anything* with our partners.

Agreement about parenthood. Both partners must have similar feelings about whether or not children are wanted. It is also important to agree about how many children are wanted.

Marriage itself will not make everything fall into place for us. Like any other new relationship, there are adjustments that take place within a marriage. Not only do we need to adjust to one another, but we also have to adjust to our friends and families. Being married gives us a new social identity, and we may find ourselves interacting differently with friends and family.

Another important change involves money. When two people marry, they are viewed as a single economic unit by the state. This means learning how to manage the family income, budgeting, and paying taxes. Not everyone spends and saves money the same way. Many couples experience conflict and anxiety over money. Learning how to compromise and communicate about financial issues is very important. It is healthier if both partners have input into financial decisions—regardless of who is earning the money.

Perhaps the biggest change has to do with our sexuality and how we express it. Once again, open and honest communication can ease this transition and help each partner to learn how to enjoy an intimate, mutually satisfying sexual relationship. Decisions have to be made about:

- how often to have sex
- when to have sex
- choice of sexual activities
- amount of nonsexual attention we give to one another

It is also important that each partner have the right to say no to sex without fear of consequences. All of us have times when we need to do this. Discussing your feelings about it helps your partner understand the situation. Nonverbal rejection can cause your partner unnecessary worry about the relationship. We all have our own preferences. Learning our partners' preferences and trying to compromise can be difficult, but a mutually satisfying sex life is a wonderful reward!

Parenthood

One of the biggest decisions we make in our adult years is whether or not to have a child. Deciding to have children brings with it a huge responsibility for another's life. How to be a parent is not something that we learned in school. Most of what we learn about parenting we learn from our own parents. We really do not get a lot of formal training.

We need to know about equality, health care, discipline, understanding behavior, dealing with anger, praising, setting limits, and belonging—whether or not we were taught them by our parents! Becoming a parent is a life-altering decision that should be considered very carefully.

Sex and Pregnancy

Being pregnant can have a big impact on a woman's sexuality. Her sexual desire may increase or decrease while she is pregnant. It can vary from month to month or day to day. Hormone levels are constantly changing. In the first trimester, nausea, breast tenderness, and fatigue may make a woman less interested in having sex. In the second trimester, she may have increased sexual desire because her body is adjusting and becoming more balanced. Overall, there is a general decrease in sexual interest throughout pregnancy, with the lowest interest in the third trimester.

If a pregnancy is proceeding normally and the woman is healthy, health care providers will generally advise that sexual intercourse can safely be enjoyed up until the last four weeks of pregnancy. Sexual intercourse should be discontinued immediately if the woman experiences vaginal bleeding, abdominal pain, or any other symptom of miscarriage, or if her water breaks.

Experimenting with your partner will allow you to figure out which sexual positions are most comfortable. It may be necessary to find or modify some positions. The so-called missionary position of man on top may be uncomfortable if you are pregnant. Side by side, woman on top, and rear entry might prove to be more comfortable. Oral sex and manual genital stimulation as well as touching each other's body and holding may also be satisfying. Condoms should be used to prevent sexually transmitted infections if either partner has been diagnosed with one.

Intimacy, eroticism, and sexual satisfaction can increase and continue during pregnancy. Being sensitive to and aware of a woman's changing body and feelings, as well as accepting the need for adjustment, can add excitement to your sexual relationship.

Why do some pregnant women enjoy sex and others don't? A decrease in sexual interest can be caused by physical discomfort during sex, feeling big and unattractive, or fear of hurting the fetus. Later in the pregnancy, an increased awareness of the fetus can make sex feel like a gathering of too many people!

Some women become more sexual during pregnancy. They may feel more womanly and less inhibited. The heightened awareness of their bodies can increase their sensuality. During pregnancy, there is increased flow of blood to the genitals. This increase can heighten sexual desire and response for some women.

Sex after the Baby Is Born

During childbirth, some women have a procedure called an episiotomy. An episiotomy is an incision through the skin and muscles in the perineum, the area between the vagina and the anus. This incision is made just before delivery and before the baby's head comes out. It's done to help prevent the baby from naturally tearing the skin and tissue in areas that would cause more complications.

Not every woman has an episiotomy. Some health care providers do not believe it is necessary, while others say that it helps a woman heal more quickly after labor. How rapidly a woman heals affects how soon she may have sex after childbirth.

In general, health care providers suggest waiting about four to six weeks before resuming sexual intercourse. This allows the body to heal and the uterus and vagina to return to their prepregnancy size. There is also a time after childbirth called the postpartum period, a time of both physical and psychological adjustment for a woman and everyone in her family. It is a time of intense emotional highs and lows. A father may soon become jealous of the closeness between a mother and newborn. A new mom might feel that she has to care closely for the baby and doesn't want to be distracted by others. She may not be interested in sexual activity.

Breast-feeding is another way a mother forms a close bond with an infant. This is a very special relationship. Breast feeding has very practical benefits. It helps weight loss for the new mom and causes the body to release a hormone called oxytocin. Oxytocin causes contractions of the uterus during breast-feeding, which help the uterus return to its normal size. These contractions can be sexually pleasurable. Some women feel guilty over these sexual feelings, but they are perfectly normal and natural.

Breast-feeding can also affect sexual intercourse. A decrease in estrogen can inhibit vaginal lubrication. This can make sex painful. The interactions of hormones in some breast-feeding women may cause decreased sexual desire. In addition, a woman's breasts and nipples may be tender and sore. Some women are self-conscious because their breasts leak milk. Other women feel that the close skin-to-skin contact they have with their infants while breast feeding is enough physical contact for them. Still other women simply do not have the energy for sex. Lack of sleep and unrelenting fatigue tend to decrease a woman's interest in sex.

New parents have to make a lot of adjustments. The first few months of parenthood are filled with fatigue from interrupted sleep due to feeding and changing diapers. Some new moms and dads have low sexual interest after childbirth. Decreased interest can have physical or emotional causes like tiredness, lack of privacy, or feeling self-conscious about one's body. Communication and understanding from both new parents can help make this transition smoother.

Being an adult has many responsibilities whether or not we have partners and whether or not we have children. Not only are we responsible for taking care of our emotional and physical health, but we must also consider others. We may make commitments that we must keep. We have to take full responsibility for all of our actions. We must continually educate ourselves. Above all, respecting ourselves and others is something that we should never fail to do. These are all essential keys to our sexual health and happiness.

OUR SEXUAL JOURNEY THROUGH MIDLIFE

When we reach midlife, our lives are about half over. We have come a long way from our childhood years. Many people mistakenly think that after they get married or live with someone for many years, life will get boring. This does not have to be true. Our sexuality does not stop growing, changing, or being expressed just because we are older than 29! Our middle adult years are a new and exciting leg of our sexual journey through life. Midlife, or middle age, is generally considered to range from 40 years to 55 years old. The two biggest myths surrounding our midlife sexuality are (1) older people are no longer interested in sex and don't have sex anymore, and (2) older people are *unable* to enjoy sex.

In this section, we will explore the physical changes that accompany middle age. We will also look at some of the concerns of our midlife years. Our sexual desires are no longer as exclusively focused on the attributes of youth and attractiveness as they were when we were younger. We become more concerned with our potential partners' sense of themselves. Self-worth begins to matter more than physical appearance.

Physical Changes during Midlife

At this time of life, we reach a stage in which our bodies change in ways that may be unexpected and dramatic. This stage of change is called the **climacteric.** The climacteric marks the physiological changes that occur in our transition into midlife. Both women and men go through a climacteric. It is a more definitive stage for women because they pass through a transition from being fertile to infertile. Men do not experience this transition. Men are fertile until death. Women experience greater physical changes in their middle life. The changes for men are less noticeable and cause fewer side effects.

Menopause

The first stage of a woman's climacteric is called **perimenopause.** It is the period of transition that leads to menopause—the time in midlife when a woman has her last period. Menopause was for a long time a mystery and not really spoken about. We have heard the expression "changes" to describe menopause. That is quite accurate.

A woman in perimenopause is going through a process of physical change. The process usually begins in the mid-40s. But like the rest of our sexual journey, all women arrive at menopause at different times. Because a woman's life expectancy is about 80 years of age, most women experience the second halves of their lives and their journeys after menopause!

At around 40, ovaries begin to slow down the production of estrogen. Menstruation continues but starts to become irregular.

POSSIBLE SYMPTOMS OF MENOPAUSE THAT MAY AFFECT A WOMAN'S SEXUALITY

fatigue

hot flashes

insomnia

dizziness

vaginal dryness

difficulty with balance

changes in sexual desire

extreme sweating

diminished pleasure from touch

diminished secondary sex characteristics—loss of fullness of breasts, buttocks, vulva, hips, and pubic hair

thinning of vaginal tissue

itchy or burning skin

sensitivity to clothing or touch

numbness or tingling in hands or feet

conditions associated with premenstrual syndrome

In addition, the shortage of estrogen can cause severe headaches, short-term memory loss, difficulty concentrating, depression, and increased anxiety.

Eventually, ovaries stop producing mature eggs. When this happens, estrogen production decreases dramatically. The liver, adrenal glands, and fatty tissue, however, continue to produce small amounts of estrogen. Decreased amounts of estrogen affect a woman's sexuality.

Since each woman experiences menopause differently, her symptoms will differ from those experienced by other women. These symptoms are caused by the decrease in estrogen production and can range from mild to severe. They are most acute in the two years before the last menstrual period and the two years after. In her early 40s, a woman may notice the first changes in her menstrual flow and her sleep patterns. In addition, she might start having night sweats and hot flashes, when the body temperature rises quickly from hormone surges. A woman may desire less sexual activity during periods of night sweats and hot flashes.

Though menopause can be a time of concern, knowing what to expect and that most symptoms are not permanent and that it is a natural and healthy process can alleviate fear. There are also permanent physical changes that can take place. These include an increased growth of facial hair and a deepening of the voice. The clitoris becomes larger, and the vagina also changes. The vaginal walls become thinner and dryer. Without natural lubrication, intercourse can become painful. Vegetable oils or an over-the-counter lubricant like Astroglide® or Replens® can be helpful with this problem.

Some women will lose muscle tone in the vaginal area. They may lose a small amount of urine while coughing, sneezing, or jumping—this is called stress incontinence. This is especially common for women who have experienced several vaginal childbirths. The Kegel exercises on the next page can strengthen the walls of the vagina to enhance orgasm and prevent urine loss.

KEGEL EXERCISES FOR STRONGER ORGASM AND STRESS INCONTINENCE

Kegel exercises are done by tightening and relaxing the muscles used to stop urination. Strengthening these muscles can prevent and improve urinary incontinence, improve sexual sensations, and aid recovery from childbirth. Because they are internal muscle exercises, Kegel exercises can be done anywhere, anytime. Do at least five in a row several times a day:

1. Tighten muscles a little and hold for five seconds.
2. Tighten a little more and hold for five seconds more.
3. Tighten as much as possible and hold for five seconds more.
4. Relax the muscles in reverse steps, holding five seconds at each step.

To benefit from Kegel exercises, you must isolate the correct muscles. For women to be sure they are isolating the correct muscles, they may insert two fingers into the vagina the first time they try the exercise. They should be able to feel pressure around their fingers when they squeeze the correct muscles. Once the correct muscles have been located, it is unnecessary to insert the fingers to do the exercise.

Men who do Kegels must be sure to constrict the urethra as well as the anal sphincter.

The sexual response cycle of a woman is also affected by menopause. All phases of the cycle continue but a little less intensely. There is an old saying, "If you don't use it, you'll lose it." This can apply to the sex organs as well. The more sexually active a woman remains, the more lubrication she will produce naturally.

Some women are relieved that they no longer have to worry about contraception, pregnancy, or menstruation. Others may mourn the loss of their reproductive years and/or their menstrual experience. Many women, however, enjoy increased freedom and sexual intimacy after menopause.

HORMONE REPLACEMENT THERAPY

Following menopause, a woman can use pills, patches, or creams to restore estrogen and other hormones that have diminished during perimenopause and after menopause. Estrogen alleviates hot flashes, maintains skin tone, thickens vaginal walls, and increases vaginal lubrication. It can help a woman maintain sexual interest and response. It is primarily indicated for prevention of cardiovascular disease and osteoporosis, a weakening of the bones due to calcium deficiency.

Progestins are often included in hormone replacement therapy (HRT) to decrease the potential overgrowth of the lining of the uterus that may be caused by estrogen. Testosterone can be used to increase sexual desire. Women who use estrogen may be at higher risk for endometrial cancer unless a progestin is also included in the HRT. Deciding whether or not to use HRT is a decision that should be made by each woman with advice from her health care provider.

The Male Climacteric

Men also experience changes with midlife. These changes result from a decrease in testosterone production. A man's hormones are actually at their peak when he is 17 to 20 years old. When a man reaches his 40s, he may start to experience a decline in sexual responsiveness.

These changes are more likely to be caused by stress and anxiety than they are by age. It might take him longer to develop an erection. He might require more direct genital stimulation during foreplay in order to get an erection. In addition, the angle of his erection decreases, and his orgasm becomes slightly less intense.

Kegel exercises can enhance orgasm for men. However, for many men there is no perceptible decline in erection or ejaculation until the 60s or later. Testosterone supplements may be helpful for some men, but side effects include decreased size of the penis and testicles as well as hair loss.

There are physical changes as well. The penis, testicles, and scrotum all decrease in size. The prostate gland becomes larger and can interfere with the flow of urine. Smaller amounts of semen are produced. But the sperm in the semen is still perfectly capable of fertilizing an egg. Men can cause pregnancy regardless of their age.

Emotional Changes during Midlife

As adolescents, many of us were very anxious about the changes in our bodies. We wondered if the changes were okay and if we were normal. In midlife, we have those anxieties all over again.

We worry if our bodies are still attractive. We may develop performance anxiety. Men may become anxious about developing problems with their erections. These problems can be magnified by stress over money, ill health, career, sexual boredom, fatigue, or excessive drinking. One partner may blame herself or himself if the other is having problems. We can feel that we are no longer desirable or sexually attractive.

The slowing down of the sexual response cycle in women and men is natural. This slowdown may also make us anxious. But we may not feel as anxious if we understand that sex is a vital part of the lives of most middle-aged women and men. In fact, middle-aged women often have strong sexual desires, and they are more likely to reach an orgasm than younger women.

Women and men both report that midlife sexuality can bring a whole new world of sexual satisfaction: They have less fear of unintended pregnancy. Their children are likely to have left home, giving the older parents more privacy. They may even have financial freedom.

Marital Sex during Midlife

Sex patterns may change during the course of a married life. Although the frequency of sexual activity decreases with age, most married people 45 years and older still have sex once a week. After 15 or more years of any relationship, sex habits can be quite different from those of the first year of marriage. Time, children, and careers all contribute to personal growth. As people grow, so does their sexuality. But it is not necessary that sex become dull with age.

After being married for some time, a couple may have to make further adjustments. After women and men experience their climacterics, they might have to shift the frequency of sexual activity or the time of day they can enjoy sex with one another. Their choices of sexual activity may also change to allow for the changes that are taking place in their bodies.

The amount of nonsexual attention partners give each other may also undergo change. Communicating about fears and anxieties and educating one another about midlife changes can alleviate the stress over sexuality for both partners in a midlife relationship. Many partners are able to begin expressing more affection and pleasure with one another as their children leave home and allow them more privacy.

Sexual Diversity—Coming Out in Midlife

Just because people get married does not necessarily mean they are straight. Many people discover that they are lesbian, gay, bisexual, or transgender later in their adult lives. Others may also come to realize that their gender identities do not reflect the social norm.

Denying their sexual feelings can lead people to attempt to act and *feel* straight by dating, marrying, and having children. Sexual experiences during our teen years and early 20s don't determine our sexual orientation. Reevaluating our sexual orientation or gender identities after a committed relationship with someone of the other gender, marriage, widowhood, or divorce can result in discovering a whole new world of sexuality, including our sexual orientation.

Many people whose sexual identities differ from social norms may be uncomfortable about themselves and their sexuality for many years and may lack the confidence to face their differences and actualize their desires until they develop the maturity that comes with midlife.

Divorce and Widowhood

Not all people who get married establish other committed relationships or live together for the rest of their lives. Some people end their relationships or marriages intentionally. Many do so legally with divorce. Others experience the death of a partner and become widowed. All these situations require a time of adaptation.

People who are divorced, leave relationships, or become widowed are usually accustomed to regular sexual expression. Suddenly, they find themselves without a sex partner. Often, women and men must renavigate their sexual journey.

Thirty-three percent of women and 40 percent of men who become divorced are between the ages of 35 and 54. Divorce and breaking up can be a response to stresses such as people growing differently from one another, midlife career and identity crises, discovery of sexual identity, and extramarital affairs.

Many people accept divorce as a positive alternative to an unhappy marriage. Others find divorce to be devastating to their emotional, social, and financial lives. Becoming the single, primary caretaker of children can be especially overwhelming.

Midlife widowhood is not uncommon. Because women have a longer life expectancy than men, there are generally more widows than widowers. A woman may feel like a fifth wheel when she socializes with couples that she and her partner knew. Finding single people of the same age may be difficult. But today, women and men who become single again in midlife are unwilling to resign themselves to a life without companionship and sexual activity.

Many people who marry again after divorce or widowhood have successful marriages. Their marriages are often based upon mutual interests, goals, and emotional compatibility. Divorced and widowed women and men who have sexual activity without being married again also express great satisfaction.

Dating and marriage after becoming single again in midlife can be difficult. Remember how anxiety-ridden we were about dating during adolescence? Dating in midlife makes a person a second-time beginner. Rules for dating and sexual relationships may have changed since we were teenagers. We may have to relearn them in the process of dating again. This may feel very clumsy at first.

Newly single men usually have less difficulty finding dating opportunities. They may date women their own age or women quite a bit younger. Although the same opportunities should be available to women, our social norms do not generally support dating between older women and younger men.

Our sexual journey does not end with parenthood or midlife. It changes pace and design as we become older adults.

OUR SEXUAL JOURNEY AS OLDER ADULTS

In American culture, we have a myth that sexuality is only related to procreation. According to this myth, once our reproductive years are over, we are no longer sexual people. Many people mistakenly believe that it is unacceptable for older people to have sexual needs or to express themselves sexually. The truth is that we all remain sexual throughout our lives, even in old age.

Physical Changes during Older Adulthood

There are two basic requirements for maintaining healthy sexual capacity in old age. The first is maintaining good physical and mental health. The second is to keep having regular sexual activity. "Use it or lose it" still applies to women and men in the later years of life. The more sexually active that people remain in their later years, the healthier and more enjoyable their sexual activities become.

In the later years of life, well-established relationships may evolve and blossom into more intimate relationships. For older adults, love relationships may slowly transform from passionate love into deep and intimate companionate love. On the other hand, old friendships may become romantic and sexual. Opportunities for sexual expression may decrease *or* increase. But the quality of sexual activity may become more important than the quantity.

As with our entire sexual journey, there are physical changes that affect the sex lives of older women and men. Understanding these changes can reduce performance anxiety and the feeling that one has become useless and unattractive.

Women go through specific physical changes that affect their sexuality. After menopause, the vaginal walls become thinner, a process that continues into the senior years. The thinner walls can't absorb the pressure from a thrusting penis as well as they could in youth. This pressure on the vaginal walls is also pressure on the urethra and bladder. These tissues can become irritated. As a result, older women may feel the need to urinate immediately after sexual intercourse.

The vagina also shrinks in width and length. The labia majora also shrink. Because of the smaller size, insertion of the penis may be difficult or painful. Women also continue to experience hormonal imbalances in their later years. These imbalances may cause the natural uterine contractions that occur during orgasm to become painful. It is important to remember, however, that a woman in her 80s has the same capacity for orgasm that she did at 30.

Physical changes affect men as well. Good circulation is essential to getting an erection, but with old age, there is usually a hardening of the arteries. This change in circulation may make it take longer to become erect. In addition, older men experience fewer morning erections. There is also a longer refractory period after orgasm for men.

It may take up to 24 hours before an older man can get another erection. Muscle tension and sex flush also diminish with age.

The volume and force of ejaculation also decrease. Sperm, however, are still viable and can fertilize an egg. Older men can generally control their orgasms better and can make sex last longer than younger men.

Many of these changes can be dealt with easily. Vaginal lubricants and extended foreplay can ease lubrication and erection problems. Women and men retain the capacity and desire for sexual expression throughout their entire lives. The natural changes of the body do not erase our ability to maintain rewarding sex lives. Our options may change, however. We depend more on sex play, such as masturbation, kissing, embracing, stroking, and oral sex, or on alternative sexual positions.

Medication can have a major impact on our sex lives. Older adults especially may be taking a variety of medication for heart problems or arthritis. Because older people are so often considered sexless, it is common for medications to be prescribed without regard to their potential side effects on sexual functioning. Some tranquilizers, antidepressants, and medications for high blood pressure or arthritis can have an inhibiting effect on sexual desire and arousal.

All side effects of medication should be discussed with our health care providers. Often adjustments and substitutions can be made. Before having surgery, especially surgery that involves the heart or the reproductive organs, it is important to thoroughly educate ourselves on the possible effects the surgery may have on our sexuality.

Emotional Changes during Older Adulthood

The factors that contribute to a general feeling of sexual well being differ for women and men. Women find satisfaction in being sexually attractive and becoming intimate with their partners. Men take pride in their sexual performance and their attractiveness to their partners, but they may be less interested in intimacy.

As women and men age, however, the need for intimacy grows, especially among men. In the later years of life, we may find new and deeper dimensions of intimacy in our relationships. Although sexual intercourse may become less frequent, our interest and pleasure in other sexually intimate activities may increase. These activities can include caressing, embracing, and kissing. Nonsexual, intimate relationships can also provide affection, closeness, intellectual stimulation, and opportunities for socializing.

Social Pressures and Responsibilities during Older Adulthood

Each stage of our sexual journey is affected by the double standards society holds regarding our sexuality. These double standards can have a powerful impact on older adults who are profoundly affected by many other losses—loss of friends through death and illness, loss of physical and financial independence, loss of contact with family, as well as declining health.

It is commonly believed that feelings and behaviors that are acceptable for young or midlife people become inappropriate for older adults, especially those in the care of others. Attitudes about masturbation form a good example. Many people who believe that it is acceptable for a 25-year-old man to masturbate also believe that it is "dirty" for a 70-year-old man to masturbate.

Double standards about gender may also prevail. Many believe, for example, that it is acceptable for an older man to have a younger wife, but they question the marriage of an older woman with a younger man.

Our double standard also holds that as women age they become unattractive, but as men age they become "distinguished." These double standards can become particularly isolating and painful in our older years when we may be preoccupied with a variety of financial and health issues that may make us less resilient.

As we age, however, the gender role differences between women and men begin to lessen at both the psychological and the social levels. The expectations of gender behavior a society holds are more pronounced in young adulthood. As older adults, we become free to move away from stereotypical behavior. Women may focus less on the relationship aspect of sexuality, and men may move away from concentrating on genital sex. There also might be a shift in power in marital relations.

Sexual Diversity during Older Adulthood

There is a powerful myth that lesbian, gay, bisexual, and transgender people face a lonely and empty old age. In reality, people with different sexual orientations and gender identities may be better equipped to cope with the adjustments of aging. They are more likely to plan for their own financial independence and to have built a supportive network of friends.

Lesbian, gay, bisexual, and transgender people have had to navigate their sexual journeys through the difficulties presented by a homophobic and oppressive society. Because of their experiences, they might be better at dealing with changes and losses that come with aging.

Being of different sexual orientation or gender identity, however, can make it difficult for an older person to express affection or have sexual contact with a partner who is hospitalized or in a nursing home facility. Though few nursing homes offer conjugal visits for heterosexual partners, far fewer offer them for the partners of lesbian, gay, bisexual, or transgender patients.

Sexuality in Nursing Homes

Expressing our sexuality in nursing homes may be the most difficult part of our sexual journey. Many facilities have been criticized for their insensitivity to human rights of aged women and men. Most nursing homes have antisex prejudices and practices. Often, married partners who engage in sexual activities are separated from one another.

Most patients are denied the right of sexual opportunity and privacy. Masturbation is frowned upon, and women and men who masturbate are often reprimanded. Patients' infatuations for their caregivers may be ridiculed or treated harshly.

Before selecting an assisted-living facility for an older adult, it's important to become knowledgeable about the practices and rules of the facility. Try to determine if there are programs on sexuality for the residents and staff. Are there private lounges for time alone? Is there an acceptance of sexual need and rights of the elderly? Can partners in a relationship share their living space? These questions and answers may influence your choice of a facility.

OTHER SEXUAL JOURNEYS

"Are we there yet?" Not quite. Our sexual journey is never quite over. To remain on course, we may have to make adaptations at various times of our lives.

Sex in Asexual Environments

At some time in our lives, we may live in environments that can be considered asexual. These environments include hospitals, prisons, the military, and religious organizations. Privacy is a major concern in these environments. So is the role of celibacy.

In a prison, privacy is a privilege. Masturbation might be the only option for sexual expression. Some people might refrain from all sexual expression in that environment. Others may turn to homosexual relationships. Straight women and men in prison may have sex with others of the same gender to satisfy their need for human physical contact. Most will return to having sex with the other gender after they are released. Same-gender rape is one of the risks of prison life.

Sexual expression may also be limited in the military. Privacy is also scarce, and masturbation must be accomplished quietly. There is often personal leave time off of the base that can allow for sexual expression. Some military people are married and have the privilege of living with their spouses on the military base. Other people in relationships can see partners or spouses periodically when they are on leave.

Sexual diversity in military life can be difficult. Currently, the military cannot ask personnel whether they are homosexual. However, if someone's homosexuality is revealed, there is a great chance that person will receive a dishonorable discharge. Although homosexual activity is against the military code of conduct, significant numbers of lesbian, gay, bisexual, and transgender people are enlisted, or *want* to enlist. Each must make a personal decision about the level of risk she or he is willing to take to serve the country.

Religious life is also a unique sexual environment. Many religious people take vows of chastity or celibacy. This means that they promise not to be sexually active. But this does not mean that religious people are not sexual. Celibacy is one of the many ways we can express sexuality. Although difficult for most women and men, celibacy can be a personally rewarding and insightful way of life. Celibate women and men may enjoy deeply intimate, nonsexual relationships with others.

We know that **sexual repression** can cause mental health problems. It may seem ironic, then, that sexual expression is usually repressed in mental health settings. Partnered sex play, same-sex erotic attachments, and masturbation are all forbidden in most long-term, mental health care facilities. Romantic attachments between women and men are often ridiculed and discouraged. Moreover, many of the mood-altering medications used in these settings decrease sexual desire and arousal among the residents.

We need to remember that the mentally ill are also entitled to sexual expression, access to birth control, and safer-sex information. If it becomes necessary for friends or members of our families to spend long periods of time in institutional settings, we can try to evaluate those settings for humane and enlightened attitudes toward human sexuality.

Paraphilia and Uncommon Sex Practices

Most people tend to be suspicious of sexual behaviors that are uncommon. While it is true that some paraphilias, such as **pedophilia,** are harmful, many people also think negatively about *harmless* paraphilias and other uncommon sex practices. Years ago, for example, Americans generally thought that oral and anal sex were revolting. Since World War II, however, the majority of sexually active Americans have come to enjoy oral sex, and about 30 percent have experimented with anal intercourse. Once considered paraphilias, oral and anal sex are now increasingly common sexual behaviors.

Although uncommon sex practices can alienate others, including potential sex partners, there are opportunities in which they can be enjoyed with partners who are comfortable with them. Instead of "flashing" people on the street, for example, exhibitionists who like to show off their bodies or engage in sex in front of others can join clubs to meet their needs with other people who want to share this practice. There are organizations for foot **fetishists,** transvestites, mate-swappers, and others. There are also clubs where members can learn safe sadomasochistic role play. Sex clubs and organizations for various uncommon sex practices can be found in magazines or on the Internet.

People who lead perfectly ordinary lives and have successful jobs and family responsibilities may enjoy uncommon sex practices. It is important to be honest about our sexual preferences with our partners in order to achieve sexual satisfaction with their consent and understanding.

Enjoying uncommon sex practices does not make us deviant or dysfunctional. If, however, we can be aroused only by a paraphilia that harms others or involves them without their consent, we must seek professional counseling as soon as possible.

For more information about paraphilias and uncommon sex practices, see Chapter 3, "Our Sexual Bodies," and Chapter 5, "Our Sexual Feelings—the Psychology of Sex."

Wherever we are on our sexual journey, we may want to keep in mind that we are all very different. Our journey may not be the same as anyone else's. We won't travel at the same speed or arrive at any milestone at the same time or in the same way. Our sexual journey is not a race. There is no need to hurry, and there is no prize for being the first to get there. Accepting that each of us is unique will only make the journey that much more enjoyable and fulfilling.

CHAPTER 5

Our Sexual Feelings—the Psychology of Sex

The fact that we are all human beings is infinitely more important than all the peculiarities that distinguish humans from one another.
—Simone de Beauvoir (1908–86)

THE SEX DRIVE

All of our sexual feelings are created in the brain. This makes the brain our largest sex organ. Two separate areas of the brain are most responsible for our sexual feelings—the **hypothalamus** and the **cerebral cortex.**

The tiny hypothalamus at the back of our brain gives us our basic urges: to find food, to flee danger, to fight to protect ourselves, and to have sex. These are the basic urges we share in common with all other animals.

The large cerebral cortex at the front of our brains records the information we learn and the experiences we have. It helps determine how we think, feel, and act about sex. It is also the area of the brain that allows us to be aware of sexual sensation. The hypothalamus generates our **sex drive,** sometimes called the **libido.** Some scientists believe that the hypothalamus also helps shape our sexual orientation as part of our sex drive.

The cerebral cortex civilizes our libido. It is where our personal experiences and social and sexual norms live within us. It manages our sex drive by processing sexual information, making sexual decisions, recalling sexual memories, developing sexual fantasies, and evaluating sexual risks. It holds the information that shapes our sexual attitudes, feelings, and behaviors.

The **psychology** of sex is our understanding of how the sex drive, sexual sensations, fantasies, memories, and thinking work together in our minds to affect our sexual behavior.

SEXUAL INHIBITION

Although many animals enjoy homosexual sex play, their sex drives are largely driven by their fertility cycles. Usually, female animals are interested in sexual intercourse with males only during the time that they can become pregnant. This period in the female animal's fertility cycle is often called **estrus.** Male animals become sexually excited most often when a female gives off an odor that indicates she is in estrus. This kind of sexually exciting odor is called a pheromone.

In many kinds of animals, the females all go into estrus at around the same time. The air becomes saturated with pheromones that arouse the males' sexual instincts. This season of sexual excitement in the male animal is called **rut.**

Scientists are still not sure what role pheromones play in human sexuality. We do know for certain, though, that women and men have no periods of estrus or rut. It is one of the major differences between humans and other animals—our sex drive is not limited to reproduction. We can seek and enjoy erotic or sexual pleasure at any time, regardless of fertility. Our human sex drive also makes it possible for us to enjoy a wide variety of erotic and sexual behaviors. In this way, the human sex drive is not as biologically limited as other animals' sex drives are. Although we have a greater capacity for sexual pleasure than most other animals, our sex drives can be much more inhibited.

The inhibitions that constrain the human sex drive are usually not triggered by built-in biological factors as they are in other animals. Our sexual inhibitions are usually social. They are recorded in the cerebral cortex. It is within this part of the brain that our sexual identities and lovemaps develop. They are formed by our biology as well as our life experiences with our families and the social and sexual norms of our communities. This is where our feelings about our sexual selves reside. These feelings affect how we have sex, how much variety in sexual behavior we can enjoy, and how much pleasure we can receive.

Many of the feelings we have about sex are inhibitions. Many of these inhibitions help us protect ourselves and our communities. For example, most of us feel inhibited from forcing other people to have sex with us. On the other hand, many of the inhibitions we feel only serve to prevent us from enjoying ourselves sexually. For example, we may want to have our partners touch a certain part of our bodies, but we may not know it's okay to ask.

Many of our sexual inhibitions are associated with our body image, our self-esteem, jealousy, homophobia, and our ability to be intimate.

Body Image

We all have a mental image about how we look. This mental picture is part of our **body image,** and it has a great influence on our sexuality and our sex lives. Our feelings about our bodies form the other part of body image.

A good body image is a gift that our families and friends help give us. It can allow us to feel secure about our sexuality and our sex lives, whether we're big or small, fat or thin, muscular or soft, light or dark. A poor body image is a handicap that we may receive from families and friends who ridicule or humiliate us and give us negative feelings about our sex organs and masturbation. Poor body image can make us feel insecure about our sexuality and our sex lives, no matter how beautiful we are.

Sexual inhibitions can make us feel bad about our bodies, and poor body image can magnify our sexual inhibitions. They form a vicious circle. Each intensifies the other. Just as our families and friends contribute to our sense of body image with their approval or disapproval, so does the society in which we live. Television and other media play a crucial role in reflecting and establishing social norms about body image. The standards it sets for women and men are impossible for most of us to meet.

Popular magazines show "perfect" women and men and include articles on how to achieve a "perfect" body. Advertisers barrage us with millions of images of what it is to be beautiful and sexy. A healthy, fit, and trim body is a wonderful thing, but the media message is that beauty does not include people with disabilities, unwanted facial hair, acne, soft bellies, or small breasts. In fact, there are thousands of beautiful, sexy, and beloved women and men in the world with disabilities, unwanted facial hair, acne, soft bellies, and small breasts.

We are likely to forget that fact, though, when we compare ourselves to the images in film, on television, and in print. Advertisers benefit from the insecurities we feel about our bodies as we compare ourselves to the standards they set. The more we become insecure about our image, the more likely we are to buy a product to cure our "problem." And the more likely we are to become sexually inhibited.

Although there is no single cause, sexual inhibition and poor body image can contribute to serious eating disorders—**anorexia, bulimia, and binge-eating disorder.** These disorders are attempts some people make to take control of their lives, especially their sexuality. Although much more common in women, eating disorders are increasing among young men. Women with anorexia go without eating to achieve what they believe is socially approved thinness. Unfortunately, they come to believe they can never be thin enough and starve themselves. One out of five dies of heart failure or other complications associated with malnutrition. Anorexic women develop many other serious life-threatening conditions. They may also lose their menstrual periods, fertility, breast tissue, vaginal lubrication, and sexual desire.

In order to achieve thinness, bulimic women and men binge on large amounts of food and then purge themselves by fasting for long periods, using laxatives, or inducing themselves to vomit.

Binge-eating is compulsive overeating. It is done to relieve stress and anxiety, including sexual anxiety. Becoming obese may heighten sexual inhibitions and provide an excuse to avoid sexual contact.

Eating disorders can be treated with psychotherapy and professional medical guidance. Even after an eating disorder is put under control, however, a person may struggle with the consequences for a lifetime.

While most of us will not develop a serious eating disorder, worrying about our bodies is very common and can cause sexual inhibition and conflict. Are we pretty enough for the partner we desire? Are we handsome enough? Are we the right size and shape? Are we tall enough? Are we too tall? Are we the right color? Are our genitals attractive? We can make ourselves very unhappy with these concerns. They can also inhibit our sexual pleasure if they linger in our minds during sexual activity.

Self-Esteem

"Self-esteem" is another expression for self-confidence. It is our respect for ourselves. It allows us to feel strong, capable, and worthwhile. Self-esteem is an important part of body image, and body image is an important part of self-esteem. Self-esteem is also often a gift we receive from family and friends. We can develop it on our own if we don't receive it from them, but that is much more difficult than receiving it as a gift.

Like body image, self-esteem has a great influence on our sexuality. It can help us to feel secure about our sex lives. Lack of it can make us feel sexually inhibited. The more sexually inhibited we are, the more lacking in self-esteem we are likely to be.

Self-esteem is important in all of our relationships, especially those that are more intimate, including those that are sexual. In order to have a relationship with another person, we have to allow ourselves to be vulnerable. We take an emotional risk whenever we begin a relationship because we know it may not work out. It takes self-esteem to take such risks. It also takes self-esteem to negotiate, set limits, and make healthy compromises in the relationships we have.

Women and men without self-esteem are liable to "take what they can get," make few demands, and find themselves exploited or abused. They are also likely to exploit whomever they can to make up for their own poor self-esteem. It's another vicious circle.

Self-esteem is undermined by many life experiences, including **corporal punishment,** loss of a loved one, sexual abuse, neglect, and harsh parenting that fosters negative attitudes about sex. It can also be caused by alcohol and substance use, disability, and chronic illnesses such as depression and diabetes.

Lack of self-esteem can inhibit our sexual pleasure by causing us to worry about whether we are loved, whether we are attractive, whether we are worthwhile, and whether we have a right to our opinions and desires. Lack of self-esteem makes it difficult to express our sexual desires and to protect ourselves sexually. It is also one of the causes of jealousy, which can threaten valuable relationships.

Self-esteem allows us to feel good about ourselves and ask for what we desire, and empowers us to take good care of our sexual health. If we have lost our self-esteem through our life experiences, we can rebuild it through counseling and careful self-examination.

Jealousy

Jealousy is our anxiety about a partner's love and commitment. It can play an important role in the development of sexual inhibition and conflict. Jealousy does not occur in all cultures. It is most likely where marriage is seen as a way to have guilt-free sex, security, and social recognition.

Jealousy mostly occurs in women and men with low self-esteem who are unhappy with their lives. It is based on the impossible idea that we must fulfill all the needs of our loved ones and that our loved ones must fulfill all of our needs. It does not allow for the fact that people we love have many needs that we cannot fulfill, and we have needs that they cannot fulfill.

If we have self-esteem, we can appreciate when other people confirm our feelings that our loved ones are attractive, capable, sensitive, caring, intelligent, and amusing. If we have little self-esteem, we need constant reassurance from our loved ones that we have all those attributes. Jealousy can eat away at a sexual relationship and create sexual inhibitions and conflicts.

Internalized Homophobia

Homophobia is the fear of homosexuality. Our society has developed such negative attitudes about homosexuality that many people have come to fear homosexuality within themselves—whether they are lesbian, gay, bisexual, straight, or transgender. This fear is called **internalized homophobia.** It can cause sexual inhibition in women and men, although it may occur more often in men.

Internalized homophobia is so powerful that up to 30 percent of lesbian, gay, and bisexual adolescents attempt suicide. It can also cause severe depression. Community groups for lesbian, gay, and bisexual people can be very helpful in building support and self-esteem for these young women and men. Professional counseling is also helpful.

Internalized homophobia may make it very difficult for gay men and lesbians to develop intimate relationships with their sex partners. It can also create such fear that they will go without sex, pretend to be straight, or force themselves to have frustrating and disappointing sexual relationships with people of the other gender.

Straight men who worry that some of their sexual desires and fantasies may be homosexual may be less able to develop intimate relationships with women. They may develop "tough guy" or "macho" attitudes in their sexual relationships with women. Men with internalized homophobia may also be more likely to commit **gay-bashing** and other forms of sexual assault. Internalized homophobia can be treated with professional counseling and psychotherapy.

Coming out is the process of accepting and being open about one's sexual orientation and gender identity. It is also the process of challenging social and internalized homophobia. There are many stages. The first is coming out to one's self. This may happen during adolescence, but it may not happen until a person is older. The next steps involve coming out to other people—friends, family, neighbors, schoolmates, coworkers, and others.

The coming-out process helps build self-esteem and a capacity for intimacy, but it can be very stressful. The people we come out to are all influenced by homophobia in one way or another. A few of them can help make the process easy, but many won't. Despite its stresses, coming out offers great relief from internalized homophobia, although it is not a cure-all. Many people who have been "out" for most of their lives still suffer sexual and social inhibitions associated with internalized homophobia. Ridding ourselves of it may be a process that continues most of our lives.

Intimacy

Intimacy is the closeness and familiarity we feel as we share our private and personal selves with someone else. It is the foundation of our most personal relationships with other people, whether or not the relationships are sexual.

Intimacy is based on trust. It is another gift our parents can give us. If we are cuddled as infants, if we are treated with respect and grow up in an environment with healthy attitudes about sex, and if we learn to trust that the people closest to us will not hurt us, we can more easily develop the ability to be intimate with our sex partners, as well as with other people. If we are able to be intimate with our sex partners, we will be able to share our feelings, express our desires, make healthy compromises, and disagree with them without fear. We will also be able to appreciate their feelings and point of view.

Many women and men discover that they are unable to be as intimate with their sex partners as they are with other people in their lives. They may find that they are unable to enjoy sex as much with someone with whom they are intimate. This kind of sexual inhibition can be very damaging to long-term relationships like marriage. Inability to be intimate with a sex partner can result from sexual inhibitions that are associated with body image, self esteem, and internalized homophobia. Women and men with highly developed social skills may still be unable to be intimate. Problems with intimacy can be treated with psychotherapy.

OUR SEXUAL INHIBITIONS AND CONFLICTS

We live in a culture that has been fearful and repressive about sexuality for thousands of years. Because of its emphasis on the dangers of sex and sexuality, we may feel many inhibitions that clash with our sex drives. The clash between sex drive and inhibition is called **sexual conflict.** It can interfere with our self-esteem, our sexual pleasure, and our sexual relationships.

We are in conflict with ourselves whenever our sexual impulses and desires don't match what we feel is okay according to our family values and social norms. For example, we may not know it's okay to enjoy sex as older adults. We are much more likely to believe that sex is for the young and beautiful. If we accept this common myth, we may inhibit our natural sexual impulses as older adults. This sexual conflict can cause us to become less happy with our lives. Sexual conflicts within ourselves about what is okay and what is not okay can occur at any age.

The sexual conflicts most people feel are somewhere in between **sexual discomfort** and sexual dysfunction. But even the discomforts caused by these conflicts can have an enormous impact on our sex lives. The following are some of the common sexual dysfunctions that may be caused by negative feelings about sex or by other people's feelings about sex. Although we may not have these dysfunctions, understanding them may help us understand some of the discomforts that we do have.

Inhibited Sexual Desire

An uninhibited, positive appreciation of various erotic and sexual behaviors is called **erotophilia,** which means "liking the erotic." Fear and anxiety about the erotic is called **erotophobia.** Most of us are somewhere in between.

Many people, however, feel such fear and anxiety that they seem to turn off their sex drives. They lose interest in sex. They don't seek opportunities for sex, and they don't take advantage of opportunities that they have. This is called **inhibited sexual desire** or **hypoactive sexual desire.**

Fear of sex is one of the major causes of inhibited sexual desire, but it is not the only cause. Other causes include depression, anger with a sex partner, divorce and other losses, stress, illness, and difficulty accepting one's sexual orientation. No matter the cause, inhibited sexual desire is considered a sexual dysfunction. Like other sexual dysfunctions, it can be diagnosed and treated with professional counseling that includes psychotherapy and sex therapy. This combined therapy is called psychosexual therapy. Anti-anxiety medications may be helpful in some cases.

Sexual Aversion

Some people feel such fear and anxiety about sex that the very idea of having sexual contact is repelling. They will avoid sex and certain kinds of sexual contact, even though their sexual desire may be uninhibited. They can be repelled by any kind of touch. Their disgust can make them ill. Their fear of sexual contact can sometimes cause sweating, nausea, vomiting, or diarrhea. The fear of sexual contact is called **sexual aversion disorder.** People with sexual aversion disorder may be able to enjoy certain sex acts, on certain occasions, and under certain circumstances.

Sexual aversion disorder can be caused by sexually fearful or repressive parenting, sexual abuse, pressure from sex partners, or gender identity problems. Problems with self-esteem and body image can open us up to developing sexual aversion. Psychosexual therapy may be very beneficial for women and men who have sexual aversion disorder.

Although most of us do not have a sexual aversion disorder, many of us may have anxieties and inhibitions that make sexual contact less pleasurable for us than it might be.

Gender Dysfunctions and Sexual Inhibitions

Gender identity is not the simple matter it may seem. Our sexual organs and hormones are biological elements of our gender, just as are the sex drive and, perhaps, our sexual orientation. Our *feelings* about our sexual selves begin to take shape when we are given our **gender assignment.** We are "assigned" our gender at birth. It is usually based on the physical appearance of our sex organs. The doctor or midwife announces we're either girls or boys. The decision is written on a birth certificate and becomes a legal statement of our gender. Gender assignment is very important in a society that sees female and male as being opposite—a society like ours.

The majority of people are born with clearly differentiated sex organs—they are either female or male. A much smaller number of people, however, are born with undifferentiated, or ambiguous, sex organs that are not clearly female or male. Some are born with both. Sometimes the external sex organs are both female and male. Sometimes the internal organs are both. Sometimes the internal organs are of one gender, but the external organs are of the other. A person who has clearly differentiated genitals of both genders is called a **hermaphrodite.** This occurrence is very rare.

Some hermaphrodite children and children with ambiguous sex organs become adults without distinct gender assignments. Some may become adults before they realize that their exterior sex organs are not the same gender as their interior sex organs. Some infants are given reconstructive surgery at birth to assign a gender that is clearly female or male. The surgery seems to have been helpful in some cases, but there are also cases in which the surgically assigned gender is in conflict with the person's gender identity and feeling. And in other cases, surgical gender reassignment has led to a loss of sensation—especially when the size of the clitoris has been surgically reduced. Whatever the cause, ambiguous gender has profound effects on a person's sexual identity in a society that has low tolerance for gender confusion.

After our gender assignment is made, we continue to rely on society to reflect our mental pictures of our sexual selves. We spend the rest of our lives learning what behaviors are proper for the female and what behaviors are proper for the male. But our sexual orientation, lovemaps, gender roles, and gender scripting may affect our gender identities in ways that conflict with our family values and social norms.

Many people find comfort in the feminine and masculine gender scripts dictated by social norms. Many other people are made uncomfortable by them. Many people accept their gender roles. Many people don't. They may become sexually inhibited by their conflict about gender identities.

Some feel that they have aspects of both genders. This sense of sexual self is called **androgyny.** Some feel they have nothing in common with either gender. Transgenders or transsexuals may become more comfortable with themselves through psychotherapy, hormonal treatments, cosmetic surgery, and support from family and friends. Despite these supports, however, transgenders face serious emotional struggles because of the sexual norms of our culture. Those that choose surgery to reassign their genders undergo a process that is difficult and expensive.

Most of us do not experience such severe conflict with our culture's **gender norms.** But each of us is so unique that we may feel conflict between the gender norms of our communities and some of our own sexual desires. For example, women may not know that it is okay to be sexually aggressive, and men may not know it's okay to be passive. Many women and men try very hard to overcome the gender inhibitions they may feel by becoming hyperfeminine or hypermasculine.

Hyperfemininity is the exaggeration of gender-stereotyped behavior that is believed to be feminine. Hyperfeminine women, as well as some gay men and male-to-female transgenders, exaggerate the qualities they believe to be feminine. They believe it is their job to boost men's egos by being passive, naive, innocent, soft, flirtatious, graceful, nurturing, and accepting.

Hypermasculinity is the exaggeration of gender-stereotyped behavior that is believed to be masculine. Hypermasculine men, as well as some lesbian and female-to-male transgenders, exaggerate the qualities they believe to be masculine. They believe it is their job to compete with other men and dominate women by being aggressive, worldly, sexually experienced, hard, physically imposing, ambitious, and demanding.

Hyperfeminine women often seek out hypermasculine men for sexual relationships. Hypermasculine men often seek hyperfeminine women. They are likely to have rocky relationships, however. Hyperfeminine women are more likely to accept physical and emotional abuse from their sex partners. Hypermasculine men are more likely to be physically and emotionally abusive to their partners.

Although most of us are not hyperfeminine or hypermasculine and do not have a gender disorder, many of us may have anxieties and inhibitions about femininity and masculinity that make sex less pleasurable for us than it might be.

Inhibited Sexual Arousal

At various times in their lives, most women and men are unable to become sexually aroused. The causes include fatigue, alcohol use, anxiety about impressing a sex partner, anger with the sex partner, stress, boredom, and illness. Women and men with sexual arousal disorder, however, are unable to become aroused over long periods of time.

Women and men with inhibited sexual arousal may be unable to become sexually aroused and unable to enjoy sex play, despite their sexual desires. Women may be unable to become lubricated for intercourse; men may be unable to become erect. If they are able to lubricate or become erect, people with sexual arousal disorder may not be able to enjoy the physical sensations of sexual activity.

Women with inhibited sexual arousal may be able to become aroused with some partners or sex-play activities they desire, but they may not be able to become aroused with others that they desire. Women who cannot lubricate may yet be able to have vaginal intercourse by using other lubrication.

Inhibited arousal disorder in men is also called **erectile dysfunction.** Men may be unable to become erect with their partners, or they be unable to maintain their erections during intercourse. Most men with erectile dysfunction can become erect, however, during masturbation. Erectile dysfunction most often occurs after a long period of normal sexual arousal. It becomes increasingly common in men over 60. Erectile disorders can be very frustrating for gay and straight men because they may be rejected by their partners.

The causes of inhibited sexual arousal in women and men are usually psychological. They are very like those of inhibited sexual desire: fear and anxiety about sex, anxiety about pleasing the partner, depression, anger with a sex partner, divorce and other losses, stress, illness, and difficulty accepting one's sexual orientation. Women who have been sexually abused, especially during childhood, are likely to experience inhibited sexual arousal. They may feel helplessness, guilt, shame, or anger, or they may even experience flashbacks of the abuse that prevent them from becoming aroused.

No matter the cause, persistent inhibited sexual arousal is considered a sexual dysfunction. Fantasy, relaxed sex play, open and frank communication with sex partners, and the use of outercourse can be very relaxing for women and men with inhibited sexual arousal and can help them overcome their anxieties and inhibitions. Like other sexual dysfunctions, it can also be treated with professional counseling that includes psychotherapy and sex therapy. Anti-anxiety medications may be helpful in some cases.

Although most of us do not have a sexual arousal disorder, many of us may have anxieties and inhibitions that make sexual arousal more difficult than it might be. Open communication with our partners can help reduce our anxieties and inhibitions.

Performance Anxiety

Performance anxiety is the fear of being unable to please a partner. In men, it is the fear of erectile dysfunction. It is also one of the causes of erectile dysfunction. Poor body image, lack of self-esteem, problems in relationships, and fear and anxiety about sex can contribute to performance anxiety. If a man can believe that occasional failure to become erect is common, he is more likely to break the vicious circle of inhibited erection leading to performance anxiety leading to inhibited erection.

Performance anxiety can lead to a habit of thinking about, comparing, grading, and monitoring our sexual performance while we are having sex with a partner. This is called **spectatoring.** We can become so preoccupied spectatoring that we inhibit our sexual arousal. Spectatoring, like performance anxiety, seems to be more common in men than women, but it may be that a man's failure to become erect is more obvious than a woman's failure to become aroused.

Most of us will experience inhibited sexual arousal from time to time. It is important that we accept this as a normal part of our sex lives and not let ourselves become so anxious that we make sex less pleasurable for us than it might be.

Inhibited Orgasm

The inability to have an orgasm is very common in women and very uncommon in men. It is the most common reason for women to seek sex therapy. About one-third of women experience **inhibited orgasm.** Up to 10 percent of women have never had an orgasm. This is called **anorgasmia.** Most women with inhibited orgasm have previously reached orgasm during sexual intercourse, but no longer can. They may be able to have an orgasm while masturbating, but not during intercourse with their partners. Some women may not even know they can have an orgasm. Many women with anorgasmia enjoy their sexual experience and do not feel that orgasm is important for their sexual pleasure.

Often, women are unable to reach orgasm during intercourse because intercourse does not last long enough, stimulation by the penis is not effective, or there is not enough manual stimulation of the clitoris by the woman or her partner. Inhibited orgasm is the failure to reach orgasm even though there has been sufficiently intense stimulation.

Inhibited orgasm in men is often called **retarded,** or **delayed, ejaculation.** These are somewhat misleading terms, however, because ejaculation and orgasm are different events, although they most commonly occur at the same time. In fact, some men with inhibited ejaculation have orgasms without ejaculating. Inhibited ejaculation and orgasm can be very frustrating for both partners. It may take a man with delayed ejaculation up to 40 minutes of thrusting before he can ejaculate. For some men, ejaculation is entirely inhibited. Men with inhibited orgasm may "try harder" to ejaculate and reach orgasm. This will only make matters worse. Inhibited ejaculation is more common among gay men than it is among straight men.

Some women and men who have inhibited orgasm believe that the best way to end sex play or please their partners is **fake orgasm.** Ultimately, however, this kind of deception is not healthy, especially in a committed relationship. It may become a habit that leads to diminished sexual pleasure, and the partner of the "faker" may never learn how to help her or him reach orgasm.

Certain medications and physical conditions can also inhibit orgasm in women and men. The most common reasons for inhibited orgasm are sexual guilt, shame, performance anxiety, anger with the partner, and spectatoring. Fear of causing pregnancy can inhibit ejaculation and orgasm in men.

Masturbation can help anorgasmic women to reach orgasm. Fantasy, relaxed sex play, and open communication between partners may help some women and men overcome inhibited orgasm. Psychosexual therapy may be beneficial to others.

Most us will experience inhibited orgasm from time to time. Like occasional inhibited arousal, this as a normal part of our sex lives. We need not become so anxious about it that we make sex less pleasurable for ourselves than it might be.

Rapid Orgasm and Premature Ejaculation
Rapid orgasm is rare in women, but it does occur. It happens when a woman reaches orgasm more quickly than her partner and then loses interest in continuing sex play. It is so rare that it is not included in the diagnostic manual for psychotherapists.

Men who have **premature ejaculation** ejaculate before they want to. They are unable to control their responses to the stimulation that triggers ejaculation. Some may ejaculate at the sight of their partner undressing, before sex play even begins. Also called **early ejaculation,** this is the most common sexual dysfunction among men. Up to 30 percent of men experience early ejaculation at some time. Premature ejaculation is often difficult for a man's partner because it may deprive her or him of continuing sex play and orgasm. Men who have early ejaculation may feel guilt and anxiety and may at some point decide to avoid sexual contact.

Fear and anxiety about sex, alcohol and drug use, depression, and other psychological conditions may cause premature ejaculation. Early anxiety can be treated with psychosexual therapy. Open communication and increased focus on sensation during sex play can help men delay ejaculation.

Some partners are taught to use the **squeeze technique:** The man's partner brings him to full erection manually. As he approaches ejaculatory inevitability, his partner squeezes his penis between thumb and forefinger, just below the glans. The partner applies considerable pressure to the penis for 10 to 30 seconds until the erection is reduced by 10 to 30 percent. The penis is released for 30 seconds before being manually brought to erection again, and again, just before ejaculation, the penis is squeezed and pressure is applied. This procedure is used until the man can go 15 to 20 minutes before ejaculation. After several days of this therapy, in which the man postpones ejaculation for more than 15 minutes, he is allowed to insert his penis into his partner.

Many men will experience early ejaculation from time to time. It is important that we accept this as a normal part of our sex lives and not let ourselves become so anxious that we make sex less pleasurable for us than it might be.

Painful Intercourse—Dyspareunia and Vaginismus

Painful intercourse occurs in women and men. It is often caused by infection and conditions like **vaginitis.** It is much less common in men, who may experience painful intercourse because of a physical condition such as a tight foreskin.

Dyspareunia is painful intercourse for women that may be caused by hormonal imbalances, especially those that happen after menopause. Dyspareunia also happens in up to one out of five women because her partner tries to have intercourse with her before she is fully aroused. Some women are so sexually inhibited that they are unable to let their partners know that they are in pain. Some are in poor relationships and fear telling their partners. Others have such fears and anxieties about sex that they mistakenly suppose that sex is naturally painful.

Vaginismus occurs when a woman's fear and anxiety about vaginal intercourse cause the muscles around her vagina to go into spasm when her partner tries to insert his penis. Vaginismus was extremely common in the nineteenth century when women were taught to fear intercourse. Today, it is much less common. It results not only from fearful attitudes toward sex but also from sexual abuse, rape, brutal early sexual experiences, or painful pelvic examinations.

Dyspareunia may be relieved by open communication with partners who are prepared to be more attentive to a woman's need for complete arousal before intercourse begins. Physical causes may be relieved by the use of medication, lubrication, or estrogen therapy. Vaginismus may be relieved by psychosexual therapy.

Sexual dysfunctions are often a combination of physical and psychological problems. Those caused by physical conditions often develop psychological challenges. That is why psychotherapy is an important component of holistic treatment of sexual dysfunctions and inhibitions.

For more information about the physical and medical causes of sexual dysfunction, see Chapter 6, "Our Sexual Health—Taking Care of Our Bodies."

SEXUAL CONFLICT AND OUR LOVEMAPS

Our childhood experiences, especially the sexual ones, have lasting effects on our sex lives. They are recorded in the cerebral cortex and added to our lovemaps. For example, if a child is kissed and hugged, kissing and hugging may become an important part of the child's lovemap. This is because our lovemaps are most open to impression during childhood.

We are likely to feel sexual inhibitions or conflict at some point in our lives. The ones we feel as children can have a lasting effect on us, too. For example, if a child is spanked, especially when erotically aroused, spanking may become an important part of the lovemap.

Common and Uncommon Lovemaps

If we grow up to have lovemaps that allow us to be sexually aroused by kissing and hugging and sexual intercourse in ways that are socially approved, we are said to have **normophilia.** This means that our sexual "likes" are considered common or "normal" by our society. We are said to have paraphilia if we grow up to have lovemaps that allow us to be sexually aroused only by other likes.

Paraphilic lovemaps include activities, relationships, conditions, or objects that are considered uncommon. For example, while many people with normophilic lovemaps occasionally enjoy and are aroused by playful spanking while they have sex, people who cannot become sexually aroused without being spanked or having fantasies of being spanked are said to have a paraphilia called **masochism.**

Not all the causes of paraphilia are clearly understood. Some children who have felt severe disapproval or have been harshly punished for their sexuality or sexual desires may grow up to develop paraphilias. For example, a child who is sexually aroused and treated angrily by a parent may grow up to fear rejection in sexual relationships. As an adult, it may be safer to develop erotic attachment to shoes than to the people wearing them. This paraphilia is called fetishism.

Having a shoe fetish is only one of hundreds of possible fetishisms. Some people develop a fetish for various parts of the body, such as the foot. Some develop a fetish for lacy underwear. The lingerie industry is based on the idea that women in brief lacy underwear are sexually arousing. Some people can't have an orgasm unless their partners are wearing silk underwear. Other people just like the look or feel of silk underwear.

There are hundreds of different paraphilias. Most paraphilias are much more common in men than in women. Perhaps this is because men may be more likely to be aggressive in their sexual expressions than women. Perhaps because women are less likely to be aggressive, their paraphilias may be less obvious and more difficult to identify.

Sexual Addiction

In our sexually repressive culture, we have little concern for the well-being of women and men who have sex less often than most people. But we have grave concerns about women and men who have sex more often than most people. Having sex very infrequently, or not at all, is called **hypophilia.** Having sex more often than most people is called **hyperphilia.** The desire for women to have sex very frequently with many different partners is called **nymphomania.** A similar desire in men is called **satyriasis** or **Don Juanism.**

Some mental health professionals consider nymphomania and satyriasis **sexual compulsions,** or **sexual addictions,** if the search for sex partners:

- results from an obsession that is like being in a trance and involves the development of rituals to intensify sexual arousal
- interferes with important responsibilities and commitments, such as getting to work, home, or school, maintaining good health, and forming nonsexual social relationships
- seems utterly hopeless to control

Recovery groups, such as **Sexual Compulsives Anonymous,** can be very helpful for women and men who want to control what they believe to be sexual addiction. However, accurate diagnosis and treatment for sexual addiction through psychosexual counseling may also be very important for people who are concerned that they may be addicted to sex.

Paraphilias That Rely on Consent

Most paraphilias, like fetishism, are not dangerous and rely on the involvement of consenting partners. Here are some other common paraphilias that rely on consent:

Pictophilia. Sexual arousal becomes dependent on viewing pornographic pictures, movies, or videos, with or without a partner.

Transvestophilia. Sexual arousal becomes dependent on wearing clothing, especially underwear, associated with the other gender.

Sadism. Sexual arousal becomes dependent on sexual role play or fantasy that includes giving punishment, discipline, or humiliation.

Masochism. Sexual arousal becomes dependent on sexual role play or fantasy that includes receiving punishment, discipline, or humiliation.

Sadomasochism (S and M). This is sexual role play that is often called **dominance and submission (D and S).** It may include **bondage and discipline (B and D),** in which one partner is tied up or leashed. In this kind of sex play, one person has power over the other. Many normophilic couples also play erotic power games. They are similar to the games we played as children. Tag, hide-and-seek, and cops-and-robbers are games that use power for fun.

Dominant and submissive erotic play is very different from harmful relationships in which one person actually bosses, threatens, or harms the other. D and S or S and M games are based upon trust and consent. Couples talk about what they want to have happen before they play their roles. They may wrestle, tease, or spank one another, or they may play master and servant. They set limits by using a **safe word** that they decide upon before sex play begins. If one partner uses the safe word, it means the partner is no longer enjoying the activity and it must stop.

Consensual paraphilias may be unusual to many people, but they provide others with sexual pleasure. Many people with similar paraphilias belong to groups that offer emotional support and information so that members can live comfortably with themselves and learn to safely express their unique sexuality. They play out their sexual activities in a safe, healthy, and consensual manner.

Some paraphilias that rely on consent are dangerous. For example, people with **asphyxophilia** depend on strangulation for sexual arousal. They may rely on partners to strangle them, or they may rely on self-strangulation—**autoerotic asphyxiation**—up to the point of passing out. If the strangulation does not stop in time, they may be killed.

Paraphilias That Rely on Lack of Consent

There are also paraphilias that are based on lack of consent. These paraphilias can be very harmful, and engaging in them is illegal. People with these paraphilias should seek professional counseling.

Exhibitionism. Sexual arousal becomes dependent on exposing the sex organs to those who the exhibitionist thinks will be surprised.

Voyeurism. Sexual arousal becomes dependent on watching people undress or have sex play unaware that they are being watched.

Kleptophilia. Sexual arousal becomes dependent on stealing things.

Biastophilia. Sexual arousal becomes dependent on sexually attacking a nonconsenting, surprised, terrified, and struggling stranger. This is a kind of rape, but most rapes are committed by normophilic men.

Pedophilia. Sexual arousal for an adult becomes dependent on having sexual contact or fantasies of sexual contact with a child. *Pedophiles* are more likely to be heterosexual than homosexual.

SEXUAL ASSAULT AGAINST CHILDREN

Sexual abuse of children and rape are two of the most disturbing sexual activities in our culture. They are both forms of sexual assault. They are sometimes committed by people with paraphilias, but they are often committed by people who can be sexually aroused by other activities.

Sexual assault is the use of force or coercion, physical or psychological, to make a person engage in sexual activity. Sexual assault is a physical violation of a person's body. It is also a psychological violation of the mind. It is not committed only for sexual pleasure. It is a way to exert power over someone smaller or weaker. Sexual assault is often violent. Many women, men, and children die as a result.

Sexual assault against children and adults can have long lasting and damaging effects on their psychological health and lovemaps. Because the lovemaps of children are especially vulnerable, the effects of sexual assault may be especially powerful.

Attitudes toward sexual relationships between adults and children vary from culture to culture. It is not universally believed that these relationships are unhealthy. However, any sexual activity between an adult and a child in the United States is considered assault because children are viewed as being incapable of giving consent. Although a child may appear to be seductive and want to have sexual contact, it is the adult's responsibility to protect the child against it, regardless of the circumstances or relationship. Child sexual abuse is a vicious circle. Many victims become sexual abusers as adults.

Child sexual molestation or child sexual abuse, **statutory rape,** pedophilia, and incest are terms that refer to an adult having sexual contact of any kind with a child or an adolescent below the age of consent. This includes touching or fondling, oral–genital stimulation, anal stimulation, and sexual intercourse.

Signs of Child Sexual Abuse

Physical signs of child sexual abuse include weight gain or loss, abdominal pain, vomiting, urinary tract infections, or pain in the genital areas.

Behavioral signs may include sleeping problems, nightmares, withdrawal from others, loss of toilet training, or frequent bathing. When they are being sexually abused, children may become preoccupied with their sexuality. They may indulge in excessive masturbation or sex play. Children who are sexually abused may also abuse younger children.

The emotional effects of sexual abuse include low self-esteem, guilt, shame, and depression. Suicide attempts, eating disorders, drug and alcohol abuse, intimacy problems, and sexual dysfunction can also be responses to child sexual abuse.

Incest

When sexual abuse of children happens within the family, it is called incest. Incest is a controversial topic. Some adults report that their incestuous relationships as children were positive. This is especially true of those who recall exploratory sex play with siblings of about the same age. Many others recall that these relationships were confusing and harmful.

Incest, especially between parent and child, can have serious emotional effects on children. They may become less able to feel safe and secure, even when they become adults. Like other children who are abused, they may feel such guilt and shame that they grow up having difficulty with intimacy, self-esteem, body image, and sexual pleasure.

These aftereffects may be especially confusing. Children may experience some erotic pleasure and some comfort by being so close to a parent. At the same time, they may fear and distrust the parent whom they love and with whom they want to feel safe. They may be so ashamed and confused by their feelings that they don't know what to do or where to turn. They may try to keep it all a secret within themselves.

Children and adults who suffer the effects of incestuous relationships may benefit from professional mental health care to relieve the shame, guilt, anger, and sexual conflict they feel.

TIPS FOR REDUCING THE RISK
OF CHILD SEXUAL ABUSE

- Show that you can listen to whatever your child needs to say without getting angry.
- Help your child understand sexuality by having open, easy, and frequent conversations about it.
- Talk with your child every day and take time to become acquainted with your child's activities and feelings.
- Encourage your child to share concerns and problems with you.
- Teach your child that children's bodies belong only to them.
- Help your child learn that no one has the right to touch children without their permission. And help your child learn to make decisions and choices by offering alternatives instead of commands as often as possible.
- Let your child know that some adults may want to do things with children that may hurt them or make them feel uncomfortable.
- Let your child know that adults who want children to keep secrets from their parents are doing something wrong. Children must not keep such secrets from their parents or other people that they trust, even if an adult threatens to hurt a child or the child's parents.
- Explain that it is wrong for adults whom children know and trust, even adults in their own families, to do things with children that may hurt them or make them feel uncomfortable.
- Be sure to keep from frightening your child. Children should know that most grown-ups will not sexually abuse them and that most adults are deeply concerned about protecting children from harm.
- Make sure that your child knows that you must be told as soon as possible if someone does something confusing such as talking about secrets, touching, giving gifts, or taking naked pictures.
- Reassure your child that children are not to blame for anything that adults do to them.

Recovering from Child Sexual Abuse

Child sexual abuse is sometimes recalled only when the survivors reach adolescence or adulthood. Children may not have understood what was happening to them. They may have felt that something was "wrong," and they may have been very uncomfortable with the activity at the time, but they have tried to forget it.

Recovery from the effects of child sexual abuse can be a long process. Not every survivor of sexual abuse will react in the same way. Although the psychological responses may affect daily life, they may be difficult to identify. Adult survivors may go through many traumatic events as they learn how to deal with the facts and effects of the past abuse.

Recovery from child sexual abuse may include professional help. It is also important to talk with loved ones in order to deal with all the feelings that arise from child sexual abuse. They can provide the essential support system that is needed. Having someone listen, believe, and care is essential for a survivor to begin to feel safe and worthwhile during recovery.

HELPING CHILDREN WHO SAY THEY'VE BEEN ABUSED

- Believe the child. Children rarely lie about sexual abuse.
- Praise the child for telling you about the experience.
- Don't let the child take the blame. Children fear being at fault and responsible for what's happened.
- Be as calm as you can and don't let your response increase the child's sense of shame, confusion, and guilt. If you can avoid describing the event as being "bad," you may help the child recover more quickly.
- Find a specialized agency that evaluates sexual abuse victims—a hospital, child welfare agency, or community mental health therapy group. If a medical examination is necessary, ask for a referral to a health care provider who has experience and training in recognizing and treating sexual abuse.
- If other children in the community may be harmed, talk with other parents so they can talk with their children and be on the lookout for unusual behavior or physical symptoms in their children.

SEXUAL ASSAULT AGAINST ADULTS

Sexual assault is among the most underreported crimes, and most rapists are not convicted. Sexual assault is committed by women and men in same-gender and opposite-gender relationships. Most rapists are straight men in their late adolescence or early twenties. Most victims are women. Sexual assault includes:

- *acquaintance rape*—when someone the assailant knows is forced to have sexual intercourse
- *marital rape*—when one spouse forces the other to have sexual intercourse
- *stranger rape*—when the attacker is not known by the person who is attacked
- *gang rape*—when two or more people sexually assault another (also known as fraternity or party rape)

It is difficult for people to report that they have been sexually assaulted by someone they know. They do not want to believe anyone they trust or love could hurt them in this way.

MEN WHO COMMIT SEXUAL ASSAULT

Here are some of the attributes common in men who commit sexual assault:

- They often lack self-confidence from an early age.
- They are often hypermasculine, or very "macho."
- Many were victims of sexual abuse as children or adolescents.
- Many witnessed violence in their families.
- Many committed assault during their childhood and adolescence.
- Many are hostile toward women and believe aggression, dominance, and physical violence are part of male sexuality.
- Many rely on peers to support their feelings that rape and sexual assault are justified if the women in their lives don't behave the way the men want them to.
- Many have problems with erection and ejaculation while committing sexual assault, although not with consenting partners.

REDUCING THE RISK OF SEXUAL ASSAULT

Here are some ways to avoid sexual assault:

- Have and use locks on doors and windows, and change the locks in a new home.
- Do not open your door to strangers. Ask for identification when service people come to the door, and call the company to verify that they are on legitimate business.
- Always show self-confidence with your body language and speech when you are in public.
- Have first dates with groups of friends or in public places.
- Do not tell new acquaintances that you live alone. Use only initials on your mailbox and in the phone book.
- Avoid controlling or demanding men who may try to control your behavior by planning all the activities and making all the decisions.
- Share dating expenses. Men who are willing to share expenses may be less likely to use sexual coercion to "get what they pay for."
- Lock your car when you drive and when you park.
- Avoid dark and deserted areas and always be aware of your surroundings so that you can try to get away if someone pursues you.
- Have house or car keys in hand before coming to your door.
- If your car breaks down, attach a white cloth to the antenna, lock yourself in, and wait for a uniformed officer in an official car. If other people ask to help, tell them to call the police or a garage, but do not unlock the car door.
- Carry a device for making a loud noise. Sound an alarm at the first sign of danger.
- Don't lead anyone to believe you are more sexually available than you want to be.
- Avoid using alcohol or other drugs when you definitely do not wish to be sexually intimate with your date.
- If assaulted, try to get away, but don't struggle if the struggle seems to arouse your assailant (see "biastophilia," page 162).

WHAT TO DO IF YOU ARE SEXUALLY ASSAULTED

- Tell someone you trust, immediately. Before you change your clothes or wash, call your local rape-crisis hot line or women's center—look under "rape" in the telephone book. They will send someone to help you.
- Get medical help. Have someone you trust with you. You may need emergency contraception as well as treatment for any injuries or infections you may have received. You may also be asked to agree to be physically examined for rape evidence.
- Decide whether you want to report the rape to the police or other authorities. If you do, you may have to recount what happened in detail.
- Take time to recover. You may want to take a few days off from work or school and find a safe place to stay for a few days.
- Get counseling. Recovery takes time and lots of support. You may choose to join a rape recovery group as well.
- Don't blame yourself for what happened. No matter how you behaved, no one deserves to be raped.

Recovering from Sexual Assault

The effects of sexual assault include physical and psychological problems. Psychological effects include loss of self-esteem, impaired body image, eating disorders, anxiety, depression, and sexual inhibition and conflict. The victim may lose interest in sexual contact, be unable to become sexually aroused, or have flashbacks of the assault while trying to have sex with someone who is loved and trusted. Victims may feel dirty, ugly, and unloved. These painful responses are common. They may stress the victims' relationships with their partners.

Rape trauma syndrome is the physical and emotional pain that begins during sexual assault and continues afterward. The acute phase begins with the assault and can last for several weeks. A woman may appear calm and controlled, or she may be very expressive. Her feelings may include anger, sadness, shame, shock, fear, anxiety, guilt, and a loss of control.

The acute phase is followed by the **long-term reorganization phase,** which may last a year or more. During this time, a woman tries to reorganize and regain control of her life. She may want to move, change her phone number, or look for a new job.

HELPING THE RAPE SURVIVOR

- Believe her. One of the great fears of rape survivors is that they will not be believed, or that their experience will be minimized as "not important."
- Listen patiently so she can tell her story at her own speed.
- Comfort, soothe, and calm her. She may want to be held while she cries or may not want to be touched.
- Don't ask questions that put the blame on her—for example, "Why didn't you scream?" and "Why did you go to his room?" Reassure her that the rapist, not she, caused the rape.
- Provide her with a secure place to sleep and companionship after she returns to her home.
- Suggest that she call a rape-crisis center. Reassure her that all calls are confidential and are not reported to the police.
- Encourage her to preserve evidence of the assault. A rape-crisis center can give information about preserving evidence and having a physical examination before she washes her hands, face, and body or brushes her teeth.
- Encourage her to get medical attention and go with her to the hospital, clinic, or doctor's office.
- Help her organize her thoughts but let her make decisions on how to proceed.
- If you are her lover, reassure her that you do not consider her "dirty." Let her decide when sex play can begin again. Don't pressure her to prove that everything is "normal" between you.
- Help her get psychological and legal help. Help her set up appointments, baby-sit, dog-walk—whatever—and get her to where she needs to go.
- Remain available in the weeks and months following the rape.
- Educate yourself about rape trauma to help you deal with your friend's recovery.
- Get help for yourself to deal with your feelings about your friend's experience. A rape-crisis center, women's center, or university counseling center will be able to suggest someone who can help you.

Adapted with permission from *I Never Called It Rape: The* Ms. *Report on Recognizing, Fighting, and Surviving Acquaintance Rape,* by Robin Warshaw (New York: Harper and Row, 1988).

The silent assault victim does not tell anyone about her experience and will go through the process of rape trauma syndrome without the support of professionals or friends. Survivors who express their feelings to supportive professionals, families, and friends may be able to recover more completely and quickly.

Some women go through rape trauma syndrome a long while after the assault. The trauma may cause the survivor to deny the incident, even to herself. She may not be able to deal with her memories and feelings, and they become hidden within her, unremembered. She may feel hurt, sad, angry, and sexually inhibited and not know why.

Sexual Assault by Women against Men

Men who report being sexually assaulted by women were pressured by guilt or threat of breakup. Some described being too drunk or incapacitated to be able to control the situation. Others report being threatened with physical violence, blackmail, or demotion.

Sexual assault against men by women is much less common than sexual assault against women. There are more than 9,000 cases of sexual assault by women against men reported each year, but sexual assault against men is often unreported. Men encounter disbelief when reporting a woman as a rapist. They may fear public and private humiliation. They may feel that they have failed to be masculine enough to defend themselves. Some fear they will be perceived as effeminate or homosexual.

The emotional effects of sexual assault for men are anger, fear, shame, guilt, and disruptions in sexual, social, and family relationships, as well as in sleeping and eating. Professional counseling can help relieve these effects. Rape-crisis centers assist men as well as women.

FEELING GOOD ENOUGH FOR GOOD SEX

Most of us want to enjoy our sex lives. We want to be able to feel uninhibited, aroused, and confident. We also want intimacy and trust in our relationships. Many of us, however, have sexual inhibitions and life experiences that make it difficult to fulfill these desires. Professional counseling can benefit anyone, but there are a lot of things we can do ourselves, and with our partners, to improve our sex lives.

Get to Know Our Own Bodies

Most people masturbate because it feels good. Although it is normal and healthy to do so, many feel guilty about it. We must give ourselves permission to enjoy our bodies and explore what it is that gives us pleasure. This isn't easy in a society that has condemned masturbation for hundreds of years, but we must try.

Recognize and Allow Sexual Fantasies

Sexual fantasy is any sexually arousing thought or image. It often involves thinking about the sexual things we might like to do or have happen to us. It can be a brief flicker in our minds as we glimpse someone who might be a perfect fit to our lovemaps. It can be an erotic inner script we use to heighten our pleasure when we have sex alone or with a partner. Fantasy can help alleviate inhibited arousal, inhibited orgasm, and other sexual inhibitions.

Sexual fantasy is another natural and healthy human function that many of us tend to censor. Overcoming our own self-censorship may be difficult. As with masturbation, many of us have been taught that sexual fantasy is dangerous. It is not. Having a fantasy is very different from acting it out. Perhaps we should set aside a few moments every day to let our sexual fantasies rise up in our minds. We may want to share some of them with our partners. Talking about our sexual fantasies with our partners is a good way to overcome sexual inhibition.

Choose Trustworthy Partners

We all deserve sex partners who are honest, share our values, have respect for us and themselves, and will treat us as equals. Some of us, however, have lovemaps that turn us on to potential partners who may not be good for us. We may have to learn a lot about ourselves to learn how to be turned on by someone who will be good for us. This may take some professional counseling.

In the meantime, we may want to do without partners who are domineering, manipulative, secretive, or uncommunicative. We can also do without partners who make judgments about us, ridicule us, or gossip about us. Of course, trust is a two-way street. We have to be the partners we want our partners to be.

Be Open with Partners

We want our partners to know what we want and what we don't want. Talking openly about our desires with our partners may be difficult at first. We may have many sexual inhibitions about doing so. But if we try to make it part of the way we deal with our sex partners, it will become easier and easier to do.

Many people use sexual role play to explore their fantasies and diminish their sexual inhibitions. Those of us who "played doctor" as children already have experience in sexual role play. We can use it in our adult sexual lives, too. Being open with our sex partners increases the intimacy we share with them, increases our self-esteem, and allows us to feel sexually capable.

Be Mentally and Physically Alert

Fatigue, alcohol, drugs, and anxiety can sap our sexual pleasure. Although having sex is one way to relieve stress, to get the most out of our sexual experiences we should feel good in our bodies and minds. We may want to rethink our sex habits if our sexual inhibitions lead us to put off sex until we've had too many drinks. The same thing goes for putting off sex until we've exhausted ourselves by getting everything else done first. A sleepy cuddle can be one of life's great treasures, but it is also important to let ourselves be sexual when we're feeling our best, our most energetic, and wide-awake.

Be Aroused

We do not need to have sex to please a partner. We may choose to have sex if we are sexually aroused by our partners and we believe we will enjoy having sex with them, but it is *always* our choice. We can increase our sexual inhibitions, damage our self-esteem, and decrease the intimacy we share with our partners if we "fake it" or "just let it happen" when we are too tired, too ill, too bored, too stressed, or too drunk to become aroused.

Sometimes our sex play with our partners may become too habitual and predictable to be arousing. Spending more time in nongenital touching and caressing may be very helpful.

Have Sex in Safe Places

Many first sexual experiences take place in environments that are not entirely safe or secure from intrusion. As young people, we may have avoided the intrusion of adults by having sex in cars or in dark and hidden public places that may have been dangerous. As adults, we may have anxiety about the intrusion of our roommates, children, or members of our families.

Anxieties about intrusion can be distracting and sexually inhibiting. Not only must we find time to have sex, we must also find a private place to enjoy ourselves. If we have sexually active children, we may want to consider their safety and well-being as we decide whether or not they will be allowed to have sex at home.

Getting to know our own bodies, allowing ourselves our sexual fantasies, choosing and being open with trustworthy partners, being alert and aroused when we decide to have sex, and deciding to have sex in safe places are not goals we can accomplish quickly. They take a lifetime of learning. Learning them is one of the great pleasures and rewards that life has to offer. From time to time, we may want professional counseling as we make our sexual journey through life. But it is ourselves who are our best teachers and guides for our sexual journey. We need only to listen carefully to what is already in our hearts and minds.

Developing and maintaining healthy feelings and attitudes toward sex and sexuality are important ways to preserve our sexual health. Taking care of our bodies is equally important. Turn to Chapter 6 for an in-depth discussion of sexual health, hygiene, and safer sex.

Our Sexual

Health—

Taking Care

of Our Bodies

Our bodies are our gardens,
to the which our wills are gardeners.
—William Shakespeare (1564–1616)

TAKING CARE OF OUR BODIES

According to the World Health Organization, sexual health includes the physical, emotional, intellectual, and social aspects of sexuality combined in ways that are positively enriching and that enhance personality, communication, and love. People who are sexually healthy protect themselves from illness and unintended pregnancy, are aware of their sexual behavior and attitudes, and accept responsibility for their sexual behaviors. They also believe that a healthy sexuality is part of a healthy life.

As sexually healthy people, we accept and appreciate our bodies, the way our bodies are made, and we are generally pleased with our appearance. We understand that we have to know how our bodies function in order to keep them working well. We promote sexual health by eating well, exercising, abstaining from tobacco and drugs, using alcohol moderately if at all, and getting regular medical checkups—in short, taking good care of our bodies.

As sexually healthy people, we learn what is normal for our bodies, and we ask questions or get help from a health practitioner whenever we notice that something is wrong. We are also comfortable enough with our own bodies to discuss our health, as well as our pleasure, with our partners.

Nothing is more crucial to our sexual health than taking responsibility for what we do with our bodies. Identifying our values, acting on them, and accepting the consequences of our actions help us maintain our sense of ourselves and protect our bodies. We need to recognize risks that are dangerous and self-destructive. And we need to know how and where to get the information we need. We need to think about our sexual health as often as we think about the other aspects of our health.

Our sexual feelings have a great deal to do with how well we take care of our bodies. They have a profound impact on the choices we make. For example, a woman who has a poor body image may harm her health by having sex just to fulfill the need to feel desirable. A man who has low self-esteem may risk infection by having unprotected sex because a partner requests it.

One of the most important skills in maintaining our sexual health is communication. A study of married women with chronic illnesses found that many lost their desire to have sex because they believed their husbands saw them as sick and undesirable. Researchers found, in fact, that these women's husbands wanted to have sexual relations with their wives—they just never talked about it with their wives.

Being able to talk openly with our partners can also help us feel safe and secure. We can negotiate our sexual limits and decide together what we feel comfortable doing and what we'd rather not do. Telling our health care providers what's on our minds helps us protect our bodies. If you have a clinician or counselor who makes you feel uncomfortable about sexual issues, you may want to find another.

FIVE EASY STEPS TO A HEALTHY SEX LIFE

1. Use a condom every time! Condoms offer the best protection against sexually transmitted infections for people having sexual intercourse who are *not* in safe, monogamous relationships.
2. Talk with your partner before the heat of passion. Be open. Let your partner know your health concerns and sexual health history, and encourage your partner to be open, too. Be direct. Talk about your sexual needs and expectations. Be persistent. Don't let your partner remain silent on these issues.
3. Keep medically fit. Have a checkup for infections every year. Protect your immune system by eating well, getting enough rest, and limiting your use of alcohol, tobacco, and other drugs. Finally, talk with your clinician about your health concerns.
4. Do the following if you think either you or your partner has an infection: See a clinician for testing, diagnosis, and treatment. Find out if your partner(s) needs to be examined and treated, too. Use all the medication that is prescribed—symptoms often disappear before an infection is cured. Do not take anyone else's medicine and do not share yours. Do not have sex until your infection is under control—then when you resume having sex again, use a condom every time!
5. Stay in charge. Remember that alcohol and other drugs weaken good judgment and self-control. Don't let them jeopardize your responsible decision making.

Don't let embarrassment become a health risk. Many people find it very difficult to talk about their sexual health. Some even find it shameful. But discomfort and shame can get in the way of common sense—and can keep people from taking good care of themselves and their partners. Keep yourself healthy by choosing a practitioner with whom you can be comfortable while discussing these issues. Speak frankly and openly with your clinician about your sex life and your sexual health concerns. Some clinicians don't ask, so take charge and speak up.

Staying sexually healthy is like taking care of a car. There are things we can do to keep it running properly, such as having it tuned up periodically. There are some things over which we may have no control, such as potholes in the road. But the better our car's condition, the better we can deal with the potholes. The same is true of our sexual health. We must develop good sexual health habits to keep our bodies in tune. Good sexual health habits include keeping informed about sexual issues, maintaining good sexual hygiene, having regular medical checkups, and developing sound habits of safer sex.

GOOD SEXUAL HEALTH HABITS FOR WOMEN

Genital Hygiene for Women

In our society, it is common to talk with children and adults about cleanliness. But because we are uncomfortable with sexual communication, we often avoid talking about sexual hygiene. It is important to learn that sexual cleanliness does not mean elimination of all natural odors. In fact, some natural odors can have erotic effects. However, cleanliness does mean the elimination of odors caused by bacteria and other microorganisms that can grow on the body.

Washing very gently between the folds of the vulva with warm water and a mild soap is all women need to do to keep their genitals clean. If you are sensitive or allergic to even mild soaps, a soft rubbing around the folds of your labia while sitting in a tub of warm water should do the trick. All you really want to do is remove sweat and bacteria from around the vulva outside your vagina.

The inside of the vagina cleans itself—mucus, semen, menstrual blood, and discarded cells from the walls of the vagina flow out. The vaginal walls and the cervix also produce fluids that are white or yellowish in color. These secretions are normal and healthy. The smell, taste, and thickness of the fluid changes with your cycle. They also change when something is wrong, so it's a good idea to know how your vagina usually smells. You won't know how your healthy vagina smells if you cover it up with perfumes and deodorants or wash your smell away with douches. These products are unnecessary. If you are healthy and wash regularly, you will simply smell like a woman with a healthy vagina.

Many different bacteria and organisms live in a healthy vagina, including some that can cause vaginitis. They don't usually cause any problems because there are not too many of any one kind. Regular douching or irritating perfumes can upset this balance and cause vaginal infections. Vaginitis is an inflammation of the vagina that is caused by a change in the normal balance of vaginal bacteria. A common symptom is heavy and unusual vaginal discharge that is often grayish and frothy and may have an unpleasant odor. Having vaginitis can actually cause the bad odor you may be trying to avoid with douches and sprays. If you have any of these symptoms, don't hesitate to contact your health care provider.

SOME HEALTHFUL VAGINAL HYGIENE TIPS

- Bathe regularly with mild soap and rinse well with clean water.
- Bathe before, and especially after, sex.
- Wash your hands before touching your vagina.
- Always wipe from front to back, vulva to anus, after bowel movements or urinating. Wiping the other way could spread fecal bacteria to your vagina.
- Wear clean underwear with a cotton crotch. Other materials like nylon hold in heat and moisture—great for bacteria, bad for a healthy vagina.
- Avoid using feminine hygiene sprays and deodorants, douches, bubble bath products, colored toilet paper, and other people's washcloths or towels on your genitals.
- If you really want to douche, use plain water.
- Ask your partner to practice good hygiene.

Menstrual Hygiene

Having your period can seem messy. But this is a healthy time for a woman's body because the uterus is shedding its unused lining. Most women use sanitary pads or tampons to soak up the flow.

Pads and tampons hold the flow inside an absorbent material such as cotton until you can throw them away. Pads stay in place by sticking inside the underwear. A tampon fits inside the vagina. The walls of the vagina hold it in place. Each tampon has a string that hangs outside of the vagina. The tampon is removed easily by pulling the string.

Tampons or pads and regular bathing are all a woman or girl needs to stay clean during her period. Deodorant tampons and pads are not necessary for good sexual hygiene. The chemicals may be irritating to some women.

Tampons should be changed four or five times a day to reduce the possibility of an infection from bacteria growing on the tampon. This type of infection is called **toxic shock syndrome.** It is rare, but very dangerous. This is also the reason that women should not have intercourse with the tampon in place. If it is pushed far into the vagina and forgotten, bacteria will multiply.

It is possible to have vaginal intercourse during menstruation, but diaphragms or cervical caps should not be used. Infections can develop if the flow is blocked and held in the vagina for extended lengths of time. Women who are practicing **periodic abstinence** for contraception should not have unprotected vaginal intercourse during menstruation—the days of menstruation are "unsafe days."

Regular Medical Checkups

It is important to have annual medical checkups by a practitioner to maintain total health and to keep your practitioner aware of the changes you may experience. It is also important to have specific sexual health checkups. **Gynecology** is sexual and reproductive health care for women. Routine gynecological care:

- prevents illness and discomfort
- allows for early detection of cancers of the breast and cervix—when they are more curable
- can detect sexually transmitted infections and other conditions before they cause serious damage

- can help prevent sterility
- eases pregnancy and childbirth

You should have a routine gynecological (GYN) exam every year if you are sexually active or over 18. You may need to have checkups even more often if you have:

- plans to become pregnant
- a sexually transmitted infection or a sex partner who has one
- a history of sexual health problems
- a sexually related illness
- a mother or sister who developed breast cancer before menopause
- an abnormal **Pap test**

You should visit your clinician, no matter how old you are, if you have:

- unusual vaginal or pelvic pain
- abnormal vaginal bleeding or discharge
- severe lower abdominal pain
- pain, swelling, or tenderness of the vulva, vagina, uterus, or ovaries
- itching of the vulva or vagina
- been exposed to a sexually transmitted infection
- growths on or thickening of the breast or armpit
- puckering, dimpling, or other changes in the skin of the breast
- newly retracted nipples or bleeding or discharge from the nipple
- changes in size or shape of the breast
- increased pain, discomfort, or emotional distress before your period

Regular GYN exams include:

- talking about your personal, family, sexual, and medical history
- laboratory tests and screening for sexually transmitted infections and other conditions
- counseling
- a **pelvic exam**
- a breast exam
- assessment and treatment of health problems

Schedule your routine GYN exam for a time when you will not have your period—unless you have bleeding problems your clinician wants to observe. Menstrual fluid can affect the results of some lab tests. Don't douche for at least 24 hours before the appointment or use any other vaginal preparation. They can mask many vaginal conditions.

Bring a list of all the questions and problems you want to talk about. Include:

- vaginal discharge
- spotting between periods
- heavier-than-usual flow
- bleeding after sex
- pelvic pain or other problems

Before you are examined, you will be asked to fill out a questionnaire. All information is confidential and remains known only to you and your clinician. Information in your medical chart is not accessible to anyone without your written permission. The questionnaire will include some of these questions:

When was the first day of your last period?
How often do you have periods—every 28 days, 25 days, 35 days?
How long do they last?
Do you have any bleeding between periods?
Are you currently sexually active—one or more sex partners during the last six months?
Do you feel any pain when having sex?
Is there any bleeding after sex?
Do you have any unusual genital pain, itching, or discharge?
Do you have any other medical conditions?
What medical problems do other members of your family have?
Do you suspect you are pregnant?
Are you trying to become pregnant?
Are you using birth control? Have you had any side effects?

You may also be asked for a urine sample to tell if you're pregnant or have diabetes, kidney infections, or other diseases. Emptying your bladder may also help you be more comfortable during the exam. It will also be easier for the clinician to examine you because your cervix and uterus are located behind your bladder.

Your clinician will examine your breasts for lumps, thickening, irregularities, and discharge. You will be asked if you do your monthly breast self-exams regularly and whether you have noticed any changes in your breasts since your last GYN exam. Breast lumps are often discovered by a woman or her sex partner. Most are not cancerous. But report anything unusual to your clinician as soon as possible. Your clinician may also suggest that you have a **mammogram**—x-ray photographs of the breasts that can detect cancerous tumors up to two years before they can be felt.

The Pelvic Exam

There are four parts to a pelvic exam. You will be asked to lie down, let your knees spread wide apart, and relax as much as possible. Usually, the exam lasts just a few minutes. You'll feel less tense if you do the following:

- Breathe slowly and deeply with your mouth open.
- Let your stomach muscles go soft.
- Relax your shoulders.
- Relax the muscles between your legs.
- Ask the clinician to describe what's being done as it's happening.

The External Genital Exam

The clinician visually examines the soft folds of the vulva and the opening of the vagina to check for signs of redness, irritation, discharge, cysts, genital warts, or other conditions.

The Speculum Exam

In the **speculum exam,** the clinician inserts a duckbill-shaped **speculum** into the vagina to separate the walls of the vagina so that the cervix can be seen. You may feel some pressure or discomfort, especially if you are tense or if your vagina or pelvic organs are infected.

The clinician checks for any irritation, growth, or abnormal discharge from the cervix. If you request them, tests for gonorrhea, **HPV (human papilloma virus), chlamydia,** or other infections may be taken by collecting cervical mucus on a cotton swab.

The clinician will also use a tiny brush to gently collect cells from the cervix for a Pap test. You may have some slight staining or bleeding after the sample is taken. The cells are tested for the presence of precancerous or cancerous cells. Pap tests can detect:

- the presence of abnormal growth in the cervix
- infections and inflammations of the cervix
- thinning of the vaginal lining from lack of estrogen

The Bimanual Exam

In the **bimanual exam,** the clinician, wearing a lubricated examination glove, inserts one or two fingers into the vagina. The other hand presses down on the lower abdomen. You may find it somewhat uncomfortable. Deep breathing through the mouth helps. If you feel pain, tell the clinician.

The clinician can feel the internal organs of the pelvis between the two fingers in the vagina and the fingers on the abdomen and examine them for:

- the size, shape, and position of the uterus
- an enlarged uterus, which could indicate a pregnancy
- tenderness or pain that may indicate infection
- swelling of the fallopian tubes
- enlarged ovaries, cysts, or tumors

The Rectovaginal Exam

Many clinicians complete the bimanual exam by inserting a gloved finger into the **rectum** to check the condition of tissues that separate the vagina and rectum. They also check for possible tumors located behind the uterus, on the lower wall of the vagina, and in the rectum. Some clinicians complete the **rectovaginal exam** with one finger in the anus and another in the vagina for a more thorough examination of the tissue in between. You may feel as though you need to have a bowel movement. This is normal and lasts only a few seconds.

After the exam, you will discuss the results with your clinician, arrange for any follow-up or consultation that may be needed, and ask any further questions you may have. This is another opportunity to discuss your concerns about sex and sexuality, birth control, pregnancy, abortion, sexually transmitted infections, loss of urine, inherited disorders, infertility, signs of cancer, breast self-exam, or menopause.

If the lab tests indicate anything unusual, you will be contacted when the results are completed. Pregnancy test results are usually ready during your visit. Other test results may take three to 14 days.

Vaginitis

Vaginitis is a condition in which the walls of the vagina become irritated or infected, causing discharge, itching, irritation, and discomfort. Vaginitis may also cause vaginal bleeding, pain in the lower abdomen, and pain during sexual intercourse. About 75 percent of women will have at least one vaginal infection in their lifetime, and 22 million will have repeat infections. The five most common types are atrophic vaginitis, vaginal yeast infections, chemical vaginitis, **BV (bacterial vaginosis),** and trichomoniasis.

Atrophic Vaginitis

This vaginal irritation causes no discharge. It is brought about by a low level of estrogen caused by menopause, removal of the ovaries, pelvic radiation treatments, certain kinds of chemotherapy, and childbirth, especially when followed by breast-feeding. Low estrogen levels also make vaginal tissue become thinner and drier. Women may also notice spotting caused by tearing of the dry skin.

Sexually active women with atrophic vaginitis experience painful intercourse and may need to use lubricants or engage in other types of sex play. Estrogen vaginal creams or oral tablets can rebuild the vaginal tissue, restore lubrication, and decrease irritation.

Yeast Vaginitis

Many different bacteria and organisms live in a healthy vagina. They don't usually cause any problems because there are not too many of one kind. Yeast vaginitis is an inflammation of the vagina that is caused by a change in the normal balance of vaginal bacteria or yeasts. The most common cause is an overgrowth of yeasts from a family called **candida.** Symptoms include:

- thick, cottage cheese-like vaginal discharge
- a yeasty odor
- itching or irritation of the vagina and/or the vulva

Persistent or recurrent vaginitis may lead your clinician to evaluate you for diabetes or other diseases—although these are not common causes. Women may also have chronic vaginitis because of the altered balance of bacteria in their lower bowels. The abnormal balance of bacteria in the bowel may create an overgrowth of yeast that is reflected in the vagina. Fecal bacteria may also enter the vagina through sweat, wiping, and sexual activity. If the bowel bacteria are not in

TREATMENT OF YEAST VAGINITIS

- Use **over-the-counter** antifungal creams, ointments, or suppositories or oral medications if your yeast infection has been verified by a clinician.
- Eat plain yogurt with live acidophilus culture, or take tablets containing the culture.
- Wear breathable underwear, panty hose with a cotton crotch, or loose-fitting pants.
- Do not share towels.
- Do not sit around in a wet bathing suit.
- Always wipe away from the vagina after bowel movements or urination.
- Some women find it soothing to apply yogurt directly to the vagina. Some soak a tampon in yogurt and insert it.

Additional treatments for recurrent yeast vaginitis:

- Avoid simple sugars and carbohydrates such as candy, cake, and ice cream.
- Limit or avoid foods containing yeasts, molds, or ferments such as cheese and bread.
- Use antifungal medicines, such as caprylic acid, citrus seed extracts, or garlic products. These can be found in most health food stores.
- Use antibiotics only if necessary.

healthy balance, the vaginal bacteria may become altered with a resulting chronic vaginitis. Bacterial imbalances are commonly the result of overuse of antibiotics and a high-sugar diet.

Chemical Vaginitis

Objects and chemicals left in the vagina may cause irritations that lead to vaginitis. Do not leave tampons, toilet tissue, contraceptives, or other objects in the vagina longer than necessary. Some women have very sensitive skin in the vulvar area—often because of a recent infection. The skin may be further irritated by scented toilet paper or tampons, vaginal sprays, and soap and shampoo residue. Other possible irritants are latex condoms, diaphragms and cervical caps, and **spermicides.**

Bacterial Vaginosis (BV)

BV is a condition caused by a change in the balance of vaginal bacteria. Normal **lactobacilli** decrease in number as the number of competing bacteria increase. Hundreds of thousands of women in the United States develop BV every year. It is not usually sexually transmitted, but it may be aggravated by sexual intercourse. It is not a *true* vaginitis because it is not an "inflammation" and does not cause irritation or itching. Common symptoms of BV include heavy and unusual vaginal discharge that is often thin and gray and may have a "fishy" odor, especially after intercourse.

The disturbed balance of vaginal bacteria that causes BV can be created by antibiotics or the presence of fecal material—as in diarrhea. It can be further intensified by introducing new bacteria through intercourse and the presence of a man's ejaculate.

BV is diagnosed by microscopic examination of the vaginal discharge. Ironically, it is treated with antibiotics, either in vaginal gel or in pill form.

Trichomoniasis
See page 210.

GOOD SEXUAL HEALTH HABITS FOR MEN

Always wash your hands *before* as well as after you urinate. The penis should be washed with soap and water at least once a day. If you are uncircumcised, pay particular attention to pulling the foreskin back and washing all the surfaces as well as the underside of the foreskin. Washing before and after sex may reduce the risk of exchanging some infectious organisms with your partner. Urinating after having sexual intercourse may help flush out bacteria that may cause urethritis— inflammation of the urethra.

Testicular Exam

Cancer of the testicles is highly curable if discovered early. A simple, once-a-month examination can save your life. On the same day of each month, examine your testicles. This is best done after a shower. While sitting down, take one testicle at a time in both your hands and feel for any small bumps, surface irregularities, or enlarged areas that are not the same in both testicles. There are also other serious conditions besides cancer that have similar symptoms. If you find anything, you should see your health care provider immediately.

Some Conditions That Affect the Sex and Reproductive Organs of Men

Jock itch is a very common fungal skin infection in the genital area that is caused by wearing tight clothing, by sweating, and by not drying the genitals carefully after bathing. The fungus is called *Tinea cruris* and can cause a reddish, scaly rash that can become inflamed, very itchy, and painful. Jock itch can be easily treated with over-the-counter, antifungal creams and ointments, such as Cruex®.

Prostatitis is an enlargement of the prostate gland that results in a dull persistent pain in the lower back, testes, scrotum, and glans of the penis. There may also be a thin discharge of mucus from the penis, especially in the morning. More than 30 percent of men develop prostatitis. It is commonly caused by a buildup of bacteria and congestion due to infrequent ejaculation. It can also be caused by sexually transmitted or other infections. Antibiotics and long, warm baths can alleviate the condition in younger men.

In older men, prostatitis may lead to blockage of the urethra, causing a reduced stream of urine, burning sensations while urinating, chills, and fever. Older men may need to have their blocked urethras surgically cleared.

Prostatitis is not the same as **"blue balls,"** a similar discomfort that men may feel if they have been unable to ejaculate after being sexually stimulated. Masturbation to ejaculation is a good remedy for "blue balls."

Epididymitis is an inflammation of the epididymis in a testicle. Mild infections may cause a slight swelling and tenderness of the epididymis. Untreated, the infection can involve the entire testis and cause sterility. More than 500,000 men develop these infections every year. Half of these infections are caused by sexually transmitted infections such as chlamydia and gonorrhea. The other half are caused by abnormalities in the urinary tract, other infections, and illnesses such as tuberculosis. Using condoms is a good way to protect against epididymitis. To prevent sterility, monthly self-examination is very important for sexually active men.

Varicoceles are enlargements of the spermatic vein that supplies blood to the testis. They occur in one out of 10 men. A varicocele can reduce blood flow and increase the temperature of the testicle, causing infertility. Varicoceles can be surgically removed.

Cryptorchidism happens when one or both of the testicles do not descend from the lower abdomen during puberty. It happens in one out of 50 men and may not be noticed until much later in adulthood—especially if a boy is very shy and private about being seen naked. The testes can be brought into the scrotum with hormones or surgery; otherwise they will degenerate and the secondary sex characteristics of the man may not develop.

Balanitis is an inflammation of the glans and foreskin that can be caused by infections, irritations, drugs, sexually transmitted infections, or other factors, including a tight foreskin. Depending on the cause, balanitis may be treated with antibiotics.

Priapism is a continuous partial erection without sexual stimulation that is caused by dysfunctional blood flow into the corpus cavernosa. Priapism is usually sudden and painful and can cause permanent damage to erectile tissue. African-American men are more susceptible to priapism than European-American men because of their susceptibility to sickle-cell anemia, which affects the blood and circulatory system. Men who experience priapism should seek medical care immediately.

Yearly Physical Exams

All men should have annual physical exams by their medical practitioner. There is no yearly exam for men that specifically focuses on the sexual system. It is therefore important to discuss with your practitioner any sexual concerns you may have during your annual visit. Sexually active men who are not in monogamous relationships should ask to be screened for sexually transmitted infections at least once a year. Many of these infections have no symptoms for long periods of time and can be passed from one partner to another without anyone knowing it.

If you experience pain during erections or notice a distortion of the penile shaft, tell your practitioner. You may have a rare condition called **Peyronie's disease,** which is caused by fibrous growths inside the penis. Be sure to inform your practitioner about all your health concerns, especially your sexual concerns.

SAFER SEX

Safer sex is for all women and men who may be at risk for sexually transmitted infection. In today's world, practicing safer sex is one of the best things we can do for our sexual health. Safer sex is anything we do to lower our risk of getting sexually transmitted infections—infections that are spread through sexual contact, including vaginal, anal, and oral intercourse. Some can be spread through touching and kissing. Safer sex is also about getting more pleasure as we reduce our risks.

Approximately 12 million new cases of sexually transmitted infections are diagnosed each year in the United States. Most of these infections have dangerous consequences and require professional medical treatment. Some can cause sterility. Some increase the risk of getting certain cancers. And others, such as hepatitis B, syphilis, and HIV, can be fatal.

Nobody is immune to sexually transmitted infections. But most people who have one don't know it, because they don't notice the symptoms or they don't have any symptoms. Millions of people don't know they're infected until serious and often permanent damage has occurred or they pass the infection to someone else. But one out of four of us will have a sexually transmitted infection in the course of our lifetimes. Safer sex can protect us and our partners.

Most of us have taken risks to have sex—risks that include unintended pregnancy as well as sexually transmitted infections. When it comes to infection, the risks we take can be dangerous. Many sexually transmitted infections:

- last a lifetime
- put stress on relationships
- cause sterility
- cause birth defects
- lead to major illness and/or death

We know that safer sex reduces our risks. But many of us don't make the effort, because we think safer sex will be less satisfying. It does not have to be. Some of us think safer sex is only about condoms. It's not. We may think it's only about AIDS. It's not. Safer sex is about a lot more. It's also about sexual pleasure. Exploring safer sex can make sex more satisfying. It can:

- improve partner communication
- increase intimacy and trust
- prolong sex play
- enhance orgasm
- add variety to sexual techniques and pleasure
- reduce the risk of illness, pain, and discomfort
- relieve anxiety about unintended pregnancy and infection
- strengthen relationships

There are three basic steps to prepare ourselves for safer sex:

1. **Be honest with ourselves about the risks we take.** Do we have more than one partner? Do we really know whether or not a partner is carrying an infection? Do we have vaginal or anal intercourse without a condom? Have we been tested for sexually transmitted infections, including HIV?

2. **Decide which risks we are willing to take—and which ones we aren't willing to take.** Are we ready to be pregnant or to father a child? Do we want to take our chances with AIDS, hepatitis, or another serious infection?

3. **Find ways to make our safer sex play as satisfying as possible.** What can we do that's fun and safe? What do our partners like?

There are two basic rules for safer sex:

1. **Keep our partners' body fluids out of our bodies.** The body fluids to be most careful about are blood, semen, pre-ejaculate, vaginal fluids, and the discharges from sores caused by sexually transmitted infections. We must keep our partners' body fluids out of our vaginas, urethras, anuses, mouths, eyes, and any open cuts or sores. We shouldn't touch the sores caused by sexually transmitted infections.

2. **Keep our own body fluids out of our partners' bodies.** To protect our partners, we must not allow our body fluids to get into their bodies. We shouldn't have sex with our partners if we have sores or other contagious symptoms. We must get tested for sexually transmitted infections every year, and get and complete the correct treatment if we become infected.

Sex in Monogamous Relationships

Is it safe to have sex with only one partner? Maybe. The ideal for many people is to do so. Women and men don't need to worry about getting sexually transmitted infections:

- if neither partner ever had sex with anyone else
- if neither partner ever shared needles
- if neither partner was ever infected

Most of us have more than one sex partner during our lives. We may not plan it that way, but it happens. We may also get an infection from one partner and carry it to another. The partners who gave it to us:

- may not have known they were infected
- may have *hoped* they wouldn't infect us
- may not have been totally honest about their sexual histories

Some of us have only one partner, but our partner may "cheat." Many women who got HIV from having sex thought they were their sex partners' only sex partners.

We may want to give up safer sex because we've decided with our sex partners to have sex with no one else. But first we must be sure that neither partner is infected. Some infections, such as HIV, may take 10 years or more before symptoms develop. The early symptoms of many infections may go unnoticed. That's why mutually monogamous partners must be sure to be tested for sexually transmitted infections before they give up safer sex.

Establishing trust in a sexual relationship is very important. We should be able to talk openly and honestly with our partners about our sexual histories and theirs. We should know whether our partners have had infections, and they should know about any infections we've had, before we agree to have unprotected sexual intercourse. Unfortunately, however, nearly one out of three people will lie about their feelings in order to have sex with someone else. A similar number will lie about their sexual histories. Only slightly fewer will lie about whether or not they have HIV!

When it comes to safer sex, we must rely on ourselves, not on our partners. Unless we have a very long, committed relationship that is built on open communication, we are the only people we are absolutely sure we can trust. Believing you are your sex partner's only sex partner will not make it true. Here are some questions to think over:

- Do I know how my partner spends time away from me?
- Is my partner always open about everything with me—including the past?
- Does my partner get upset if I want to have a "serious" talk about our relationship?
- Does my partner keep secrets from me?
- Does my partner ever say, "I'm just going out," or, "It's none of your business"?
- Is my partner always respectful to me?

If you have a relationship that is secretive, has little open communication on serious health issues, and is lacking in equality and respect, you may very well be at risk for sexually transmitted infection.

We all want partners we can trust. The key is to make sure our partners earn our trust. We should never just give it away. Whether or not our partners have HIV won't matter if we accept responsibility to protect ourselves. We shouldn't take someone's word for something so dangerous until we've been through an awful lot together—and even then we must be careful.

Women are at greater risk of getting an infection than men are. The vagina and rectum are more easily infected than the penis. A woman's chance of being infected by a man with HIV is twice as great as a man's chance of being infected by a woman with HIV.

Moreover, women generally have fewer symptoms than men. They are less likely to know that they are infected. Lots of damage can be done, even if there are no symptoms. Many women develop **PID (pelvic inflammatory disease)** because they don't know they have gonorrhea or chlamydia. PID increases the risk of sterility and **ectopic pregnancy.**

Safer Sex Techniques

Having sex with an uninfected, long-term, faithful partner is considered safe. Outside of this kind of relationship, there are two important safer sex techniques—outercourse and use of a condom.

Sex play without penetration is called outercourse. A lot of people have vaginal intercourse because they think they're supposed to. For a long time, women and men were taught that "good sex" only meant having an orgasm during vaginal intercourse. Nothing could be less true.

Most women don't have orgasms from vaginal stimulation. Most of them have orgasms when the clitoris is stimulated—whether or not they are being penetrated by a penis. Men also enjoy outercourse—even if they're shy about letting their partners know. Outercourse can provide intense sexual satisfaction for women and men, and it is considered a low-risk activity for most serious sexually transmitted infections.

Outercourse includes:

- masturbation
- mutual masturbation

For more information about outercourse, the condom, and the vaginal pouch, see Chapter 7, "Planning Our Families."

- erotic massage
- body rubbing
- kissing
- deep kissing
- oral sex
- role play

Unprotected vaginal and anal intercourse pose the highest risks for the most dangerous infections. Lower-risk sex play includes outercourse and:

- vaginal intercourse with a condom or vaginal pouch
- anal intercourse with a condom or vaginal pouch

The latex condom is the best protection for enjoying sexual intercourse when there is any risk of sexually transmitted infection. Not only does it prevent semen and pre-ejaculate from getting into the vagina, anus, or mouth, but it also protects the penis from being exposed to infection.

The latex condom is the only contraceptive method that is proved to be **prophylactic**—protecting against the most serious sexually transmitted infections. The vaginal pouch or plastic or animal condoms also offer some protection. The diaphragm, cervical cap, and spermicides offer limited protection against certain infections. Other methods of birth control offer none. This means we need to correctly use a latex condom or vaginal pouch every time.

CONDOMS WORK!

In a 1987–91 study of couples in which one partner had HIV, all 123 couples who correctly used condoms every time for four years prevented transmission of HIV. In 122 couples who did not use condoms every time, 12 partners became infected.

A similar 1993 study showed that using condoms every time prevented HIV transmission for all but two out of 171 women with male partners with HIV. However, eight out of 55 women whose partners didn't use condoms every time became infected.

NOT ALL SEXUALLY TRANSMITTED INFECTIONS ARE TRANSMITTED THE SAME WAY

You need to know a little bit about how you might get an infection in order to evaluate your risks. Here are the basics:

If you have unprotected vaginal or anal intercourse, you are at high risk for:

- trichomoniasis
- gonorrhea
- chlamydia
- syphilis
- chancroid
- human papilloma viruses (HPV), which can cause genital warts
- HPVs that are associated with cervical cancer
- herpes simplex virus (HSV), which can cause genital herpes
- pelvic inflammatory disease (PID), which can cause sterility
- hepatitis B virus (HBV)
- cytomegalovirus (CMV)
- pubic lice
- scabies
- human immunodeficiency virus (HIV), which can cause AIDS

If you have unprotected oral sex, you are at high risk for:

- gonorrhea
- syphilis
- chancroid
- HSV
- HBV
- CMV

If you have sex play without sexual intercourse, you are at risk for:

- HPV
- CMV
- HSV
- pubic lice
- scabies

Lots of other diseases, from the flu to mononucleosis, can also be transmitted sexually.

Many people, especially women, gay men, and the transgendered, have been taught to be ashamed of their sexual feelings and behaviors. Many of us feel shy and insecure about our bodies. Those of us who are sexually inexperienced may be nervous and confused about what is going to happen and what we are supposed to do. Anxious feelings about sex can interfere with our ability to stand up for our sexual rights and our commitment to practice safer sex.

Anyone who feels guilty or embarrassed by talking about sexual needs and limits may also be unable to ask a sex partner to use a condom. Many people are so concerned about jeopardizing their relationships that they fear saying anything that may offend or scare off potential sex partners. They may prefer taking health risks rather than risk being left alone.

To protect ourselves, we need to develop negotiation and refusal skills so that we can talk about our sexual needs and limits. To do this, we can role-play with friends or practice what we want to say in front of a mirror. It may sound silly, but learning *how* to say what we want or don't want may be a lot easier when we're not being pressured by someone who is sexually excited.

Men who cannot use a condom due to erectile problems can ask their partners to use a vaginal pouch. Some people, however, have controlling partners who refuse to allow them to protect themselves with condoms or vaginal pouches. These people may have an especially difficult time negotiating the use of protection against sexually transmitted infection if they fear violence as a consequence. This kind of relationship is destructive on many levels, and the sexual, emotional, and physical health of the "victim" is often best served by leaving the relationship as soon as possible.

These relationships point to the urgent need for new and more discreet ways to allow people to prevent sexually transmitted infections and pregnancy, without a partner's knowledge. Meanwhile, people in such difficult relationships may go through a period when they have to make tough choices. If they are being forced to have unprotected sex, it may be best for them to discreetly use a spermicide. While using spermicide alone is risky, it may be better than using nothing. At least it can lower the risk of infection with gonorrhea and chlamydia, although it may be less effective against HIV.

A SAMPLE SCRIPT FOR CONDOM NEGOTIATION TO GET YOU STARTED

If your partner says: It doesn't feel as good with a rubber.

You can say: I'll feel more relaxed. If I'm more relaxed, I can make it feel better for you.

If your partner says: But we've never used a condom before.

You can say: I don't want to take any more risks.

If your partner says: Don't you trust me?

You can say: Trust isn't the point. People carry infections without knowing it.

If your partner says: I'll pull out in time.

You can say: You can get infections from pre-ejaculate, too.

If your partner says: I thought you said using condoms made you feel cheap.

You can say: I decided to face facts. I like having sex and I want to stay healthy and happy.

If your partner says: Rubbers aren't romantic.

You can say: What's more romantic than making love *and* protecting each other's health at the same time?

If your partner says: But it just isn't as sensitive.

You can say: Maybe that way you'll last even longer and that will make up for it.

If your partner says: I don't stay hard when I put on a condom.

You can say: Not if I help put it on.

If your partner says: I'll try, but it might not work.

You can say: Practice makes perfect.

If your partner says: But I love you.

You can say: Then you'll help us protect each other.

Sex can be exciting, satisfying, caring, and rewarding—especially when we plan ahead and wait until we're ready. If we know what we're doing and if we stay in charge, we can have happier, healthier, and more satisfying sex lives.

Alcohol and Safer Sex

Alcohol is a popular social drug that many people think enhances sexuality. Illegal party drugs, such as pot, cocaine, and ecstasy, have the same reputation. Some people feel more attractive or think they have better sex when they are drinking or getting high. In reality, pot and alcohol are depressants. Used in moderate amounts, they have a tranquilizing effect. At best, they reduce the social inhibitions that could interfere with sexual restraint, but, like ecstasy, they can inhibit sexual arousal.

Alcohol affects everyone differently and tends to affect women more quickly and powerfully than men. This is believed to be due to many factors. Women have fewer enzymes to break down alcohol and less fluid content in their bodies, and they experience more complicated hormonal changes.

Alcohol should never be mixed with any other drug or medication. Long-term, heavy drinking can increase the risk for heart disease, circulatory problems, peptic ulcers, cancer, brain damage, and cirrhosis of the liver. A lot of heavy drinking can cause permanent damage physically and emotionally. Being drunk can lead to unintended pregnancy, sexually transmitted infections, and date rape, as well as injuries, car accidents, and fights. It also increases the risk of suicidal behaviors that may result in death.

Even the lowest levels of alcohol consumption during a pregnancy have been known to affect the fetus. The period of highest risk occurs around the time of **conception.** Drinking alcohol during pregnancy can cause **fetal alcohol syndrome** (FAS). Children with FAS have abnormalities affecting growth, the central nervous system, and facial features. **Fetal alcohol effects** may also occur in the absence of FAS. Children with fetal alcohol effects have learning and behavioral problems as well as hearing and birth defects.

SEXUALLY TRANSMITTED INFECTIONS

There are more than 30 different kinds of sexually transmitted infections that are spread through vaginal, anal, and oral sex. Some can be spread by touching or kissing. One out of four Americans will contract a sexually transmitted infection during his or her lifetime. About 12 million new cases are diagnosed each year in the United States. In many cases, there are no symptoms until serious and permanent damage has occurred.

SYMPTOMS OF SEXUALLY TRANSMITTED INFECTIONS

See your health care provider if you have any of the following symptoms in the genital area:

abnormal or smelly discharges from the vagina, penis, or rectum	chancres	rashes
	growths	sores
	irritations	swellings
bleeding	itches	tenderness
blisters	odors	ulcers
boils	pains	urine changes
buboes	polyps	vaginitis
cervicitis	pus	warts

Other symptoms may also be associated with sexually transmitted infections. No matter the cause, see your health care provider if you have any of the following symptoms:

appetite loss	general weakness	night sweats
bowel problems	growths	pain in the joints
chills	hair loss	run-down feeling
coatings of the mouth, throat, or vagina	headaches	sore throat
	hearing loss	swollen glands
coughs	jaundice	vision loss
diarrhea	light-headedness	vomiting
discolored skin	mental disorders	weight loss that is
fatigue	muscular pain	constant, rapid, or
fevers	nausea	unexplained

Some sexually transmitted infections can be passed from a woman to her developing fetus during pregnancy or during childbirth. Some can result in the death of the fetus in the womb. Others can cause serious birth defects, developmental disabilities, and other health problems for newborn infants—problems that can last a lifetime or even cause death. All pregnant women, and women who want to become pregnant, should consider being tested for sexually transmitted infections.

Common Sexually Transmitted Infections—
an Alphabetical Listing

Chancroid

Chancroid (*SHANG-kroid*) is an especially dangerous sexually transmitted bacterium because the sores it causes increase the chances of getting HIV. Once very common, reported cases of chancroid have fallen to fewer than 1,500 per year in the United States. This may be due to increased condom use among American men.

Common Symptoms

- First, a small boil or ulcer appears, usually on the genitals. But it doesn't heal like a common pimple.
- Later, the ulcer becomes an open sore. There may be pus and pain.
- Many people also develop swollen lymph glands in the groin—buboes.
- Women may have no sores, but they may have painful urination or bowel movements, painful intercourse, rectal bleeding, or vaginal discharge.

Untreated, chancroid can infect and swell glands located in the groin. (These swollen sores are called buboes.) Men are more commonly infected than women. Symptoms usually appear within a week of infection.

How Chancroid Is Spread: Vaginal, anal, and oral intercourse.

Diagnosis: Chancroid sores can be confused with herpes, syphilis, and other conditions. Microscopic examination of the discharge from the sore may be necessary.

Treatment: Both partners can be treated successfully with oral antibiotics.

Protection: Condoms offer very good protection.

Chlamydia

Chlamydia (*cla-MIH-dee-ah*) is a microscopic parasite that can cause sterility in women and men.

In women, chlamydia infects the cervix and can spread to the urethra, fallopian tubes, and ovaries. It can cause bladder infections and serious pelvic inflammatory disease (PID), ectopic pregnancy, and sterility.

In men, chlamydia infects the urethra and may spread to the testicles, causing epididymitis, which can cause sterility. Chlamydia can also lead to Reiter's syndrome—especially in young men. Reiter's syndrome includes eye infections, urethritis, and arthritis. One in three men who develop Reiter's syndrome become permanently disabled.

In infants, chlamydia can cause pneumonia, eye infections, and blindness.

Chlamydia is the most common and most invisible sexually transmitted infection in the United States. Four million American men and women become infected every year.

Common Symptoms
- discharge from the penis or vagina
- pain or burning while urinating; urinating more than usual
- spotting between periods or after intercourse
- excessive vaginal bleeding, abdominal pain, nausea, fever
- painful intercourse for women
- inflammation of the rectum
- inflammation of the cervix
- swelling or pain in the testicles
- bleeding after vaginal intercourse

Seventy-five percent of women and 25 percent of men with chlamydia have no symptoms. Many women discover they have chlamydia only because their partners are found to have the disease. Other women discover they must have had it for some time when they are treated for the infertility that it can cause.

Symptoms appear in seven to 21 days—if they appear. If your partner is a man and he has a urinary tract infection, you may have chlamydia.

How Chlamydia Is Spread
- vaginal and anal intercourse
- from the birth canal to the fetus
- rarely, from the hand to the eye

Diagnosis: Can be confused with gonorrhea and other conditions. Laboratory tests of tissue samples or urine are necessary for correct diagnosis.

Treatment: Both partners can be treated successfully with antibiotics.

Protection: Condoms offer very good protection.

Cytomegalovirus (CMV)

Cytomegalovirus (*sigh-tow-MEG-a-low-VI-rus*), or CMV, is an infection that is transmitted through many bodily fluids. It is also sexually transmitted. Every year, CMV causes permanent disability, including hearing loss and mental retardation, for 4,000 to 7,000 babies. It is the most common infection in the United States that is spread from a woman to the developing fetus—from 10 to 20 percent of infants born to women with CMV will become infected. CMV is also very dangerous for people with weakened immune systems. It can cause blindness and mental disorders. CMV can remain in the body for life.

Common Symptoms

- swollen glands, fatigue, fever, and general weakness. CMV causes 8 percent of the cases of mononucleosis.
- irritations of the digestive tract, nausea, diarrhea
- loss of vision

There are usually no symptoms with the first infection. But reinfection with CMV, or infection with other sexually transmitted infections such as HIV and hepatitis B, may reactivate the virus and cause illness.

How CMV Is Spread: In saliva, semen, blood, cervical and vaginal secretions, urine, and breast milk by:

- close personal contact
- vaginal, anal, and oral intercourse
- blood transfusion and sharing IV drug equipment
- pregnancy, childbirth, and breast-feeding

Between 40 and 80 percent of Americans get CMV through contact (usually through saliva) with other children by the time they reach puberty. Adults, however, usually get CMV through sexual activity.

Women who want to become pregnant and who may have the virus should consider testing for CMV.

Diagnosis: Blood test.

Treatment: There is no cure. Symptoms may be managed with a variety of intravenous drugs, including foscarnet and ganciclovir. Treatment is not successful during pregnancy.

Protection: Condoms can provide protection during vaginal, anal, and oral intercourse, but kissing and other intimate touching can spread the virus.

Gonorrhea

Gonorrhea (*gone-o-RHEE-a*) is a bacterium that can cause sterility, arthritis, and heart problems. In women, gonorrhea can cause PID, which can result in ectopic pregnancy or sterility. During pregnancy, gonorrhea infections can cause premature labor and stillbirth. To prevent serious eye infections that are caused by gonorrhea in newborn babies, drops of silver nitrate or antibiotics are routinely put into the eyes of infants immediately after delivery. More than 1 million cases of gonorrhea are reported every year in the United States.

Common Symptoms

- *women:* frequent, often burning urination; menstrual irregularities; pelvic (or lower abdominal) pain; pain during sex or pelvic examination; a green or yellow-green discharge from the vagina; swelling or tenderness of the vulva; and even arthritic pain
- *men:* a puslike discharge from the urethra or pain during urination

Eighty percent of the women and 10 percent of the men with gonorrhea show no symptoms. If they appear, they appear in women within 10 days. It takes from one to 14 days for symptoms to appear in men.

How Gonorrhea Is Spread: Vaginal, anal, and oral intercourse.

Diagnosis: Microscopic examination of urethral or vaginal discharges. Cultures taken from the cervix, throat, urethra, or rectum.

Treatment: Both partners can be successfully treated with oral antibiotics. Often, people with gonorrhea also have chlamydia. They must be treated for both infections at the same time.

Protection: Condoms offer very good protection.

Hepatitis B Virus (HBV)

Although 90 to 95 percent of adults with HBV recover completely, the virus can cause severe liver disease and death. Unless they are treated within an hour of birth, 90 percent of the infants born to women with HBV will carry the virus. Pregnant women who may have been exposed to HBV should consider being tested before giving birth so that their babies can be vaccinated at birth or treated if they become ill. Like many other viruses, HBV remains in the body for life.

HBV is the only sexually transmitted infection that is preventable with vaccination. But about 200,000 Americans get HBV every year because they have not been vaccinated. There are now about 1.5 million people with HBV in the United States.

Common Symptoms
- extreme fatigue, headache, fever
- nausea, vomiting, lack of appetite, tenderness in the lower abdomen

Later Symptoms: dark urine, clay-colored stool, yellowing of the skin and whites of the eye (jaundice), and weight loss.

HBV may show no symptoms during its most contagious phases. If symptoms appear, they appear within four weeks.

How HBV Is Spread: In semen, saliva, blood, **feces,** and urine by:
- intimate and sexual contact, including kissing, vaginal and anal intercourse, oral sex and oral/anal sex.
- use of unclean needles to inject drugs
- passing from a woman to her fetus during pregnancy

Health care workers may be infected when accidentally stuck by a needle containing the infected blood of a patient. Hepatitis B is highly contagious.

Diagnosis: Blood test.

Treatment: None. In most cases, the infection clears within four to eight weeks of rest. Some people, however, remain contagious for the rest of their lives.

Protection: Condoms offer some protection against HBV during vaginal, anal, and oral intercourse, but the virus can be passed through kissing and other intimate touching. *Children and adults who do not have HBV can get permanent protection with a series of HBV vaccine injections.*

Herpes

There are two forms of genital herpes—herpes simplex virus-1 and herpes simplex virus-2. Although herpes-1 is most often associated with cold sores and fever blisters, both forms of herpes may be sexually transmitted. Rarely, a primary outbreak of herpes during pregnancy may cause miscarriage or stillbirth. If active herpes infections are present during childbirth, newborn infants may suffer serious health damage, including developmental disabilities and, rarely, death. Transmission to a newborn is more common during the first episode of a herpes infection and less common during a recurrent herpes outbreak. More than 30 million Americans have genital herpes, and 500,000 new cases are diagnosed every year. **HSV (herpes simplex virus)** remains in the body for life.

Common Symptoms

- a recurring rash with clusters of blistery, painful, or itchy sores appearing on the vagina, cervix, penis, mouth, anus, buttocks, or elsewhere on the body
- a primary outbreak that may result in pain and discomfort around the infected area of sores, itching, burning sensations during urination, swollen glands in the groin, fever, headache, and a general run-down feeling

Symptoms usually appear from two to 20 days after infection, but it may be years before an outbreak occurs.

Recurrences are sometimes related to emotional, physical, or health stresses. During recurrences, it is important to observe strict rules of day-to-day hygiene. Wash hands frequently and do not touch the sores. If the sores are touched inadvertently, wash hands immediately. Be particularly careful when handling contact lenses and touching the eyes.

How HSV Is Spread

- touching, sexual intimacy (including kissing)
- vaginal, anal, and oral intercourse
- rarely, during childbirth

HSV may be passed from one partner to another or from one part of the body to another, whenever contact is made with an active herpes virus.

HSV is most contagious from the time the sores are present until they are completely healed and the scabs have fallen off. Unfortunately, recent studies show that some people may be contagious when they have no symptoms. Mucous membranes of the mouth, anus, vagina, penis, and eyes are especially susceptible to infection.

Diagnosis: Can be confused with syphilis, chancroid, and other infections. Examination of the sores and laboratory culturing of fluid samples taken from the sores are important. Definitive diagnosis may not be possible if the sores are dried or scabbed. If you think you have herpes, it is important to have a diagnosis early in the outbreak.

Treatment: No cure. Symptoms can be relieved and the number of recurrences reduced with drugs such as valacyclovir and acyclovir.

Protection: Partners should refrain from sexual intimacy from the time they know the blisters are going to recur until after the scabs have completely fallen off the healed sores. Condoms offer some protection when the virus is not active.

Human Immunodeficiency Virus (HIV)

HIV infections weaken the body's ability to fight disease and can cause acquired immune deficiency syndrome (AIDS)—the last stage of HIV infection. HIV is the most dangerous sexually transmitted infection, and it affects people of all ages. It is now the leading cause of death for American women and men between 25 and 44 years of age. About 40,000 women and men are infected each year. About 1 million Americans have had HIV since the beginning of the epidemic. Like many other viruses, HIV remains in the body for life.

Common Symptoms

- constant or rapid unexplained weight loss, diarrhea, lack of appetite
- fatigue, persistent fevers, night sweats, dry cough
- light-headedness, headaches, mental disorders
- a thick, whitish coating of yeast on the tongue or mouth— "thrush"
- severe or recurring vaginal yeast infections
- chronic PID
- purplish growths on the skin

There may be no symptoms for 10 years or more. In one study, about 5 percent of men with HIV have not developed symptoms for 20 years.

How HIV Is Spread: In blood, semen, vaginal fluids, and breast milk by:

- anal, vaginal, and oral intercourse
- sharing contaminated needles for injecting IV drugs
- transfusion of contaminated blood products
- childbirth
- breast-feeding

Diagnosis: There are blood tests to detect HIV antibodies. Diagnosis of AIDS is based on the presence of one or more of a variety of conditions and "opportunistic" infections related to an HIV infection.

Treatment: No cure or vaccine. Many AIDS-related conditions—such as pneumonia, cancers, and a variety of infections that take advantage of weakened immune systems—can be managed to some extent with a variety of treatments. However, AIDS is fatal, and at this time, no one has recovered.

Protection: Condoms offer very good protection.

Human Papilloma Virus (HPV)

There are 90 different human papilloma (*pap-ill-LOW-mah*) viruses. They cause a variety of warts and other conditions. A few HPVs cause genital warts, but most genital HPV infections are not visible and have no symptoms. Some of these are associated with cancer of the cervix, vulva, or penis. Every year, about 1 million Americans are infected with genital HPVs—40 million women and men are now infected.

Common Symptoms

- warts on the genitals, in the urethra, in the anus, and, rarely, in the throat
- genital warts that are soft to the touch; may look like miniature cauliflower florets, and often itch
- untreated genital warts that occasionally grow to block the openings of the vagina, anus, or throat and become quite uncomfortable

It usually takes from two to three weeks after infection for warts to develop. In women, genital warts grow more rapidly during pregnancy or when other vaginal infections are present.

How Genital HPVs Are Spread

- vaginal and anal intercourse
- very rarely, during childbirth

Diagnosis

- microscopic examination of tissue sample
- clinical evaluation of warts during a physical or gynecological exam
- use of special magnifiers—**colposcopes**—to detect genital HPVs that cannot be seen with the naked eye during pelvic exams
- Pap tests, which may reveal precancerous conditions caused by genital HPVs. Early treatment prevents cancer of the cervix.

Treatment: Though HPV can recur, genital warts can be treated in a number of ways. They may be removed by carefully applying, and often reapplying, a prescription medication, podofilox, to the wart. Clinicians offer other treatments, including:

- standard surgery
- laser surgery (vaporizing the wart with a beam of high-powered light)
- cryosurgery (freezing the wart with liquid nitrogen)
- application of podofilox, podophyllin, or trichloroacetic acid
- injection with interferon

Protection: Condoms may offer some protection, but the viruses may "shed" beyond the area protected by a condom.

Molluscum Contagiosum

Hundreds of thousands of cases of the virus **molluscum contagiosum** (*mo-LUS-kum con-TAY-gee-OH-sum*) are diagnosed every year. The virus is often transmitted by nonsexual intimate contact. In children, it may be spread by more casual contact and is often found on various parts of the body, such as the abdomen.

Common Symptoms: Small, pinkish-white, waxy, round, polyplike growths in the genital area or on the thighs. There is often a tiny depression in the middle of the growth. Symptoms usually appear between two and 12 weeks after infection—but it can take years.

How Molluscum Contagiosum Is Spread: Vaginal, anal, and oral intercourse, as well as other intimate contact.

Diagnosis: Microscopic examination of tissue taken from the sore.

Treatment: Growths may be removed with chemicals, electrical current, lasers, or freezing.

Protection: Condoms may offer some protection, but the virus may "shed" beyond the area protected by the condom.

Pelvic Inflammatory Disease (PID)

PID is a condition that harms a woman's reproductive system. PID occurs throughout the pelvic area, in the fallopian tubes, the uterus, the lining of the uterus, and the ovaries. Treated or untreated, PID can lead to sterility, ectopic pregnancy, and chronic pain. The more episodes of PID a woman has, the greater are her chances of becoming sterile. PID is not always the result of a sexually transmitted infection, but in many cases it is. The sexually transmitted infections that most commonly cause PID are gonorrhea and chlamydia. More than 1 million new cases of PID are diagnosed every year in the United States. It is believed that millions of others go undiscovered.

Common Symptoms

- fever, chills
- nausea, vomiting
- pain during intercourse
- pain in the lower abdomen
- spotting and pain between menstrual periods or during urination
- unusually long or painful periods, and unusual vaginal discharge

Diagnosis

- pelvic exam
- laboratory examination of vaginal and cervical secretions
- laparoscopy, in which an optical instrument is inserted through a small cut in the navel to look at the reproductive organs

Symptoms can be confused with those of appendicitis and other infections. Diagnosis can be difficult if patients are too embarrassed to admit sexual activity.

Treatment: Antibiotics, bed rest, and sexual abstinence. Surgery may be required to remove abscesses or scar tissue, or to repair or remove reproductive organs.

Protection: Condoms offer very good protection against the sexually transmitted infections commonly associated with PID.

Pubic Lice

Every year, millions of people treat themselves for **pubic lice.** These tiny insects are also called crabs or cooties.

Common Symptoms

- intense itching in the genitals or anus usually begins five days after infestation. Some people don't itch and don't know they are infested. People who are insensitive to the itching may experience very heavy infestation before they seek treatment. They may experience: mild fever, run-down feeling, or irritability.

How Pubic Lice Are Spread
- contact with infected bedding, upholstered furniture, clothing, and toilet seats
- intimate and sexual contact

Self-diagnosis: Seen with the naked eye or with a magnifying glass, pubic lice look like tiny crabs. They are pale gray but darken in color when swollen with blood. They attach themselves and their eggs to pubic hair, underarm hair, eyelashes, and eyebrows. Their eggs are white and are deposited in small clumps near the hair roots.

Treatment: Follow the directions on the package insert of an over-the-counter medication. Some of the brands available are Kwell®, A-200®, NIX®, and RID®. Repeated head-to-toe applications may be necessary. Pregnant women and infants must use products especially designed for them, like Eurax®. Everyone who may have been exposed to pubic lice should be treated at the same time. All bedding, towels, and clothing that may have been exposed should be thoroughly washed or dry-cleaned.

Protection: Limit the number of intimate and sexual contacts.

Scabies

The **scabies** (*SKAY-beez*) mite burrows under the skin. It can hardly be seen with the naked eye. It belongs to the same family as the spider. It is not usually sexually transmitted. Schoolchildren often pass it to one another.

Common Symptoms
- intense itching—usually at night
- small bumps or rashes that appear in dirty-looking, small curling lines, especially on the penis, between the fingers, on buttocks, breasts, wrists, thighs, and around the navel

How Scabies Is Spread
- close personal contact
- bedding and clothing

Often, symptoms are not visible. It may take several weeks for them to develop.

Diagnosis: Although people can diagnose themselves, diagnosis is often difficult. Microscopic examination of a skin scraping or biopsy by a clinician may be necessary.

Treatment: Follow the directions on the package insert of an over the-counter medication such as Kwell® or Scabene®. Repeated neck to-toe applications may be necessary. Everyone who may have been exposed to scabies should be treated at the same time. All bedding, towels, and clothing that may have been exposed should be thoroughly washed or dry-cleaned.

Protection: Limit the number of intimate and sexual contacts.

Syphilis

Untreated, the syphilis (*SIFF-i-lis*) organism—a **spirochete**—can remain in the body for life and lead to disfigurement, neurological disorders, or death. The number of reported cases of syphilis in the United States has dropped below 120,000. This may be because of effective antibiotics and increased condom use among American men.

Common Symptoms: Syphilis has several phases that may overlap one another. They do not always follow in the same sequence. Symptoms vary with each phase, but most of the time there are no symptoms.

- *Primary phase.* Painless sores or ulcers—chancres—often appear from three weeks to 90 days after infection. They last three to six weeks. They appear on the genitals, in the vagina, on the cervix, lips, mouth, or anus. Swollen glands may also occur during the primary phase.

- *Secondary phase.* Other symptoms often appear from three to six weeks after the sores appear. They may come and go for up to two years. They include body rashes that last from two to six weeks—often on the palms of the hands and the soles of the feet. The rashes are so often confused with other diseases, including measles and drug rashes, that syphilis was once called "the great imitator." There are many other symptoms, including mild fever, fatigue, sore throat, patchy hair loss, weight loss, swollen glands, headache, and muscle pains.

- *Latent phase.* No symptoms. Latent phases occur between other phases or can overlap them.

- *Late phase.* One-third of people with untreated syphilis experience serious damage of the nervous system, heart, brain, or other organs, and death may result.

How Syphilis Is Spread
- vaginal, anal, and oral intercourse
- kissing
- during pregnancy

Syphilis is especially contagious when sores are present early in the disease—the liquid that oozes from them is very infectious. People are usually not contagious during the latent phases of the first four years of syphilis infections. Untreated syphilis remains latent for many years or a lifetime, but can be spread from a pregnant woman to her fetus.

The effect of syphilis on a fetus is very serious. If untreated, the risks of stillbirth or serious birth defects are high. Birth defects include damage to the heart, brain, and skeleton as well as blindness. It is very important for pregnant women to consider testing for syphilis early and, sometimes, throughout their pregnancies. Pregnant women with syphilis should be treated to prevent damage to the fetus.

Diagnosis
- microscopic examination of fluid from sores
- blood tests
- examination of spinal fluid

Treatment: Antibiotics are successful for both partners—but damage caused by the disease in the later phases cannot be undone.

Protection: Condoms offer very good protection during vaginal, anal, and oral intercourse.

Trichomoniasis
Trichomoniasis (*trick-oh-mo-NEYE-ah-sis*), or "trich," is a protozoan— a microscopic one-celled organism. It is a common cause of vaginitis. Up to 3 million Americans develop trichomoniasis every year.

Common Symptoms
- frothy, often unpleasant-smelling discharge
- itching in and around the vagina
- blood spotting in the discharge
- swelling in the groin
- urinating more often than usual

Only rarely do men have symptoms. Sometimes women have no symptoms. It takes from three to 28 days for symptoms to develop.

How Trichomoniasis Is Spread: Vaginal intercourse.

Diagnosis: Microscopic examination of vaginal discharge.

Treatment: Antibiotics are successful for both partners.

Protection: Condoms offer very good protection.

Urinary Tract Infection

UTI (**urinary tract infection**) is caused by bacteria that have spread from the rectum to the vagina or penis and then to the urethra and bladder. UTIs may be sexually transmitted. They include infections of the bladder (also called **cystitis**), the **ureters** (the tubes that lead from the kidneys to the bladder), and the urethra (the tube that carries urine from the bladder to outside of the body). Severe cases, left untreated, may cause kidney infection.

Common Symptoms
- burning pain during urination
- the urge to urinate when the bladder is nearly empty
- a frequent urge to urinate, especially at night
- involuntary loss of urine
- lower abdominal pain
- blood and pus in urine
- fever

UTIs are very common in women and men who are sexually active. They affect women more often than men because a woman's urethra is shorter than a man's, and bacteria may get into the bladder more easily. A woman's urethra is also closer to the anus than a man's.

How UTIs Are Spread: Any kind of sex play that brings fecal material into contact with the vagina and urethra. Unprotected anal intercourse carries a very high risk for urinary tract infection.

Diagnosis: Consult your clinician to confirm diagnosis and treatment. Some women who use a diaphragm are susceptible to frequent UTIs. *Adjusting to the bacterial environment caused by having new partners may lead to a bladder infection called honeymoon cystitis.*

Treatment
- antibiotics
- Pyridium®, which may relieve symptoms but will not cure the infection

Protection: To prevent urinary tract infections or discourage them from returning:

- Drink eight or more glasses of water a day. Avoid soft drinks, which can promote the growth of bacteria.
- Drink unsweetened cranberry juice.
- Urinate immediately before and after intercourse.
- Avoid using a sexual position that seems to trigger UTIs.
- Keep the pubic area clean and dry.
- Use condoms or vaginal pouches during vaginal or anal intercourse.
- Wipe from front to back after bowel movements and urinating to avoid the spread of bacteria to the urethra.

Some women who are susceptible to frequent UTIs take antibiotics to prevent infections when they have sexual intercourse.

If You Think You Have a Sexually Transmitted Infection...

See your health care provider immediately. Early treatment can make all the difference.

If you do have an infection, let your sex partner(s) know so he or she can be tested and treated, too. Otherwise, the infection can be passed back and forth between partners.

Don't have sex, especially sexual intercourse, until your health care provider has given you a diagnosis and treatment and has said it is safe to have sexual contact once again.

For information, testing, and treatment for sexually transmitted infections, you may make a confidential appointment at the Planned Parenthood health center nearest you by calling toll free 800-230-PLAN.

INFORMATION HOT LINES

The U.S. Centers for Disease Control and Prevention funds toll free hot lines to provide information about sexually transmitted infections and AIDS. The hot lines are operated by the nonprofit American Social Health Association.

The hot lines are staffed by professional health counselors. They can answer basic questions, provide the addresses of testing sites and low-cost clinics, suggest support groups, discuss options for financial assistance, and send you free information. Anything you say will remain confidential.

National STD Hot Line: 800-227-8922. The STD hot line is open from 8:00 a.m. to 11:00 p.m. eastern time Monday through Friday. At other times, you'll reach a tape that invites you to call back during business hours. Free pamphlets on various infections and other topics are offered in English or Spanish. This toll-free number will not appear on your phone bill.

National AIDS Hot Line: 800-342-AIDS (800-342-2437). The English-language AIDS hot line is open 24 hours a day, seven days a week. The Spanish-language SIDA hot line is open 8:00 a.m. to 2:00 a.m. eastern time, seven days a week. TTY lines for the hearing impaired are open Monday through Friday, 10:00 a.m. to 10:00 p.m. eastern time. This toll-free number will not appear on your phone bill.

National Herpes Hot Line: 919-361-8488. The herpes hot line is open from 9:00 a.m. to 7:00 p.m. eastern time. A free information packet is sent in an unmarked envelope. The National Herpes Hot Line is also run by the American Social Health Association. This number is *not* toll-free and *will* appear on your phone bill. French-speaking counselors are available.

Herpes Resource Center: 800-230-6039. The Herpes Resource Center offers educational materials and newsletters for purchase. Counseling referrals are available. The center also provides access to a network of more than 90 local herpes support groups in the United States and Canada. This toll-free number will not appear on your phone bill.

Planning

Our

Families

BIRTH CONTROL

Women and men often have sex for pleasure. Less frequently, but as important, they have sex in order to begin a pregnancy and have a baby. Most people want to have children, but want to have them when they are most ready. During our reproductive years, vaginal intercourse can result in pregnancy, whether or not it is intended.

Planning a pregnancy, having a child, and building a family are some of the great pleasures, rewards, and challenges in life. Unintended pregnancy, however, can be very problematic. There are only three alternatives—raising a child, adoption, or abortion. Most women would prefer to avoid having to make one of these choices.

Contraception provides a way for women and men to avoid unplanned pregnancy. The more common name for contraception is birth control. There are many different methods of birth control available to women and men. The perfect way to avoid unintended pregnancy is to abstain from sex play entirely. This way there is no chance that sperm will spill onto the vulva, make its way into the vagina, and cause pregnancy. This method is called **continuous abstinence** or celibacy.

All other methods of birth control allow women and men to reduce the risk of unplanned pregnancy and enjoy sex with one another. Some methods can reduce the risk by nearly 100 percent. Others may be somewhat less effective, but can also reduce the risk of sexually transmitted infections. Heterosexual couples who do not use birth control when they have vaginal intercourse are very likely to start a pregnancy. In fact, 85 percent of women who use no contraceptives during vaginal intercourse become pregnant each year. It is also important to remember that every method of birth control has fewer health risks and is safer for women than pregnancy.

Your contraceptive needs may change throughout your life. To decide which method to use now, consider how well each one will work for you. These are the questions to think about as you consider each method:

How effective will it be?
How reversible will it be?
How safe will it be?
Will it protect against sexually transmitted infections?
What are the potential side effects?
How affordable and available will it be?
Will it be difficult to use?
How well will it fit into your lifestyle?
How private will it be?

HOW EFFECTIVE WILL A METHOD BE?

The key to contraceptive effectiveness is consistent and correct use. When you are looking for an effective contraceptive, it is crucial to choose one that fits the reality of your lifestyle. A condom, for example, can be 98 percent effective, but only if it is used correctly—every time.

Effectiveness rates for contraceptive methods are based on clinical studies, survey data, and scientific estimates. Clinical studies are now mandatory for methods that require a prescription and for over-the-counter methods that require approval from the U.S. Food and Drug Administration (FDA). Couples who volunteer for clinical studies report to the researchers how consistently and correctly they used the methods and whether or not they have experienced an unintended pregnancy.

Researchers use a variety of survey data to develop estimates for methods that are based on behavior and for methods whose use predates current FDA requirements for approval.

The rates of contraceptive effectiveness are measured in two ways:

- **"Method-effectiveness"** is the reliability of a method itself—when it is always used consistently and correctly. This is also called **perfect use**—the way it is intended to be used, every time.
- **"Use-effectiveness"** is the reliability of the method as it is usually used—when it is *not* always used consistently or correctly. This is also called **typical use**—the way it is used by most people.

The longer a method of contraception is used, the more effective "typical use" becomes—typical *users* usually become more effective as they become more experienced. However, the standard measure for the effectiveness of methods is the number of unintended pregnancies experienced by 100 women using the method during their *first* year of use.

For example, the *failure* rate of the condom with "typical use" is 12 percent—of every 100 women whose partners use the condom, 12 will become pregnant during the first year of typical use. On the other hand, the failure rate of the condom with "perfect use" is 3 percent—of every 100 women whose partners use the condom, only three will become pregnant with perfect use.

The table on the next page compares the "typical" and "perfect" failure rates for the contraceptive methods now available in the United States. Carefully consider the level of effectiveness and failure you can live with as you choose your method.

REVERSIBLE METHODS OF BIRTH CONTROL

Most younger women and men who choose to use contraception want to be able to have children at some future time in their lives. They want to protect themselves against unintended pregnancy now, but they also want to be able to reverse the contraceptive effects when they decide they want to have a child.

Many couples prefer a method that is quickly reversible. All barrier and behavioral methods of birth control are immediately reversible. Fertility is restored to its previous levels as soon as the contraceptive method is discontinued. With hormonal methods, however, it may take some time for the effects of the hormones to leave the body. If you are considering a hormonal method and are planning to become pregnant soon, be very sure to know how much time is needed to reverse the contraceptive effects of the methods you consider.

Behavioral Methods of Birth Control

Ever since the dawn of history, women and men have wanted to be able to decide when and whether to have a child. Many of the earliest methods of family planning they tried are still used by millions of women and men around the world. These methods are most often

COMPARISON OF EFFECTIVENESS

Number of Pregnancies per 100 Women During One Year of Use

Method	Typical Use[a]	Perfect Use[b]
Continuous abstinence	0.00	0.00
Outercourse	N/A	N/A
Norplant®	0.09	0.09
Sterilization		
Men	0.15	0.1
Women	0.4	0.4
Depo-Provera®	0.3	0.3
IUD	0.8	0.6 **ParaGard® (copper T-380 A)**
	2.6	1.5 **Progestasert®**
Emergency contraception (per use)	2.0	2.0 hormonal
	0.1	0.1 IUD insertion
The Pill	3.0	0.1 combination pills
		0.5 progestin-only mini-pills
Condom	12.0	3.0
Diaphragm	18.0	6.0
Withdrawal	19.0	4.0
Cervical cap		
Women who have not given birth	18.0	9.0
Women who have given birth	36.0	26.0
Periodic abstinence	20.0	1.0 post-ovulation method
		2.0 symptothermal method
		3.0 cervical mucus method
		9.0 calendar method
Fertility awareness methods	N/A	N/A
Contraceptive foam and suppositories	21.0	3.0
Vaginal pouch ("female condom")	21.0	5.0
No method	85.0	85.0

Effectiveness rates updated from Trussell et al. (1990) as published in *Contraceptive Technology* (New York: Irvington Press,1994).

[a] Typical Use: failure rates for women and men whose use is not consistent or always correct

[b] Perfect Use: failure rates for those whose use is consistent and always correct

N/A: Failure rates not available

used by people who have few alternatives. But many of the ancient methods are also preferred by some people who have access to the latest advances in contraceptive technology. For thousands of years, abstinence, mutual pleasuring without intercourse—outercourse, withdrawal, predicting fertility, and breast-feeding—were used by our ancestors to prevent unintended pregnancy. These methods still play important roles in family planning today.

Continuous Abstinence

If you choose **continuous abstinence,** you will not have sex play. Pregnancy cannot happen if sperm are kept out of the vagina.

Effectiveness of Continuous Abstinence
Continuous abstinence is 100 percent effective in preventing pregnancy. It also prevents sexually transmitted infections.

Advantages of Continuous Abstinence
- Abstinence has no medical or hormonal side effects.
- Many religious groups endorse abstinence among unmarried people.

Who Can Use Continuous Abstinence
Any woman or man can abstain from vaginal intercourse. Many do so at various times in their lives. Some choose to do so all their lives. Many choose to express their sexual feelings in other ways.

Possible Problems with Continuous Abstinence
- People may find it difficult to abstain for long periods of time.
- Women and men often end their abstinence without being prepared to protect themselves against pregnancy.

Cost
None.

For more information about alternatives to vaginal intercourse, see Chapter 3, "Our Sexual Bodies."

Outercourse

If you choose **outercourse,** you will have sex play without vaginal intercourse. This will keep sperm from joining egg. There are many alternatives for sex play without vaginal intercourse:
- masturbation
- erotic massage and body rubbing
- **erotica,** fantasy, role play, masks, and sex toys

Effectiveness of Outercourse
Outercourse is nearly 100 percent effective. Pregnancy is possible if semen or pre-ejaculate is spilled on the vulva.

Outercourse is also effective against HIV and certain other serious sexually transmitted infections, unless body fluids are exchanged through oral or anal sex play.

Advantages of Outercourse
- Outercourse has no medical or hormonal side effects.
- Outercourse can be used as safer sex if no body fluids are exchanged.
- Outercourse may prolong sex play and enhance orgasm.

Possible Problems with Outercourse
- It is difficult for many people to abstain from vaginal intercourse for long periods of time.
- Women and men may decide to engage in vaginal intercourse without being prepared to protect themselves against pregnancy or sexually transmitted infections.

Cost
None.

Withdrawal

If you choose **withdrawal,** the man will pull his penis out of the vagina before he ejaculates to keep sperm from joining the egg.

Effectiveness of Withdrawal
Of 100 women whose partners practice withdrawal, it is estimated that 19 will become pregnant during the first year of typical use. It is estimated that only four will become pregnant with perfect use.

Pre-ejaculate can contain enough sperm to cause pregnancy, and pregnancy is possible if semen or pre-ejaculate is spilled on the vulva.

Withdrawal is not effective against most sexually transmitted infections.

Advantages of Withdrawal
Withdrawal can be used to reduce the risk of pregnancy when no other method is available.

Possible Problems with Withdrawal
- Withdrawal requires great self-control, experience, and trust.

- Withdrawal is not appropriate for men who are likely to have premature ejaculation.
- Withdrawal is not appropriate for men who can't tell when ejaculatory inevitability occurs and they have to pull out.
- Withdrawal is not recommended for sexually inexperienced men.
- Withdrawal is not recommended for teens.

Cost
None.

Predicting Fertility for Periodic Abstinence and Fertility Awareness Methods

Periodic abstinence and **fertility awareness methods (FAMs)** are ways you can prevent pregnancy by using your fertility pattern. Understanding your fertility pattern helps you predict ovulation. You can also use this information to help you become pregnant.

If you choose **periodic abstinence,** you will not have vaginal intercourse during your "unsafe days." These are the days during which your fertile phase is likely to occur. The fertile phase lasts for about nine days—approximately six days before and three days after the day of ovulation. If you use **FAMs,** you will use a barrier contraceptive during your "unsafe days." (Sperm can live from two to seven days in a woman's reproductive system. The egg can live from one to three days.)

How Periodic Abstinence and FAMs Work
There are several ways you can predict when to abstain or use birth control.

For the **basal body temperature method:** Take your temperature every morning before getting out of bed. Your temperature rises between 0.4°F and 0.8°F on the day of ovulation. It remains at that level until your next period. You are fertile during the six days preceding ovulation.

For the **cervical mucus method:** Observe the changes in your cervical mucus. You must do so all through the first part of your menstrual cycle, until you are sure you have ovulated. Normally cloudy, tacky mucus will become clear and slippery in the few days before ovulation, and it will stretch between the fingers. When this happens, you are in your most fertile phase. You must abstain from vaginal intercourse or use a barrier contraceptive during the six days before this time. This method is sometimes called the **ovulation method.**

For the **calendar** or **"rhythm" method:** Chart your menstrual cycles on a calendar. You may be able to predict ovulation if your periods are the same every month. You must abstain or use a barrier method during your "unsafe days." It will be more difficult to predict the day of ovulation if your cycle length varies from month to month. In that case, you will have more "unsafe days." (It is best not to rely on this method alone.)

It is best to combine the basal body temperature method, the cervical mucus method, and the calendar method. Combining these methods is called the symptothermal method.

For the **post-ovulation method:** Abstain or use a barrier method from the beginning of your period until the morning of the fourth day after your predicted ovulation—more than half of your menstrual cycle.

Effectiveness of Periodic Abstinence and FAMs
Of 100 women using periodic abstinence, about 20 will become pregnant during the first year of typical use. Perfect use can give bet-

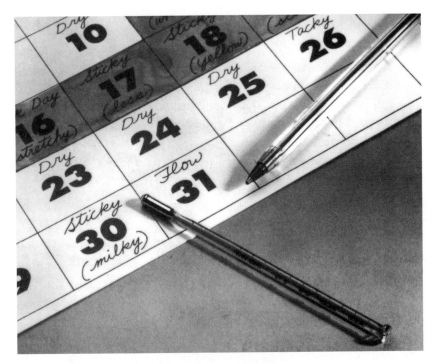

CALENDAR METHOD

ter results. Nine women will become pregnant with perfect use of the calendar method. Perfect use of the post-ovulation method, the basal body temperature method, or the cervical mucus (ovulation) method results in only one to three pregnancies. Pregnancy rates are generally higher for single women who use these methods.

Failure rates for FAMs are not available.

Periodic abstinence and FAMs provide no protection against sexually transmitted infections.

Advantages of Periodic Abstinence and FAMs

- There are no medical or hormonal side effects.
- Calendars, thermometers, and charts are easy to get.
- Most religious groups accept periodic abstinence.

Who Can Use Periodic Abstinence and FAMs

- women in good health who have had careful instruction
- women whose only sex partner is equally committed to the method

Women should *not* rely on this method if they have:

- irregular periods
- irregular body temperature patterns
- uncooperative partners

Possible Problems Using Periodic Abstinence and FAMs

- Care is needed in keeping records and interpreting signs.
- Illness or even lack of sleep can cause false temperature readings.
- Vaginal infections or use of vaginal products or medication may alter cervical mucus.
- You and your partner may be tempted to take risks during your fertile period.

Where to Learn about Periodic Abstinence and FAMS
and How Much They Cost

Expert and professional guidance is essential for women to learn how to use these methods successfully. Classes are available at Planned Parenthood and other family health, family planning, and church-affiliated centers. Classes are often free of charge. Charts are carried by family planning clinics. Temperature kits can be bought at drugstores. Kits range from $5 to $8 and up. Charts cost little or nothing. The cost in clinics or when authorized by a private doctor is covered by Medicaid in some states.

Breast-Feeding—Lactational Amenorrhea Method (LAM)

Breast-feeding prevents ovulation and causes temporary infertility. The stimulation of the nipples encourages the production of prolactin, a hormone necessary for the production of breast milk. It also inhibits the secretion of **gonadotropin,** a hormone necessary for ovulation. Without the release of an egg, pregnancy cannot take place. If you choose breast-feeding, you will breast-feed your baby on demand.

Breast-feeding as birth control is called the **lactational amenorrhea method (LAM).** LAM can be effective for up to six months after delivery only if a woman:

- has not had a period since she delivered her baby
- suckles her baby at least six times a day on both breasts
- suckles her baby "on demand" at least every four hours during the day
- provides nighttime breast-feeding at least every six hours—does not let her baby sleep through the night
- does not substitute other foods for a breast-milk meal
- does not rely on the method after six months

Supplemental feedings become *essential* for the good health of the baby after six months. The reduction in breast-feeding stimulates the return of ovulation.

Effectiveness of LAM

Out of 100 women who use LAM, two to six will become pregnant with perfect use in the first six months. Up to 40 will become pregnant with typical use in the first six months.

Some women who rely on LAM incorrectly believe that they will not ovulate until after their first period. It is important to remember that ovulation occurs *before* menstruation. If a woman relying on LAM has a period, even a very light one, she should consult her health care provider immediately and use another method of birth control.

LAM does not offer protection against sexually transmitted infections.

Advantages of LAM

Breast-feeding has many health advantages for the baby.

- Breast-feeding provides the best nutrition.
- Breast-feeding passes on some of the mother's antibodies to protect the baby from certain bacteria and viruses.

- Breast-feeding decreases the likelihood of infection from germs in water, other milk, or formula.
- Breast-feeding increases body contact and enhances comfort for the child and bonding between mother and child.

There are also advantages for mothers.
- LAM is effective in the first six months after delivery.
- LAM is inexpensive.
- LAM works immediately.
- LAM reduces bleeding after delivery.
- LAM requires no supplies or medical supervision. Women may initially benefit from consulting with a lactation expert, and they should be assisted as soon as possible if problems arise so that lactation is not disrupted.
- LAM does not affect the natural hormonal balance of women.
- LAM may offer protection against breast cancer in later years.

Disadvantages of LAM
- There are very high failure rates for women who don't use LAM correctly and consistently.
- LAM can be relied on for only six months.
- LAM does not protect against sexually transmitted infections.
- Breast-feeding on demand may be difficult within many lifestyles.

Barrier Methods of Birth Control

Barrier methods of birth control prevent the sperm from entering the uterus and swimming up the fallopian tubes to join with the egg. Spermicide, diaphragms, and cervical caps were invented to prevent pregnancy. The condom—one of the world's oldest and most popular methods of contraception—was originally devised to protect the wearer from sexually transmitted infection. The newer vaginal pouch is also designed to do both. Barrier methods are all immediately effective and immediately reversible.

The barriers provided by the condom, pouch, diaphragm, and cap are membranes that prevent sperm from entering the uterus. Contraceptive foams, creams, jellies, films, and suppositories provide chemical barriers that weaken sperm and block their movement. They can be used to increase the effectiveness of other barrier methods.

As with all barrier methods, practice makes perfect. If you decide to use a barrier method, practice inserting it or putting it on before using it with a sex partner.

The Condom

The **condom** is an over-the-counter barrier method of reversible birth control. If you choose the condom, you will wear a sheath of thin rubber, plastic, or animal tissue on the penis during intercourse. Condoms are packaged dry or lubricated.

How Condoms Work

Condoms collect semen before, during, and after ejaculation and can keep sperm from entering the vagina.

Effectiveness of Condoms

Of 100 women whose partners use condoms, about 12 will become pregnant during the first year of typical use. Only three women will become pregnant with perfect use. More protection is possible if, at the same time, a woman uses a vaginal contraceptive such as foam, cream, jelly, suppository, or film.

Latex condoms offer very good protection against many sexually transmitted infections, including HIV, gonorrhea, syphilis, chlamydia, chancroid, and trichomoniasis.

Advantages of Using Condoms

- The condom allows men to take responsibility for birth control and protection against sexually transmitted infection.
- The condom has no side effects, except for those allergic to rubber or spermicide.
- The condom is easy to obtain.
- The condom can be a reliable backup or second method.
- The condom can help relieve problems with premature ejaculation.

Who Can Use Condoms

Just about any man can use a condom. People who are sensitive to rubber may use plastic or animal tissue condoms, although these may not provide the same protection against sexually transmitted viruses as latex condoms. Condoms may be purchased by women or men, and women or men can put them on the penis as part of sex play.

How the Condom Is Used

The condom should be put on the penis before it has any contact with the opening of the vagina. Place the rolled condom on the tip of the erect penis. Pinch the air out of the half inch at the end of the condom. Pull back the foreskin and roll the condom down over the erect penis. Smooth out any air bubbles. With latex condoms, use only water-based lubricants such as K-Y® jelly and those with spermicide. Oil-based lubricants, such as Vaseline® and other petroleum jellies and mineral oils, can damage latex condoms.

After climax and before the penis softens, hold the rim of the condom against the penis as it is withdrawn from the vagina. That way, the condom is less likely to slip and spill semen into the vagina. Use a condom only once, then throw it away. A fresh one must be used every time.

If the condom breaks, withdraw the penis and condom immediately. Then remove and replace the condom. If ejaculation occurred in the vagina after the condom broke, the woman may want to consider emergency contraception (see page 253).

It is not known if inserting contraceptive foam, cream, or jelly, or douching immediately after a condom breaks, decreases the possibility of pregnancy.

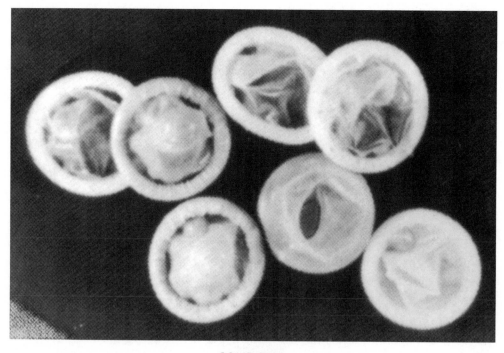

CONDOMS

Possible Problems Using Condoms
- Condoms break more often if they are not put on correctly.
- Men who do not maintain their erections throughout inter-course may find it difficult to use condoms.
- Care must be taken not to spill semen during withdrawal of the penis.
- Some couples object to the condom because it interrupts love-making. However, the condom can be put on as part of sex play.
- Some people say that sensation is reduced.

WARNING SIGNS
A man should withdraw immediately if it feels like a condom is breaking or coming off.

How to Get Condoms and What They Cost
Condoms are available from your local Planned Parenthood health center, in drugstores, family planning clinics, some supermarkets, and from vending machines. Plain condoms cost as little as 25 or 30 cents each. They may cost up to $2.50 and more if they are made from plas-tic or animal tissue or are especially shaped, tinted, flavored, or lubri-cated. The cost in clinics or when authorized by a private doctor is covered by Medicaid in some states.

The Diaphragm and Cervical Cap

Diaphragms and **cervical caps** are reversible barrier methods of birth control that are available only by prescription. Both are soft rub-ber barriers that are intended to fit securely over the cervix. Both are used with a contraceptive cream or jelly.

The diaphragm is a shallow, dome-shaped cup with a flexible rim that fits securely in the vagina to cover the cervix.

The cervical cap is thimble-shaped, smaller than the diaphragm, and fits snugly over the cervix itself.

How Diaphragms and Cervical Caps Work
If you choose the diaphragm or cervical cap, you must coat it with spermicide and insert it deep into the vagina before intercourse. Each blocks the entrance to the uterus, and the jelly or cream immobilizes sperm, preventing it from joining the egg.

The diaphragm can be inserted up to six hours before intercourse and may be left in place for 24 hours. Each time sex is repeated, more

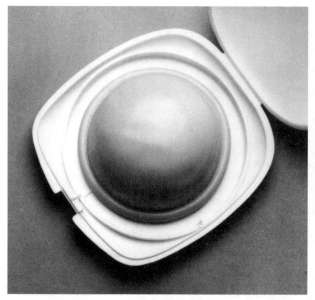

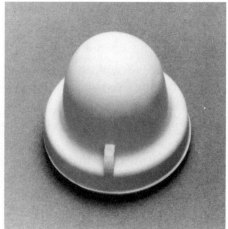

CERVICAL CAP

DIAPHRAGM

jelly or cream must be inserted in the vagina (without removing the diaphragm). The cervical cap may be left in place for up to 48 hours. Using additional spermicide with the cap is optional.

Effectiveness of Diaphragms and Cervical Caps
Of 100 women who use diaphragms, 18 will become pregnant during the first year of typical use. Six will become pregnant with perfect use. Of 100 women who have not given birth and who use the cervical cap, 18 will become pregnant during the first year of typical use. Nine will become pregnant with perfect use. Of 100 women who have given birth and who use the cervical cap, 36 will become pregnant during the first year of typical use. Twenty-six will become pregnant with perfect use. You may increase protection by checking that the cervix is covered every time you have intercourse.

Diaphragms and cervical caps may provide some protection against certain sexually transmitted infections, including chlamydia and gonorrhea.

Advantages of the Diaphragm and Cervical Cap
- Once learned, insertion is easy. Insertion can be part of bedtime routine, or it can be shared by both partners during sex play.
- If properly placed, the devices are generally not felt by either partner during intercourse.

- These barrier methods may reduce the risk of developing cervical cancer.

Who Can Use Diaphragms and Cervical Caps
Diaphragms can be worn by most women when they are not menstruating. They are *not* recommended for women who have:
  - poor muscle tone of the vagina or a sagging uterus
  - a history of toxic shock syndrome
  - recurrent urinary tract infections

Cervical caps can be worn by most women when they are not menstruating. They can be used by women whose pelvic muscles are too relaxed to hold a diaphragm in place. Some women cannot be fitted with existing sizes.

Compared to the diaphragm, the cervical cap may be more difficult and time-consuming for a professional to fit and for a woman to learn to insert and remove.

Women who are not comfortable touching their genitals will probably not like the diaphragm or cervical cap.

It is not wise to use a diaphragm or cervical cap during any kind of vaginal bleeding, including menstruation. Infection may result.

How Diaphragms and Cervical Caps Are Used
Diaphragms and cervical caps are inserted deep into the vagina before intercourse and positioned to cover the cervix. The right size must be prescribed for a proper fit. You will be shown how to put it in and take it out. Always use contraceptive cream or jelly when you insert your diaphragm or cervical cap. They must be in place every time you have sex. Leave in place for at least eight hours after the last sexual intercourse.

Women should not douche while a diaphragm or cervical cap is in place.

The diaphragm should be checked every year or two and after a weight loss or gain of 10 or more pounds to see if it is still the right size.

From time to time, the diaphragm or cervical cap should be checked for weak spots or pinholes by holding it up to a light.

Because the cap may become dislodged, women should check before and after intercourse to see if it is properly positioned.

Possible Problems While Using the Diaphragm or Cervical Cap
Most women experience no side effects. Some women are prone to develop frequent bladder infections with the diaphragm. Women

with very short fingers may need to use an inserter for the diaphragm and may not be able to use the cap. An unpleasant odor may result when cervical caps are worn for more than two days or if an infection is present. Do not wear the cap or diaphragm during vaginal bleeding or if you have a vaginal or cervical infection. Mild irritation or allergic reactions to rubber, cream, or jelly occur occasionally. Diaphragms may become dislodged when a woman is on top during intercourse.

WARNING SIGNS
Tell your clinician if:
- you or your partner have any discomfort when it is in place
- you have problems keeping it in place
- you have irritation or itching in the genital area
- you have frequent bladder infections
- you have burning sensations while urinating
- you have an unusual discharge from the vagina

How to Get Diaphragms and Cervical Caps and What They Cost
Visit your local Planned Parenthood health center, a family planning clinic, your HMO, or a private doctor for a prescription. Diaphragms and cervical caps may be purchased at a drugstore or clinic. An examination costs from $50 to $125. Diaphragms average from $13 to $25. Cervical caps are similarly priced. Diaphragms and cervical caps may cost less at family planning clinics. Contraceptive jelly or cream costs from about $4 to $18 a kit. These costs are covered by Medicaid.

Over-the-Counter Methods for Women

Over-the-counter methods for women are reversible barrier methods of birth control. They include:
- **contraceptive foams**
- **contraceptive creams**
- **contraceptive jellies**
- **contraceptive films**
- **contraceptive suppository capsules**
- **vaginal pouches (female condoms)**

If you choose one of the over-the-counter methods for women, you will insert it deep into the vagina before intercourse. Foams, creams, jellies, films, and suppositories are liquids or solids that melt after they are inserted. They contain chemicals that immobilize sperm (spermicide).

Vaginal pouches are polyurethane sheaths with flexible rings at each end. The pouch is inserted deep into the vagina like a diaphragm. The ring at the closed end holds the pouch in the vagina. The ring at the open end stays outside the vaginal opening.

How Over-the-Counter Methods for Women Work

Contraceptive foams block the entrance to the uterus with bubbles and contain a spermicide that immobilizes sperm, preventing it from joining with the egg.

Contraceptive creams, jellies, films, and suppositories melt into a thick liquid throughout the vagina. They block the entrance to the uterus and contain spermicide that immobilizes sperm.

Vaginal pouches collect semen before, during, and after ejaculation and keep sperm from entering the vagina.

Effectiveness of Over-the-Counter Methods for Women

Of 100 women who use contraceptive foams, creams, jellies, films, or suppositories, 21 will become pregnant during the first year of typical use. Five will become pregnant with perfect use. Using a condom increases effectiveness.

These over-the-counter methods may provide some protection against certain sexually transmitted infections, including chlamydia and gonorrhea.

Of 100 women who use vaginal pouches, 24 will become pregnant during the first year of typical use. Ten will become pregnant with perfect use.

The pouch provides some protection against many sexually transmitted infections, including HIV.

Advantages of Over-the-Counter Methods for Women

- All are easy to buy in drugstores and some supermarkets.
- Prescriptions or fittings are unnecessary.
- Once learned, insertion is easy and may be done by your partner as part of sex play.

Vaginal pouches allow women to take responsibility for protection against sexually transmitted infections.

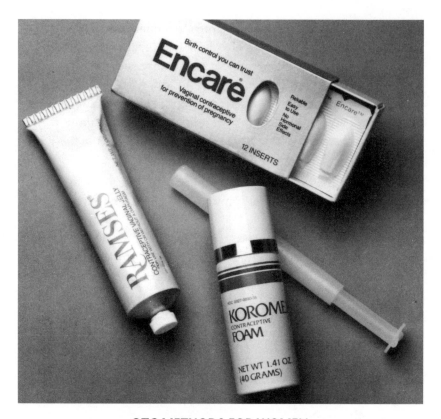

OTC METHODS FOR WOMEN

Who Can Use Over-the-Counter Methods for Women
Contraceptive foams, creams, jellies, films, or suppositories can be used by just about any woman who wants to use them.

Contraceptive pouches can be used by just about any woman who can use a tampon. Women who are not comfortable touching their genitals will probably not like the pouch.

How Over-the-Counter Methods Are Used
Detailed instructions for correct use are packaged with each over-the-counter method. Be sure to read and understand them before you use any of these products.

Contraceptive foams, creams, jellies, films, and suppositories usually require waiting 10 minutes after insertion before intercourse begins. These methods do not remain effective for more than one hour after insertion. Usually, a woman lies down or sits on her heels, then gently inserts the contraceptive deep into her vagina. More spermicide must be inserted each time sex is repeated. Women should not douche for six to eight hours after intercourse.

To insert the vaginal pouch, lubricate the closed end. Squeeze together the sides of the inner ring at the closed end of the pouch and insert the pouch into the vagina like a tampon. Push the inner ring into the vagina as far as it can go—until it reaches the cervix. Withdraw your finger and let the outer ring hang about an inch outside the vagina.

During intercourse, movement of the pouch from side to side is normal. Stop intercourse if the penis slips between the pouch and the walls of the vagina or if the outer ring is pushed into the vagina. Gently remove the pouch from the vagina, add extra lubricant to the opening of the pouch, and insert it once again.

To remove the pouch, squeeze and twist the outer ring to keep semen inside the pouch. Gently pull the pouch out of the vagina. Throw the pouch away. Do not flush. Do not reuse.

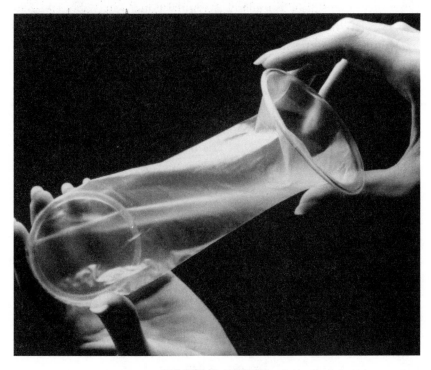

VAGINAL POUCH

Possible Problems While Using Over-the-Counter Methods
If not used exactly as directed, these products may not form a good barrier over the cervix. Some women complain of messiness or leakage.

The spermicide in contraceptive foams, creams, jellies, films, and suppositories may irritate the penis or vagina. Switching brands may solve this problem.

Some women may notice vaginal irritation using the vaginal pouch. It may slip into the vagina during intercourse. The outer ring may irritate the vulva. The inner ring may irritate the penis. Some people say that sensation is reduced.

How to Get Over-the-Counter Methods and What They Cost
Over-the-counter methods are available from your local Planned Parenthood health center, at family planning clinics, drugstores, and some supermarkets.

Applicator kits of foam and gel are $8 to $18. Refills cost $4 to $8. Large cans of foam contain between 20 and 40 applications. Films and suppositories are priced similarly. A vaginal pouch costs about $2.50. The cost in clinics or when authorized by a private doctor is covered by Medicaid in some states.

The IUD—Intrauterine Device

The **intrauterine device (IUD)** is the world's most popular method of reversible birth control for women. Nearly 100 million women use it—20 percent of all women who use birth control, including 40 percent of the women in China who use contraception. When placed inside a woman's uterus, an IUD helps prevent pregnancy. Not all IUDs are alike. There are several types, and they come in different sizes. The IUD is the most cost-effective reversible method of contraception available in the world.

The IUD is recognized by the World Health Organization and the American Medical Association as one of the safest and most effective temporary methods of birth control for women. Unfortunately, several years of negative publicity and speculation followed lawsuits brought on by the sale and use of a faulty IUD—the Dalkon Shield®—and raised many questions about the safety of all IUDs. Lawsuits sparked by the sale of the Dalkon Shield caused some man-

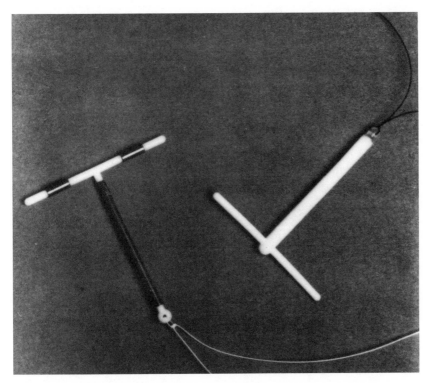

PROGESTASERT® AND PARAGARD® (COPPER T-380 A)

ufacturers to withdraw even safe IUDs from the American market. For these reasons, the variety of available IUDs in the United States is limited, and the once popular IUD is used by fewer than 2 percent of American women who use reversible contraception.

IUDs are reversible prescription methods of birth control. They are small devices made of plastic that contain copper or a natural hormone. If you choose the IUD, your clinician will suggest which is the right type for you before inserting it into your vagina. The ParaGard® (Copper T-380 A) can be left in place for 10 years. The Progestasert® must be replaced every year. Insertion and removal must be done by a clinician.

How IUDs Work
IUDs usually work by preventing fertilization of the egg. They may also work by affecting the way sperm or eggs move or by affecting the lining of the uterus in ways that prevent **implantation.**

Effectiveness of IUDs

The IUD is one of the most effective reversible methods of birth control available to women in the United States. Of 100 women who use IUDs, fewer than three will become pregnant during the first year of typical use. Fewer than one will become pregnant with perfect use of the ParaGard (Copper T-380 A). Only two will become pregnant with perfect use of the Progestasert. Fewer pregnancies occur with continued use.

You can increase your protection by checking for the IUD string regularly.

The IUD provides no protection against sexually transmitted infections.

Advantages of the IUD

- With an IUD in place, a woman does not need to think about using her birth control method every day or every time she has vaginal intercourse.
- The copper IUD does not change the hormone levels in the body.
- The cost, over time, is low compared with the costs of similarly effective methods.

Who Can Use IUDs

An IUD may be right for you if:

- you need emergency contraception
- you are not at risk for contracting a sexually transmitted infection
- you have not had PID, gonorrhea, or chlamydia within 12 months
- you are breast-feeding
- you cannot use hormonal methods like the Pill because of cigarette smoking or certain medical conditions such as hypertension

You should *not* use the IUD if:

- you have unexplained abnormal vaginal bleeding
- you have a recent history of pelvic infection
- you have a history of tubal pregnancy
- you have had an abnormal Pap test recently
- you have any disease, such as leukemia or HIV, that decreases your ability to fight infections
- you have an artificial valve in your heart
- you have sex with more than one partner or your partner does

Copper IUDs should *not* be used if you are allergic to copper, if you are having diathermy (heat) treatments, or if you have Wilson's disease.

Do *not* have an IUD inserted if there is a chance that you are pregnant. Be sure to tell your clinician if you think there is any chance that you are. A special evaluation must be done if you have a history of heart disease or certain other medical conditions.

How IUDs Are Used

Before insertion, discuss with your clinician how to watch for possible side effects or other problems. Be sure to read the package insert that comes with the IUD before you decide to have one inserted.

Your clinician will provide you with a consent form containing detailed information about the risks and benefits of the IUD you are considering. You need to read, understand, and sign this form before your clinician inserts the IUD.

Insertion is often done during menstruation. It may be somewhat painful, like bad menstrual cramps. Sometimes it is only slightly uncomfortable. The pain is usually brief and eases with a little rest and pain medication. Antibiotics may be given to reduce the chance of infection when the IUD is inserted.

A string on the IUD hangs down through the cervix into the vagina. You should feel for the string now and then, especially after menstruation, to make sure the IUD is in place. If it is not, you should use another form of birth control and call your clinician for advice. You should have a checkup within three months after insertion. You should always have annual checkups.

Ask your clinician to remove your IUD if you want to become pregnant.

Possible Problems While Using the IUD

Most women adjust to their IUDs with few or no problems. But for some women:

- cramping may be greater (mostly for a brief time after insertion)
- bleeding may occur between periods
- periods may be heavier and last longer (less so with IUDs containing hormones)
- there is slight risk of genital tract infection during the first three months of use

There is a small chance that the IUD may be expelled from the uterus. You may not know it, and pregnancy could result. Pregnancy with an IUD in place is rare, but if signs of pregnancy occur, you should have a pelvic exam immediately. If you are pregnant, the IUD should be removed as soon as possible. Removal lessens the chance of serious infections that can be life-threatening in rare cases. Removal also reduces chances of miscarriage or premature delivery. In some cases, however, removal may trigger a miscarriage. If you want to end the pregnancy, an abortion should be done early.

Some IUD users have had ectopic (tubal) pregnancies. But ectopic pregnancy occurs less frequently for IUD users than it does for women who use no method. In the rare case, however, when an IUD fails, there is a greater chance that the pregnancy will be in the tube. Ectopic pregnancies are life-threatening. They are usually removed with surgery.

Infection of the fallopian tubes happens more often in IUD users than in nonusers. But the risk of infection is greater only for women who have more than one sex partner or whose partner has other partners. Women who wear IUDs must use condoms if:

- they have more than one partner
- they take a new partner or change partners
- their partner has more than one partner

Infection, with or without symptoms, may increase the risk of tubal pregnancy, cause sterility, or, very rarely, require removal of reproductive organs. An infection that is not treated might become fatal.

Rarely, the IUD may puncture the wall of the uterus. This is usually associated with insertion. In such cases, surgery may be required to remove the IUD.

WARNING SIGNS
Tell your clinician immediately if you are not able to feel the string or if you have:

- a missed, late, or light period
- severe cramping or increasing pain in the lower abdomen
- unexplained fever and/or chills
- pain or bleeding during sex
- increased or bad-smelling vaginal discharge

How to Get IUDs and What They Cost

Visit your local Planned Parenthood health center, a family planning clinic, your HMO, or a private doctor. At this time in the United States, the variety of available IUDs is limited. Consult your clinician for more information.

The exam, insertion, and follow-up visit range from $175 to $450. These services are priced according to income at some family planning clinics and are covered by Medicaid.

Hormonal Methods of Birth Control

In the 1930s, research was launched to find a hormonal treatment to alleviate menstrual pain. The search led to the invention of hormonal contraception. The first **hormonal contraceptive** was the Pill. It became available in 1960 and is now the most popular method of reversible contraception in the United States.

Thirty-one years later, American women were offered another hormonal option—implants inserted under the skin to provide five years of contraception. Two years after the introduction of implants, an injectable method that lasts 12 weeks became available.

Throughout history, millions of women dreamed that they might live their lives free from the burdens of unintended pregnancy. While there still remains a very real need for more and better contraceptive options, the introduction of hormonal contraception changed the lives of women forever by offering them safe and highly effective methods with which to control their fertility.

The Pill

The Pill is a reversible method of birth control that is available only by prescription. It is a monthly series of pills taken once a day. The active ingredients are synthetic hormones like those produced by the body to regulate the menstrual cycle. **Combined oral contraceptives** contain both estrogen and progestin. **Mini-pills** contain progestin only.

How the Pill Works

Combined pills keep the ovaries from releasing eggs (ovulation). Mini-pills can also prevent ovulation. They also work by thickening the cervical mucus. This prevents the sperm from joining with the egg. Both types of pills can also prevent fertilized eggs from implanting in the uterus.

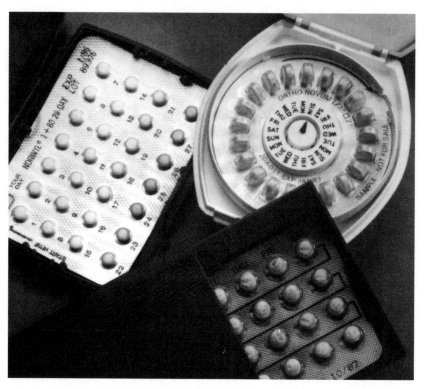

THE PILL

Effectiveness of the Pill

The Pill is one of the most effective reversible methods of birth control available to women in the United States. Of every 100 women who use the Pill, only three will become pregnant during the first year of typical use. *Women who take the Pill correctly every day* have less than a 1 percent chance of getting pregnant.

Birth control pills work best if taken at about the same time every day for the full monthly series. Pregnancy can happen if an error is made in using the Pill—especially if:

- pills are started too late in the cycle
- two or more pills are missed in a row
- pills are taken in the wrong order

The Pill may be less effective in preventing pregnancy if taken with other medicines such as those that control seizures or tuberculosis. Talk to your clinician about what to do.

The Pill provides no protection against sexually transmitted infections.

Advantages of Using the Pill
The Pill is convenient to use. Women who use the Pill have:
- more regular periods
- less menstrual flow
- less menstrual cramping
- less iron-deficiency anemia
- fewer ectopic (tubal) pregnancies
- less pelvic inflammatory disease (PID)
- less acne
- less premenstrual tension
- less rheumatoid arthritis

The Pill offers significant protection against:
- ovarian and endometrial cancers—risk reduction increases with each year of use, up to 80 percent
- noncancerous breast tumors and ovarian cysts

Who Can Use the Pill
Most women can take the Pill safely. You should *not* use the Pill if you are over 35 and smoke more than 15 cigarettes a day, especially if you are greatly overweight.

You shouldn't use the Pill if you have unexplained vaginal bleeding or if you ever had:
- cancer of the breast or uterus
- blood clots in the veins or lungs
- skin cancer called malignant melanoma that spread to another part of the body

You may need special tests to see whether you should take the Pill if you have had certain medical conditions such as liver disease, diabetes (even if it only occurred during pregnancy), high blood pressure, high cholesterol levels, or if there is a history of blood clots in your family.

For all women, except those who smoke more than 15 cigarettes a day and are over 35, the newer low-dose pills have fewer side effects and complications than pregnancy and are much safer than pregnancy.

How the Pill Is Used

If you choose the Pill, *you must take it every day,* as directed. You will be protected as long as you take them on time and don't skip any. Pregnancy can happen anytime after you stop taking the Pill.

To plan a pregnancy, stop taking the Pill and use another birth control method until your periods become regular. Normal menstrual cycles usually return in a few months.

After having a baby, get medical advice about when to go back on the Pill—especially if you breast-feed your baby.

There is no need to take a break from using the Pill, even if you have used it for a long time.

Your clinician may recommend having a medical checkup about three months after first starting the Pill. You should always have at least one checkup a year. Be sure to tell any new clinician you see that you are on the Pill.

Possible Problems While Taking the Pill

Many women adjust to taking the Pill with few or no problems. But all medications, including the Pill, pose some health risks for the women who use them.

Some minor reactions that usually clear up after two to three months of use are:

- spotting between periods
- breast tenderness
- nausea
- vomiting
- weight gain or loss
- depression

These side effects can often be avoided by changing the formulation of the Pill you use. If you experience these side effects while taking the Pill, consult your clinician to consider a prescription for a different type of Pill.

Pill users have a slightly greater chance than nonusers of developing certain serious problems that can be fatal in rare cases. These include heart attack, stroke, blood clots in the veins or lungs, and liver tumors. The chance of developing some of these problems increases with age—especially when certain other health problems are present. The risks are increased by smoking more than 15 cigarettes a day and by such conditions as diabetes, high blood pressure, high levels of cholesterol in the blood, and certain congenital conditions that increase the risk of blood clotting.

To learn more about possible problems with pill use, talk with your clinician. More detailed information about the risks of birth control pills and who should not use them also is provided in the package insert. It is essential that you read and understand this additional information.

WARNING SIGNS
Tell your clinician immediately if you have:
- unusual swelling or pain in the legs
- sudden shortness of breath
- sudden pain in the abdomen, chest, or arm
- severe headache
- sudden blurred or double vision or loss of vision in one eye
- yellowing of skin or eyes
- severe depression

How to Get the Pill and What It Costs
Visit your local Planned Parenthood health center, a family planning clinic, your HMO, or a private doctor for a prescription. Pills may be purchased at a clinic or drugstore.

The cost of an examination ranges from about $35 to $125. The cost depends on your income at some family planning clinics. A monthly package costs between $15 and $25. The cost is usually less at a clinic and is covered by Medicaid.

Norplant®
Norplant is a reversible method of birth control that is available only by prescription. If you choose Norplant, six soft capsules, each about the size of a cardboard matchstick, will be inserted under the skin of your upper arm. Each one contains **levonorgestrel**—a synthetic progestin similar to the hormone progesterone, which is produced by the body to regulate the menstrual cycle.

How Norplant Works
A small amount of the hormone is released constantly. The hormone keeps the ovaries from releasing eggs. It also thickens the cervical

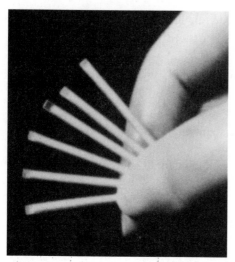

NORPLANT®

mucus. This keeps sperm from joining with the egg. Some researchers believe that Norplant may also work by preventing a fertilized egg from attaching to the lining of the uterus.

Effectiveness of Norplant
Except for continuous abstinence, Norplant is the most effective reversible method of birth control. Of every 10,000 women who use Norplant, only nine will become pregnant in the first year of use. Left in place, it can protect against pregnancy for five years.

Norplant provides no protection against sexually transmitted infections.

Advantages of Norplant
Norplant is very convenient, and it:
- gives continuous long-lasting birth control without sterilization
- does not need to be taken daily or put in place before vaginal intercourse
- can be used by women who cannot take estrogen
- can be used while breast-feeding, starting six weeks after delivery

Who Can Use Norplant
Most women can use Norplant safely. You should *not* use Norplant if you:
- are pregnant
- have unexplained vaginal bleeding
- cannot put up with irregular bleeding
- are breast-feeding in the first six weeks after delivery
- have blood clots or inflammation of the veins
- have had growths of the liver
- have had breast cancer
- have a history of a certain kind of high blood pressure—idiopathic intracranial hypertension
- have a certain kind of brain tumor—meningioma
- are sensitive to the ingredients in Norplant

You should be checked regularly by your clinician if you use Norplant and have:

- migraine headaches
- diabetes
- high cholesterol
- high blood pressure
- heart disease
- seizures that require medication
- serious depression
- conditions that may be aggravated by fluid retention
- serious liver disease

How Norplant Is Used

After taking your medical history and giving you a physical exam, the clinician will numb a small area of your arm with a painkiller and make one small cut. The six capsules will be inserted under the skin of the arm you use less. Insertion takes about 10 minutes. Protection against pregnancy begins within 24 hours.

Your clinician will advise you to have a follow-up visit within the first three months after insertion. It is best to have follow-up visits once a year after that. Be sure to tell any health care provider you may see that you are using Norplant.

Norplant must be removed after five years because it stops working. If you wish, it can be removed anytime earlier. The clinician will numb the area with a painkiller and will make one small cut to remove all six of the implants. Removal takes from 15 to 20 minutes. Implants may be more difficult to locate in some women. Removal for them may require more than one visit and/or several incisions. New implants may be inserted at this time. Pregnancy can happen anytime after the implants are removed.

Possible Problems While Using Norplant

Most women adjust to using Norplant with few or no problems. However, as with all medicines, there may be side effects for some women.

SIDE EFFECTS

The most common side effect of Norplant is not serious. It is irregular bleeding. This may include:

- irregular intervals between periods
- longer menstrual flow
- irregular bleeding or spotting between periods
- no bleeding for months at a time

Bleeding usually becomes more regular after nine to 12 months. A small number of women experience irregular bleeding throughout the five years.

There are other side effects for some women. They may include:

- scarring at insertion site
- headache
- change in appetite
- weight gain or loss
- sore breasts
- nausea
- acne
- hair loss
- increased hair on face and body
- discolored skin over the implants
- ovarian cysts

RARE SERIOUS PROBLEMS

Norplant works very much like the Pill, but it contains no estrogen. It is not yet known if problems that rarely occur with the Pill may also occur with Norplant. Smoking while using the Pill greatly increases the risks of blood clots, heart attack, and stroke in women who are over 35 years old. It is not yet known if this happens with Norplant. For now, women using Norplant are advised to stop smoking.

Although it has not been proved, some scientists believe that prolonged use of progestin-only implants or injections may slow the growth of bones in young women.

Some Norplant users have had ectopic (tubal) pregnancies. But ectopic pregnancy occurs less frequently for Norplant users than it does for women who use no method. However, in the rare case when Norplant fails, there is a greater chance that the pregnancy will be in the tube. Ectopic pregnancies are life-threatening. They are usually removed with surgery.

WARNING SIGNS

Tell your clinician immediately if:

- you have vaginal bleeding that lasts longer and is much heavier than your normal period
- your period is late after a long period of regular cycles
- you have severe abdominal pain
- you have severe headaches and blurred vision

- there is pain, pus, or bleeding at the implant site
- one of the implants seems to be coming out
- you experience nerve pain when moving the arm or hand after the insertion site has healed

How to Get Norplant and What It Costs
Visit your local Planned Parenthood health center, a family planning clinic, your HMO, or a private doctor.

Norplant costs between $500 and $750 for the medical exam, the implants, and the insertion. This amounts to a little more than $100 a year over a five-year period. Clinicians will charge an additional fee to remove Norplant—from $100 to $200. All costs are covered by Medicaid.

Depo-Provera®

Depo-Provera is a reversible method of birth control available only by prescription. It is a synthetic progestin similar to the hormone progesterone, which is produced by the body to regulate the menstrual cycle. If you choose Depo-Provera, you will have it injected into your buttock or arm every 12 weeks.

How Depo-Provera Works
The hormone keeps the ovaries from releasing eggs. It also thickens the cervical mucus. This keeps sperm from joining with the egg. It may also affect the lining of the uterus to prevent implantation.

Effectiveness of Depo-Provera
Depo-Provera is one of the most effective reversible methods of birth control. Of every 1,000 women who use Depo-Provera, only three will become pregnant during the first year.

Depo-Provera provides no protection against sexually transmitted infections.

Advantages of Depo-Provera
Depo-Provera is very convenient, and it:
- prevents pregnancy for 12 weeks
- can be used by women who cannot take estrogen
- reduces menstrual cramps and anemia
- protects against endometrial and ovarian cysts
- can be used while breast-feeding, starting six weeks after delivery
- does not need to be taken daily or put in place before vaginal intercourse

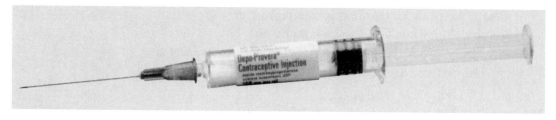

DEPO-PROVERA®

Who Can Use Depo-Provera

Most women can use Depo-Provera safely. You should not use Depo-Provera if:

- you are or might be pregnant
- you have unexplained vaginal bleeding
- you cannot put up with irregular bleeding
- you have ever had cancer of the breast
- you recently had blood clots in the legs, lungs, or eyes
- you are taking a certain medication for Cushing's syndrome
- you have serious liver disease

You should be checked regularly by your clinician if you use Depo-Provera and have:

- migraine headaches
- diabetes
- high cholesterol
- high blood pressure
- heart disease
- major depression
- a recent history of liver disease or abnormal liver tests

How Depo-Provera Is Used

After taking your medical history and giving you a physical exam, the clinician will inject Depo-Provera into your buttock or arm. Protection against pregnancy is immediate if you get the injection during the first five days of your period.

You should have a follow-up visit for another injection at the end of 12 weeks.

Possible Problems While Using Depo-Provera

Most women adjust to using Depo-Provera with few or no problems. However, as with all medicines, there may be some side effects for some women.

It is important to consider that there is no way to stop the effects of Depo-Provera. Side effects may continue until the shot wears off (at between 12 and 14 weeks).

It takes an average of 10 months for women to get pregnant after their last injection. For some, it may take only 12 weeks after the last shot to get pregnant. For others, it may take up to 18 months.

SIDE EFFECTS

The most common side effect of Depo-Provera is not serious. It is irregular bleeding and may include:

- irregular intervals between periods
- longer menstrual flow
- spotting between periods
- no bleeding for months at a time

These side effects are more common in the first six to 12 months of use. The longer a woman uses Depo-Provera, the more likely she will stop having menstrual periods. More than half of Depo-Provera users have no periods after one year of use.

Less common side effects include:

- increased appetite and weight gain
- headache
- sore breasts
- nausea
- nervousness
- dizziness
- depression
- skin rashes or spotty darkening of the skin
- hair loss
- increased hair on face or body
- increased or decreased sex drive

RARE SERIOUS PROBLEMS

Depo-Provera works very much like the Pill, but it contains no estrogen. It is not yet known if problems that rarely occur with the Pill may also occur with Depo-Provera. Smoking while using the Pill greatly increases the risks of blood clots, heart attack, and stroke in women who are over 35 years old. It is not yet known if this happens with Depo-Provera. For now, women using Depo-Provera are advised to stop smoking.

Although it has not been proved, some scientists believe that prolonged use of progestin-only implants or injections may slow the growth of bones in young women.

Some Depo-Provera users have had ectopic (tubal) pregnancies. But they occur much less frequently among Depo-Provera users than among women who use no method.

WARNING SIGNS
Tell your clinician immediately if you feel you may be pregnant or have:
- vaginal bleeding that lasts longer and is much heavier than your normal period
- severe headaches
- major depression
- frequent urination
- yellowing of skin or eyes

How to Get Depo-Provera and What It Costs
Visit your local Planned Parenthood health center, a family planning clinic, your HMO, or a private doctor. The cost of an examination ranges from about $35 to $125. The hormone costs about $50. Subsequent visits cost between $20 and $40, plus medication. Costs may be less and depend on your income at family planning clinics. All costs are covered by Medicaid.

PERMANENT METHODS OF BIRTH CONTROL

Women and men who have completed their families, or who know they do not want any children, may want a permanent method of birth control.

Permanent methods may be appropriate for mature women and men who find that:
- their partners agree that their families are complete, and no more children are wanted
- they want to enjoy having sex without causing pregnancy
- they don't want to have a child in the future
- they and their partners have concerns about the side effects of other methods
- other methods are unacceptable

- the woman's health would be threatened by a future pregnancy
- they don't want to pass on a hereditary illness or disability
- they are men who choose vasectomy to spare their partners the surgery and expense of tubal sterilization. (Sterilization for women is more complicated and costly.)

Permanent methods are not appropriate for women or men if:
- they want to have a child in the future
- they are being pressured by their partners, friends, or family
- they have marriage or sexual problems, short-term mental or physical illnesses, or financial worries, or are out of work. Permanent methods are not good solutions for temporary problems
- they have not considered possible changes in their lives such as divorce, remarriage, or the death of their children

Voluntary Sterilization

Voluntary sterilization is the most popular method of birth control in America. More than 1 million women and men choose to have the procedures every year. Sterilization is surgical birth control—it is intended to be permanent, and it is not easily reversed. Vasectomy is the surgical operation for men. It blocks the vas deferens. Tubal sterilization is the surgical operation for women. It blocks the fallopian tubes. Vasectomy is less complicated and is the less expensive of the two procedures.

Usually, people choose sterilization when they have had all the children they want. Most of them are over 30 and married. Some women and men, however, choose sterilization in their earlier reproductive years because they know they never want to have children. Others choose sterilization because they have a hereditary condition that they do not want to pass on to another generation. Still others elect sterilization when the woman is chronically ill or physically disabled in a way that would make pregnancy very difficult or dangerous.

Couples are often moved to choose voluntary sterilization after they have had to deal with a pregnancy "scare" or an abortion. Because sterilization procedures are nearly 100 percent effective, couples who do choose sterilization have very little concern about the chance of unintended pregnancy for the rest of their lives. Because sterilization is intended to be permanent, it is inappropriate for young women or men who may change their minds about having children as they mature.

Sterilization

Sterilization is surgical birth control. It is intended to be a permanent method of birth control. It is not easily reversed.

How Sterilization Works

Tubal sterilization is a surgical operation for women. It blocks the fallopian tubes. **Vasectomy** is a surgical operation for men. It blocks the vas deferens. Pregnancy cannot happen when sperm cannot reach the egg.

Effectiveness of Sterilization

Sterilization is one of the most effective contraceptive methods. Of every 1,000 women who are sterilized, only four will become pregnant during the first year. Of every 1,000 men who are sterilized, fewer than two will cause pregnancy during the first year.

Sterilization provides no protection against sexually transmitted infections.

Advantages of Sterilization

- Sterilization is intended to be permanent protection against pregnancy.
- Sterilization has no lasting side effects.
- Sterilization does not affect sexual pleasure.
- The onetime cost of sterilization is low compared to lifetime costs of most similarly effective methods.

How Sterilization Is Used

Tubal sterilization is effective immediately. Vasectomy is not. Some sperm remain in a man's system after the operation. Other birth control must be used until the sperm are used up. This usually takes at least 15 ejaculations. Semen analysis—a simple lab test—shows when there are no more sperm.

Possible Problems with Sterilization for Women and Men

- Mild bleeding may occur right after the operation.
- Mild infection may occur within one or two weeks of the operation.
- Very rarely, a fallopian tube or vas deferens reconnects and pregnancy occurs.

Side Effects of Tubal Sterilization

- There may be a reaction to the local or general anesthetic that is used.
- Very rarely, an injury to blood vessels or bowel occurs that may need surgery.

Side Effects of Vasectomy
- Bruising of scrotum at incision site may occur.
- There may be temporary swelling or tenderness near the testicles.
- Small lumps (granulomas) near the testicles formed by the sperm may occur and may require surgical treatment.

WARNING SIGNS
Pregnancy after sterilization is quite rare, but can occur years after the surgery. Contact your clinician if you have any symptoms of pregnancy, including:
- late or missed periods
- severe lower abdominal pain
- nausea and breast tenderness

What Sterilization Costs and Where to Get It
Visit your local Planned Parenthood health center, a family planning clinic, your HMO, or a private doctor. Tubal sterilization costs from $1,000 to $2,500. Vasectomy costs from $240 to $520. Medicaid and some insurance companies pay for voluntary sterilization.

EMERGENCY CONTRACEPTION

Emergency contraception is designed to prevent pregnancy after unprotected vaginal intercourse takes place. It is also called postcoital or "morning-after" contraception.

At some time in their lives, most women are faced with the fear that they might have an unintended and unwanted pregnancy. In fact, the average woman spends 75 to 80 percent of her fertile years trying to avoid pregnancy. During that time, she may forget to use a contraceptive, her contraceptive may fail, or she may be coerced into having unprotected vaginal intercourse.

You may want emergency contraception if:
- his condom broke or slipped off, and he ejaculated inside your vagina
- he forced you to have unprotected vaginal intercourse
- your diaphragm or cervical cap slipped out of place, and he ejaculated inside your vagina
- you miscalculated your "safe" days for periodic abstinence or fertility awareness methods

- you forgot to take your birth control pills
- you weren't using any birth control
- he didn't pull out in time

Contact your health care provider immediately if you have unprotected intercourse when you think you might become pregnant.

Emergency contraception is available from health care providers, Planned Parenthood health centers, and other women's health and family planning centers. It is for use only if a woman is sure she is not already pregnant. It prevents pregnancy by preventing fertilization or implantation. It will not cause an abortion.

Emergency contraception is provided in two ways:

- emergency hormonal contraception—doses of birth control pills
- insertion of an IUD

Emergency Hormonal Contraception "Morning-After" Pills

Emergency hormonal contraception is a sequence of two doses of certain oral contraceptives. The most common **"morning-after" pills** are "combination" pills that contain estrogen and progestin—synthetic hormones like the ones produced by a woman's body. Progestin-only pills—mini-pills—may be used by women who cannot take estrogen.

Women who request morning-after pills should review their medical histories with their clinicians before receiving the medication.

You should not use morning-after pills if:

- you are pregnant from a previous act of intercourse
- you have missed your period or it is late
- you are allergic to the medication

How to Use Morning-After Pills

There are several kinds of pills that can be used. Your clinician will designate the brand and dose for you. The pills are taken in two doses, 12 hours apart. You must use only one type of pill and use it for all doses.

Using Progestin-Only Pills

Progestin-only pills may be more appropriate for women who cannot take estrogen. Take 20 tablets of Ovrette® within 48 hours of unprotected intercourse and then take another 20 tablets 12 hours later.

Using Combination Pills

Combination pills that are currently used for emergency contraception include Ovral®, Lo/Ovral®, Nordette®, and Levlen®. If you take your pills from a regular 28-pill pack of combination pills, you can use any of the first 21 pills for emergency contraception.

You can also use Triphasil® or Tri-Levlen®. The first 21 pills of these pills are in three different colors—you must use only the yellow ones.

If you are using Ovral, each dose is two pills. If you are using any other kind of combination pill, each dose is four pills. The dose is repeated in 12 hours.

Don't use the last seven pills in a 28-day pack. They are only reminder pills that contain no hormones.

First dose: Swallow the pills in the first dose as soon as possible and no later than 72 hours—three days—after having unprotected intercourse.

Nausea is a possible side effect when combination pills are used. You may want to eat a snack of saltines or soda crackers or drink a glass of milk 30 minutes before taking each dose to avoid vomiting. Your clinician may prescribe an antinausea medication or suggest you use an over-the-counter product such as Dramamine®.

The side effects of antinausea medication may include light-headedness, dizziness, or feeling spacey. Please follow the precautions on the package insert.

Second dose: Swallow the second dose 12 hours after taking the first dose. If vomiting occurred after the first dose, be sure to use an antinausea medication 30 minutes before taking the second dose. Or you may want to take the second dose as a vaginal suppository.

If you vomit the second dose, do not take any extra pills—it is unlikely that they will reduce the risks of pregnancy any further. It is likely that they will increase your risk of nausea.

AFTER YOU TAKE THE PILLS

- Your next period may be earlier or later than usual.
- Your flow may be heavier, lighter, or more spotty than usual.
- If you see other health care providers before you get your period, remember to tell them that you have taken morning-after pills.

- Schedule a follow-up visit with your clinician if you do not menstruate in three weeks or if you have symptoms of pregnancy.
- Be sure to use another method of contraception if you have vaginal intercourse before your period.

SIDE EFFECTS

Side effects associated with the use of morning-after pills usually taper off one or two days after the second dose has been taken.

- Nausea, usually mild, is experienced by 50 percent of women who use morning-after pills.
- Up to one out of three women experience vomiting.
- Breast tenderness, irregular bleeding, fluid retention, and headaches may occur.

If you use emergency contraception frequently, your periods may become quite irregular and unpredictable. Repeated use is not advised.

Emergency contraception may not prevent ectopic pregnancy. Ectopic pregnancies develop outside the uterus. They must be treated or they will cause complications that may cause death.

If you think you may have an ectopic pregnancy, get medical attention immediately. Signs of ectopic pregnancy include:

- severe pain on one or both sides of the lower abdomen
- abdominal pain and spotting, especially after a missed menstrual period or a very light one
- feeling faint or dizzy

Emergency IUD Insertion

Insertion of an IUD can be done by a clinician within five to seven days of unprotected intercourse.

The Copper T-380 A IUD (ParaGard®) is used for emergency contraception. It can be left in place for up to 10 years to provide very effective contraception. Or, if you prefer, the IUD can be removed after your next menstrual period, when it is certain that you are not pregnant.

IUD insertion for emergency contraception is not recommended for women who are at risk for sexually transmitted infections:

- women with more than one sex partner or whose partners have more than one partner
- women with new partners
- women who have been raped

The side effects, advantages, and disadvantages of using IUDs for emergency contraception are the same as those associated with using IUDs for ongoing contraception.

Effectiveness of Emergency Contraception
Of 1,000 women who use emergency IUD insertion, only one will become pregnant.

Of 100 women who use emergency hormonal contraception, up to two will become pregnant.

The closer a woman is to ovulation at the time of unprotected intercourse, the less likely the method will succeed. If 100 women have vaginal intercourse without contraception during the second or third weeks of their cycle when they are most fertile, eight will become pregnant. Using emergency contraception reduces a woman's chance by about 75 percent—two out of 100 during her most fertile days.

Emergency contraception is meant for emergencies only. It is not as effective as the regular use of reversible contraception—Norplant®, Depo-Provera®, the IUD, or the Pill.

Morning-after pills only help prevent pregnancy from one act of unprotected intercourse. They do not continue to prevent pregnancy during the rest of the cycle. Other methods of birth control must be used.

Emergency contraception offers no protection against sexually transmitted infections.

Where to Get Emergency Contraception
Emergency contraception is available at Planned Parenthood health centers, public clinics and women's health centers, private doctors, and hospital emergency rooms—unless they are affiliated with religions that oppose the use of birth control.

You can get the name, address, and phone number of three emergency contraception providers nearest you by calling, toll-free, the emergency contraception hot line—800-584-9911.

TAKE-HOME PACKS
Packs of morning-after pills are available from some women's health centers for women whose medical histories are well known to their clinicians. Take-home kits allow women to use the medication in emergency situations without having to wait to see their clinicians.

What Emergency Contraception Costs

Costs vary. Costs depend on which of the following services are needed. Here are some estimates:

MORNING-AFTER PILLS

Morning-after pills kit	$8 to $15
One pack of combination pills	$20
Two packs of progestin–only pills	$50
Visit with health care provider	$35 to $150
Pregnancy test	$10 to $20
Total cost	$75 to $245

Fees may be less at family planning clinics and health centers.

IUD

The ParaGard® IUD costs about $450 for exam, IUD, and insertion. It lasts for 10 years, however, which works out to only $45 a year if left in place.

For confidential and comprehensive contraceptive information, counseling, medical services, and referrals, call the Planned Parenthood health center nearest you, toll-free, at 800-230-PLAN.

CHAPTER 8

The Laws

That

Affect Our

Sex Lives

If the right of privacy means anything, it is the right of the individual, married or single, to be free from unwarranted governmental intrusion into matters so fundamentally affecting a person as the decision whether to bear or beget a child.

—Justice William J. Brennan, Jr.,
 for the U.S. Supreme Court,
 Eisenstadt v. Baird, 1972

HOW SEX LAWS DEVELOP

Understanding Our Values about Sex

Each of us develops ideas about what is right, responsible, worthwhile, and moral. These ideas are called values. Families and communities share many values in common. Values held by most of the people in a society are called social values. Many social values are also sexual values. These reflect what behaviors and traits are considered feminine and what behaviors and traits are considered masculine. They also determine what behaviors are considered right and what behaviors are wrong.

Sexual values differ dramatically from one society to another. Among the Inuit people in the Arctic, it is acceptable for men to share their wives with other men who visit their homes. In Afghanistan, on the other hand, women and men are stoned to death for extramarital sex. In some societies, adolescent boys and girls are kept strictly separated until marriage. In others, such as the Trobriand Islands, children are encouraged to practice sexual intercourse before puberty.

Economics, politics, and religion shape the sexual values of a society as they become part of a society's customs and traditions. As economic, political, and religious needs change, so do sexual values. Some societies develop a high tolerance for the development of personal and private sexual values. Others are more restrictive and insist on conformity to the dominant social and sexual values. As a pluralistic society, the United States welcomes people from cultures all over the world. They bring a wide range of differing sexual values. Our sexual values are influenced by theirs, and theirs are influenced by ours.

Formal and Informal Values

All societies have two sets of values to guide private and public behavior. There are **formal values** based on ideals that are defined by religions, governments, and other official groups. They shape a society's laws, rules,

259

and expectations. We also have **informal values** that reflect our everyday behavior. Our informal values may not match our formal values. For example, although oral sex is against the law in many states, most sexually active people ignore those laws.

Social values have a great impact on **autonomy**—how free each of us is to exercise our own will. As we balance our public and private lives, we often question our formal and informal values: *How much freedom can an individual be allowed? When should society set limits? How do we balance autonomy with social responsibility?* These questions are particularly important when we talk about sex.

How Economic Need Has Shaped Our Sexual Values

Sexual values are often shaped by economic need. For example, so many French citizens died in World War II that the government needed to rebuild the population. It encouraged large families by lowering a family's taxes each time a child was born. Families with eight children paid no taxes.

When motherhood and large families became economically important in the ancient world, contraception and abortion became illegal. These and other sexual values that are shaped by economics become part of a culture's traditions. Often a tradition survives long after its economic roots are forgotten. As a result, contraception and abortion may remain illegal long after the economic need for large families has passed. This is one reason that women without children are traditionally stigmatized in many cultures.

Ever since the earliest agricultural times, women were expected to fulfill key roles in the economy. They were to provide labor and give birth to laborers or legitimate heirs for their families' fortunes. Traditions that developed from these economic conditions placed a higher value on the sexual freedom of men than it did on that of women.

This double standard continues today. Social judgments about women's sexual behavior continue to be more severe than judgments about the same behavior in men. For example, a man who has many sex partners may be admired as a "stud." A woman who has as many may be considered a "slut."

The double standard is the basis of sexism. Sexism is a bias held against a certain gender. Historically, most societies have favored men and boys and have been biased against women and girls. Women and girls have been given fewer privileges and opportunities than men and boys. In many cultures, they are not allowed to be educated or own property.

Sexist values are being challenged by women and men around the world. The idea that women and men have equal social, economic, sexual, and political rights is called **feminism.**

How Religion Has Shaped Our Sexual Values

Europe was dominated by a single religion for more than 1,000 years. During the Middle Ages, formal sexual values were dictated by the **sacred** laws of the Roman Catholic church. Religious law was the highest law in the land. It was based on the belief that all sensual pleasure was sinful. It determined who could marry, what kind of sex was allowed, where it was allowed, when it was allowed, and why women had to always submit to their husbands. People could be ruthlessly punished if they disobeyed. Punishment ranged from meditation, fasting, and prayerful penance to imprisonment, torture, excommunication, and execution.

Some countries worldwide are still dominated by sacred law, but over the centuries, sacred law has given way to **secular** law. Today, few people rely exclusively on religion to decide their sexual behavior. In the United States, federal, state, and local governments make laws that regulate sexual behavior. These laws are often designed to protect people against sexual abuse. Often, however, laws regulate sexual conduct between consenting adults.

Some laws, such as those that prohibit rape and prostitution, are criminal laws with criminal penalties. Other laws, such as those that prohibit discrimination and sexual harassment, are *civil* and give individuals the right to sue for damages. Criminal and civil laws are enforced by the federal, state, and local courts.

Increasingly, scientific and medical knowledge has an impact on sexual law. Lawmakers and enforcers are more likely to try to understand unusual sex practices by looking for medical or psychological explanations rather than devils or demons. People with socially unacceptable sex problems are more likely to be treated with drugs or therapy than with whips and red-hot pokers.

But the sexual values established by religious sacred laws continue to have a powerful impact on our current secular laws. They, too, have become a part of our cultural traditions. For example, religious law in the Middle Ages taught that oral and anal sex were much worse crimes than rape. Religious leaders believed that rape was a more moral behavior because it could cause pregnancy, and they believed that pregnancy was the only moral reason for having sex. Because oral and anal sex couldn't cause pregnancy, they were considered very great crimes. People were publicly executed for such behavior.

These medieval punishments left a powerful impression in cultural traditions and beliefs that lasted thousands of years. Some religious teachers still teach young people that many sexual behaviors are immoral and sinful because they don't cause pregnancy. And nearly 20 states still have laws against these sexual behaviors.

These sexual values were handed down to us from generation to generation, from the earliest church fathers, such as Augustine and Thomas Aquinas, to the **Victorians** of 100 years ago and televangelists of today. To a great degree, they are responsible for the confused attitudes toward sexuality that still have a deep hold on our society. They have taught us that sex is a dangerous, uncontrollable part of our lives, instead of a wholesome birthright that we can celebrate without fear.

Social Control of Sexual Behavior

Every society controls sexual behavior to maintain social order. For example, every society has laws or rules about who can marry, and most have laws about how people can arrange an orderly divorce. Often, however, laws about sexual behavior are unfair to certain people and do not always treat everyone equally.

Laws have traditionally favored one gender more than the other. In some societies, men are allowed to have more than one wife, but women are not allowed to have more than one husband. In our country, equal protection under the law is very important, and it is protected under the U.S. Constitution and by state constitutions. Our courts are often called upon to decide if specific laws violate this right to equal protection.

We are making great progress in equalizing the legal rights of both genders. We are also debating the legal rights of people with a minority sexual orientation, and whether or not we will extend the same opportunities and legal protections to lesbian, gay, bisexual, and transgender people as we do to the straight women and men who form the majority.

Laws are not the only ways societies try to control sexual behavior. Most societies have unwritten taboos against certain behaviors, such as incest or premarital sex. They show severe disapproval to people who violate sexual taboos. This kind of disapproval is called a **social stigma.** It is meant to instill shame and guilt. In some cultures, a whole family can be shamed by the behavior of a member.

The social pressure of a taboo can be powerfully disturbing. For example, only two generations ago, great shame was heaped upon unmarried American girls who got pregnant before marriage. They were hidden away until they gave birth and relinquished their babies for adoption, or until they had secret, unsafe, illegal abortions, or until they were shamed into getting married. Despite the hurt and shame, however, the taboos of the 1950s did little to prevent millions of teenage girls from becoming pregnant.

SEXUAL LAWS TODAY

Sexual law is a highly political issue. Some argue for more restrictive sexual laws and harsher enforcement. Others argue for more personal freedom. The sexual laws currently being debated across America include laws about:

- marriage and domestic partnerships
- divorce, child custody, and child support
- sexual health and safer sex
- sexuality education in the schools
- teenage pregnancy
- abortion and contraception
- civil rights for people who are gay, lesbian, bisexual, or transgender
- sexual assault
- sexual abuse of children
- sexual harassment
- pornography
- HIV/AIDS discrimination

Marriage and Domestic Partnerships

Each of our states has its own marriage laws. Each can decide who can marry, set the legal age for marriage, and state requirements for blood tests and marriage licenses. As of this writing, marriage can be legalized only between a man and a woman.

Bigamy

Bigamy—to have more than one spouse—is against the law in all states. There are two forms of bigamy. "Polygamy" or "Polygyny" means having more than one wife. "Polyandry" means having more than one husband. Polygamy is legal in some societies. Polyandry is no longer legal anywhere.

Domestic Partnerships

In the past, many states considered women and men who lived together for a significant period of time (different time requirements in different states) and who publicly described themselves as "husband and wife" to be common-law spouses. This gave them certain benefits held by other couples who had been married in an official way.

There are now more single people in our country than at any other time in history. Many never marry. Many divorce and do not remarry. Many singles live together in long-term, sexual relationships. This is called cohabitation. Increasing numbers of cities, states, corporations, and insurance carriers recognize these relationships and confer on couples some of the benefits otherwise available only to couples who are legally married. In some cases, same-sex couples also receive these benefits. These relationships, when recognized in this way, are sometimes called **domestic partnerships.**

Gay Marriage

In 1967, the U.S. Supreme Court overthrew all miscegenation laws in its decision *Loving v. the Commonwealth of Virginia*. The Supreme Court ruled that laws against marriage between persons of different races violated the right of equal protection. As we go to press, similar arguments are being used in the state of Hawaii, where legalized gay marriage is being debated. So many people are against gay marriage, however, that the U.S. Congress recently passed a new law, the Defense of Marriage Act, that allows states to disregard gay marriages recognized in other states. Some people think this law is a violation of the full faith and credit clause of the U.S. Constitution—which makes the official acts of one state valid in all states.

The Defense of Marriage Act also allows the government to withhold certain federal benefits from the spouses of gay marriages. These benefits include Social Security, veterans benefits, and federal pensions. President Bill Clinton signed this law in 1996.

Many states already ban same-sex marriage, and other states are considering similar laws.

Divorce, Child Custody, and Child Support

Divorce laws differ widely from state to state. The person seeking the divorce may give specific reasons, or "grounds," for wanting the divorce. These grounds traditionally required an assertion that the other spouse was guilty of some important fault and so were called fault grounds. They have included mental abuse, physical abuse, abandonment, and adultery.

In 1970, California became the first state to adopt "no-fault" divorce, which made it unnecessary to specify fault grounds, but accepted "irreconcilable differences" as an additional ground for divorce. Many states now permit divorces even when no one is "at fault."

Divorces must be granted by a court. Lawyers often help couples work out agreements regarding support, division and distribution of property, and child custody. These are sometimes called separation agreements or property settlement agreements.

Many people believe that divorce has become too easy. They want it to be more difficult for married couples to divorce—especially if they have children. Laws are now being introduced in some states to make divorce more difficult.

Child custody decisions are crucial in a divorce. Many states offer parents joint custody, in which parents can both raise their children—ordinarily in separate homes. Custody can also be awarded to only one parent. In all cases, the court is supposed to decide what is in the best interest of the child.

Judges are still more apt to give custody to mothers. Child custody is often refused a divorcing parent who is gay, lesbian, or transgender. Most states will refuse custody to a gay father. More have granted custody to lesbian mothers.

Financial Support after Divorce

During divorce proceedings, courts must consider how to provide for the financial support of the children and/or the divorcing partners. Collecting court-ordered child support can be difficult. Many fathers fail to make the required payments. Their former families are often forced into poverty and onto welfare. Poverty is less frequently a problem for fathers whose ex-wives fail to make the required payments.

Negligent parents often move to another state to avoid paying child support. Although this makes it difficult for the courts to track them, federal and state agencies are working hard to enforce child support laws around the country. To collect payments, agencies are able to withhold money—garnishee wages—from a negligent parent's salary. States may soon be able to threaten the professional licenses of working spouses to force them to pay.

Financial support of one divorced spouse by another is frequently called alimony. Alimony was designed to protect women who had never worked outside their homes and who would be left destitute after divorce, without means to support themselves and their children.

Today, the court may require the partner with the greater income or assets to support the other partner after divorce for a period of time or for the rest of the spouse's life. Usually, it is the man who pays alimony. Valuable property, such as houses and cars, must also be divided up. Some states—"community property states"—divide this property equally between the two people. Other states divide the property in a way that the court decides is favorable under all circumstances.

Adolescent Rights and the Age of Consent

All states have statutes governing the age of consent—the age at which a person is considered to be old enough to agree to have sex. A person who has sex with someone below the age of consent can be charged with rape even if the younger person was willing because, according to the statute, the younger person could not consent. This is the meaning of "statutory rape." Age of consent varies from as young as 12 or 13 in some states to 18 or older in others. Some states have double standards and set different ages for boys and girls.

The **age of majority** is the age at which one is considered an adult by law. In most states, it is 18. States also reserve the right to grant certain adult privileges to a child. This includes the right to marry without permission from parents. In such instances, other rights may be withheld until the age of majority. Such rights include, for example, the right to buy, possess, and drink alcohol. The age of consent usually arrives sooner than the age of majority.

Teenagers who live on their own without support of parents or guardians have legal autonomy and are called **emancipated minors.** Teens can become emancipated minors by joining the armed forces or getting married.

In some states, children and parents must receive court approval for emancipation. In other states, they need only show that financial independence has occurred. In some states, children may be emancipated by the court if they have been mistreated or abused by parents.

Most states grant partial emancipation to minors, under certain circumstances. In these instances, a child may seek certain kinds of medical care or social services without parental knowledge or parental consent. The following situations are so personal that an underage child has a right to find professional assistance on his/her own for:

- pregnancy
- contraception
- abortion
- drug or alcohol use
- mental health problems
- relinquishing a child to adoption

In all states, treatment for sexually transmitted infection is available to minors without parental consent.

Certain laws allow health care providers to evaluate whether a child seeking medical care is a "mature minor." To be considered "mature," the child must be capable of understanding the nature and risks of the medical procedure. Health care providers can use their best judgment to evaluate maturity in order to give assistance. Although *prior* parental consent is not required, some states expect health care providers to notify parents *after* treatment has been given.

All states recognize the importance of confidentiality between counselors and health care providers and their clients—regardless of age. But it is still not clear whether it is always legal for school guidance counselors to help underage students with emotional problems without the consent of their parents.

Most state laws protect confidentiality between students and school counselors, but require counselors to report certain problems to the authorities. These might include instances in which the student is the victim of sexual assault, child abuse, or neglect, or if the student reports a dangerous situation—for example, a crime that will be or has been committed. As often as possible, school guidance counselors encourage students to discuss personal problems with their parents.

Treatment for Minors
with Sexually Transmitted Infections

Access to treatment for sexually transmitted infections is vital to one out of five teenagers. More than half of all students in grades nine to 12 have had sexual intercourse at least once. Nearly three-quarters have had sexual intercourse by grade 12. Each year, 3 million teenagers contract sexually transmitted infections. Many of these infections have no symptoms. Left untreated, they can cause serious health problems including infertility and cervical cancer.

Minors can be treated for sexually transmitted infections without parental consent in all states. Some states set no age limits. Minors can receive treatment at Planned Parenthood health centers, other family planning clinics, and "sexually transmitted disease clinics" sponsored by hospitals or local health departments.

Public health laws require health care providers to report certain infections, regardless of the age of the patient. Sexually transmitted infections that must be reported include syphilis, gonorrhea, chlamydia, herpes, HIV, and AIDS. In most cases, names are not reported. The information is used by public health officials to track the spread of infection.

Some urban public schools are linked to special health clinics to offer teenagers assistance with sexually transmitted infections, safer sex information, pregnancy concerns, and other health-related matters. There are now more than 500 of these across the country—some located in school buildings. They have helped reduce teen pregnancy and sexually transmitted infections.

Sexuality Education

Sexuality education, also called family life education, is crucial for the sexual health of today's youth. Many parents provide this kind of education, and most of them approve of sexuality education in schools because they want their children to know about contraception and safer sex methods. Many prominent national organizations, including medical groups and religious organizations, also support sexuality education in the schools.

Despite widespread support, however, sexuality education continues to be a politicized and controversial subject. Some parents believe that family life education teachers should discuss only abstinence in the classroom. Other people believe that they should also discuss contraception and safer sex, as well as masturbation, intercourse, sexual pleasure, abortion, HIV/AIDS, and sexual orientation.

Many opponents of comprehensive sexuality education fear that it will encourage teenagers to have intercourse. A recent national study has shown that this is not true. In fact, early, comprehensive, nonjudgmental sexuality education encourages some teenagers to remain abstinent, helps other teenagers delay first intercourse by several years, and increases contraceptive use among teens who are already sexually active.

In the early 1980s, New Jersey became the first state to require family life education in grades K–12. Now almost all states either require or recommend some form of sexuality education.

Programs vary widely, however, and many states have restrictions. For example, 37 states teach about various disease prevention methods, but teachers in 12 other states must teach that abstinence is the *only* way to prevent pregnancy and infection. They are not allowed to discuss contraception or safer sex methods. Five states do not allow abortion to be discussed, and eight states require teachers to say that homosexuality is not acceptable. Only one state, Rhode Island, requires that schools teach respect for all people, regardless of sexual orientation.

Reproductive Rights

Teen Pregnancy and Welfare Laws

A 1994 study shows that increasing numbers of teenage girls are using contraception and that the rates of teen pregnancy and abortion are decreasing. Despite these trends, many states are changing their laws about public support for unmarried teen mothers and their children.

While these laws may have been designed with the teens' best interests in mind, some of these new laws may cause more harm than good. For example, some *require* a pregnant teen to live with a parent and finish high school. But if a teenager has violent or negligent parents who drink or use drugs, staying at home could be dangerous.

Some states cut off child support if more pregnancies occur. This increases the level of poverty for many teen mothers. All states now require adults on welfare, including older teens, to work after two years if they are physically able. Their welfare checks will go to their employers and be returned to them as wages. But unless states provide job training, job placement, and *affordable* child care, these circumstances may make it very difficult for young mothers to support their families.

Many people are opposed to these new laws. Some say that pregnant teenagers should not be forced to live at home, especially if they are unwanted there. They should be able to go to "safe houses" to be cared for during their pregnancies. Others believe that pregnant teens should be encouraged to relinquish their children for adoption. But for many teenage girls, having a baby makes them feel important and, they believe, gives them status.

Some teenage girls become pregnant by older men. They often look for attention and status from older partners. Many people believe that men who date teenagers should be charged with statutory rape and be forced to support the children that are born. They advocate laws that would require teen mothers on welfare to name the men or risk losing benefits.

Coercion of Pregnant Adult Women

Some courts, states, and agencies may decide that women are not taking good enough care of themselves and the fetus while they are pregnant. It may be that they are using drugs or alcohol or may not be getting proper medical care. Judges have allowed such women to be imprisoned, or have forced them to deliver their babies by cesarean section, or have separated them permanently from their children. Disabled, mentally ill, and poor women have been legally coerced into sterilization or the use of long-term contraceptives.

Women's rights groups and medical groups are protesting the use of this kind of legal force against women, whether pregnant or not. These groups believe that women's rights are being violated. They believe that there are better ways to help women in these situations.

Contraception

It was not until 1965 that the U.S. Supreme Court ruled in *Griswold v. Connecticut* that it was legal for married people in all states to use contraception. The court said that contraception for married couples was part of the "right to privacy," which is guaranteed by the U.S. Constitution. In 1972, the Supreme Court ruled in *Eisenstadt v. Baird* that unmarried people also had the right to use contraception.

It is also legal to advertise contraceptive products on television. Major television networks, however, have refused to broadcast such ads, even though smaller networks and cable stations have not lost viewers or advertisers by doing so.

Abortion

The 1973 U.S. Supreme Court decision *Roe v. Wade* found that abortion is a matter of privacy, just like contraception. However, the judges considered each of the three stages, or trimesters, of pregnancy differently. A state may not pass any laws to interfere with a woman's right to abortion during the first three months of pregnancy except to require that it be performed by a licensed physician. For the second three months, a state may make laws only to protect a pregnant woman's health and not to restrict abortion. But after the fetus is viable, a state may forbid abortion unless the pregnant woman's life or health is threatened by continuing the pregnancy. (**Viability** refers to the ability of the fetus to survive outside the woman's body and must be determined by the woman's physician.)

Other important Supreme Court decisions about abortion have been made since *Roe v. Wade,* including the following:

1976: *Planned Parenthood of Central Missouri v. Danforth.* A state cannot give a husband the right to veto his wife's decision to have an abortion. An underage woman does not need the consent of her parents in order to have an abortion.

1979: *Bellotti v. Baird.* A state can require an underage daughter to get written **parental consent** before having an abortion. However, the law must include a "judicial bypass" procedure for girls who cannot get written consent. This means that a pregnant girl has to appear before a judge in court and prove that she is mature or that an abortion would be in her best interests. Conservative judges have blocked efforts by underage girls to get abortions. Some states require parents to be notified, at least, before a minor daughter's abortion.

1988: *Webster v. Reproductive Health Services.* The reversal of *Roe v. Wade* and a return to the days of illegal abortion becomes possible. By allowing states to bar the use of public facilities for abortion, *Webster* victimized women of all economic circumstances by limiting their access to abortion services.

1992: *Planned Parenthood of Southeastern Pennsylvania v. Casey.* The right to abortion is reaffirmed, but restrictions are allowed unless they constitute an "undue burden" to the woman. Approved roadblocks to abortion include a mandatory 24-hour waiting period, a parental consent provision with a judicial bypass for minors, and the provision of state-authored anti-abortion materials.

Thirty-eight states have passed parental consent or parental notification laws since 1979, although only 27 states enforce these laws. Parental consent laws can be very dangerous. They force many pregnant girls to go to neighboring states to get abortions, to run away from home, to get unsafe illegal abortions, or to attempt self-abortion using dangerous methods. Girls who are forced to have children they do not want often abuse or neglect them.

Most girls tell their parents—usually their mothers—before they have an abortion. But some girls, such as Becky Bell, do not. In 1988, Rebecca was a 17-year-old Indiana teenager. She died from an illegal abortion. Her state required written parental notification for a minor to receive an abortion. But Rebecca did not want her parents to know about her pregnancy. She could have used the judicial-bypass provision in the law, but she was told that the judge was anti-choice. She could have traveled to the next state, Kentucky, but she had no transportation. No one knows what Rebecca did to attempt abortion, but she died from her attempt, as did hundreds of thousands of American women before abortion was made safe and legal in 1973.

Since *Roe v. Wade,* abortion continues to be a highly charged issue.

Most Americans are **pro-choice** and believe that abortion should remain safe and legal. Anti-choice activists believe that it should be illegal again. Violent assaults on doctors, clinics, and women seeking abortion have increased since the late 1970s.

Due to the number of bombings, arsons, blockades, incidents of harassment and stalking, as well as the murders of doctors and clinic workers by anti-choice terrorists, fewer doctors are willing to perform abortions now. No legal abortion services are available in 83 percent of U.S. counties, in 93 percent of nonmetropolitan areas, and in 51 percent of metropolitan areas.

Medical schools are training fewer doctors in abortion procedures. Medical students are being targeted with anti-choice propaganda and threats. One such "joke book," mailed to more than 30,000 medical students, recommended that "physicians who perform abortions should be shot, attacked by dogs, and buried in concrete."

Sexual Behavior of Consenting Adults

Many of the sex laws in America have been in place for more than 100 years. They are based on the conservative English laws that the early **Puritan** colonists brought to this country. They vary widely from state to state and are not always enforced. During the last 25 years, certain states have liberalized their sex laws. Twenty-six states have eliminated all penalties for voluntary, private sexual behavior between adults—gay or straight.

Many states continue to keep their old statutory sex laws, even though most people generally ignore them. But keeping outdated sex laws "on the books" is dangerous. These laws are often used to harass certain individuals or groups. People are easily entrapped because they are unaware that they are breaking the law. They do not know that they may be punished for private sexual behaviors that they mistakenly believe are legally acceptable. Many lawmakers fail in their attempts to get outdated laws off the books because conservative groups fight to keep strict limitations on personal sexual expression.

Fornication

Sex between unmarried people, called **fornication,** is still against the law in 12 states. Each of these states defines fornication differently. For example, cohabitation is against the law in several states. Since 2.9 million unmarried couples live together in the United States, cohabiting couples in these states may not be aware that they are breaking the law against fornication. In California, a man may not know he is committing a crime if he promises to marry a virgin and has sex with her before their wedding. But he is guilty of **sexual seduction** and can be fined and put in jail. As recently as 1996, a 17-year-old single mother in Idaho was found guilty of fornication. She was given a 30-day suspended jail sentence under a 75-year-old law. The young woman said that she did not even know what fornication was.

Adultery

Adultery is sexual intercourse between a married person and someone who is not his or her spouse. In the past, divorces were granted based on a husband charging his wife with "criminal communication" and the other man with "alienation of affection." It was not until the Fourteenth Amendment to the U.S. Constitution was passed in 1868 that wives were given the same legal right to divorce their husbands. Women were extended the same rights in divorce as their husbands had always enjoyed.

In 1969, adultery was a crime in 45 states, but by 1985, only 25 states punished people for adultery. In states such as Massachusetts, adultery is still a crime, punishable by a three year prison sentence and a fine of at least $500.

A more common term for sex outside of marriage is extramarital sex. Most extramarital sex is clandestine, or hidden from one's spouse. In some marriages, however, extramarital sex, or comarital relationships, are agreeable to both partners. These marriages are called open marriages and became popular during the 1970s.

In the United States, the incidence of extramarital sex is dropping. Prior to the 1990s, married men and women reported increasing rates of sex outside of marriage. Married women were catching up to married men in the number of their extramarital partners. More recent surveys show that extramarital sex is decreasing for both men and women.

This may be happening for several reasons. More people are marrying later in life, after they have had a variety of premarital sexual experiences. As a result, they may be more willing to commit to a sexually exclusive marriage. Others may be afraid of sexually transmitted infections, particularly AIDS.

Sodomy

In 1976, a married couple in Virginia was convicted of **sodomy,** which is defined as oral or anal sex. They were given five-year prison terms. They appealed their case to the U.S. Supreme Court. The court upheld the Virginia law, and sodomy has remained a crime in this state ever since.

The president of the American Psychiatric Association pointed out at the time that about two-thirds of sexually active American heterosexuals—80 million women and men—engage in oral or anal sex. He also reported that 20 million gay men and lesbians do likewise. If sodomy laws were enforced as they were in Virginia, 100 million Americans would be convicted.

It is not clear how the U.S. Supreme Court would now decide a case involving a criminal conviction of a heterosexual couple who had oral or anal sex. However, in 1986, in *Bowers v. Hardwick,* the Court upheld a Georgia law that punishes sodomy with 20 years in prison. In this case, two men were discovered having oral sex in their home by a policeman who was trying to serve a summons. The two men were arrested and charged with sodomy. The Supreme Court ruled that the right to privacy does not extend to sexual acts between two men or between two women, even in their own homes!

As of 1992, 19 states still had sodomy laws that applied to both straight and gay women and men, and four had sodomy laws that specifically targeted gay men and lesbians. Sodomy laws were most recently revoked in Montana in 1996.

Civil Rights for Gay, Lesbian, Bisexual, and Transgender People

The Civil Rights Act of 1964 prohibited discrimination against anyone based on race, religion, gender, or ethnic background in all states. Any enterprises having a connection with interstate commerce and businesses or institutions accepting federal funding may not discriminate in:

- education
- employment
- public transportation
- public accommodations, such as hotels and restaurants
- public services, such as getting a bank loan or mortgage
- the writing of life and health insurance policies

The act did not extend these protections to people based on their sexual orientation. As a result, in all but nine states, lesbians, gay, bisexual, and transgender people, as well as those who are perceived to be, can still be discriminated against in many ways because of their *private* sexual behavior.

Gay rights advocates have failed in their efforts to get federal protection extended in all states. In 1996, the U.S. Senate, by a margin of just one vote (50 to 49), rejected a gay rights protection bill which would have banned job discrimination for gay, lesbian, and transgender people across the country. Such people can still be treated with prejudice in employment, housing, education, and public services, including transportation and the military, because of their perceived sexual orientation, even though polls show that the majority of Americans favor ending such discrimination.

Crimes against people for their perceived sexual orientations are on the increase. Called gay-bashing, these crimes include verbal and physical assaults and murder. Although assault is against the law, police do not always respond when the victims are not perceived to be straight. In an increasing number of localities, however, such crimes are considered "hate crimes" and are prosecuted aggressively by the authorities.

Nonconsensual Sexual Behaviors

Sexual assault is *any* unwanted sexual act that involves force, threat of force, or illegal seduction. It ranges from the more serious crime of rape to unwanted touching of the sex organs. Illegal seduction is nonviolent, coercive coaxing, often directed toward children. This includes obscene telephone calls, exhibitionism, and voyeurism.

In the past, forced sex was called rape. It was the only term for sexual assault that appeared in the law. The term was only applied to men forcing women to have vaginal intercourse. Sexual assault is a broader term that also recognizes that women and men can be the perpetrators as well as the victims of sexual assault.

Sexual Assault against Adults

Sexual assault occurs most commonly between people who know each other. This is often called acquaintance rape. When two people are dating, sexual assault is called **date rape.** Sexual assault within marriage is a more recently recognized crime.

Sexual assault commonly occurs on college campuses and military bases and often involves drug and/or alcohol use. There can be one offender or a group of offenders. When more than one assailant is involved, the crime is often called gang rape. Most sexual assaults are committed by men against women. But women can also coerce men into unwanted sex.

Laws about sexual assault vary from state to state. In some locales, the victim must physically resist the assault in order to press legal charges, even if resisting may be life-threatening. Some laws require proof of assault, such as physical injury or semen in the vagina. Knowing this, some assailants use condoms to avoid depositing semen inside their victims. In some states, the use of force or the threat of force, regardless of physical injury, can constitute assault.

A victim's privacy is legally protected in many states. The victim's name or picture may not be printed in a newspaper or appear on television, without her or his permission. During trial, "rape shield" laws prevent the victim's sexual history from being discussed in court. If the assailant has been convicted of past sex crimes, however, these crimes may be brought forward as evidence.

In 1994, Congress passed the Violence Against Women Act. Under this law, women can charge their assailants in civil court. Under certain circumstances, they can also sue property owners and institutions such as colleges for not providing adequate security to prevent sexual assault. Federal judges are now deciding whether the Violence Against Women Act is constitutional.

Marital Rape

Marital rape is considered the last frontier in sexual assault law. In many societies, wives are considered the property of their husbands, who have the right to force their wives to have sex against their will. In some states, this is still true. In one study of American women, one out of every seven was raped by a husband or an ex-husband. Of 400 battered women, more than half said that they had been raped by their husbands.

New Jersey was the first state to pass a law against sexual assault in marriage. Now most states have laws that provide at least partial protection against spousal sexual assault. Usually, severe violence must be proved for assault charges to be upheld. Only 17 states provide married women full protection against sexual assault.

Sexual Assault against Children

Sexual contact between adults and children is illegal in every state. There are a number of terms used to describe sexual assault against children. These include statutory rape, sexual abuse, sexual molestation, pedophilia, incest, and "impairing the morals of a minor."

One of every four girls in our country is sexually molested by an older child or adult before age 18. One of every six boys is also molested by age 18. There are 300,000 cases of molestation, or child sexual abuse, reported each year. Most sex offenders molest many children many times. These acts can cause serious, lifelong problems for the victims. In fact, sex offenders themselves often report having been molested when they were children.

Most sexual assault of children does not involve force or threat of force. But some adult offenders may frighten or bribe children in some way to get them to keep the crime a secret. Most assaults include sexual seduction, during which the offender slowly encourages the child to participate in sexual acts. But sometimes force is used. Many children who are seduced enjoy the attention that the offender pays them and do not understand the meaning of what is happening to them.

Statutory rape is a legal term for sexual intercourse between an adult and someone who is below the age of consent. Typically, the offender is male and the victim is female. Intercourse with an underage girl is a crime even if she agrees to the act. This law is meant to protect children from seduction.

Today, many girls mature early and may appear older than they are. Some older men wrongly assume a girl has reached the age of consent. This may be more likely in states where the age of consent is 18 but partial adult privileges are granted before then. For example, girls may be allowed to drive when they are 16 or 17 but are not considered old enough to have sex. Some states give consideration to men who believed that their partners were legally capable of consent.

Incest and Pedophilia

Incest is sexual activity between members of the same family. Sex play between children in the same family is common and is not usually considered to be abusive. Exploratory sex play between cousins and brothers and sisters is not usually physically or psychologically damaging unless one child is older and bigger than the other and uses force.

Incest between adults in the same family or between adults and children in the same family is illegal. It includes all kinds of sex play, including asking children to undress. Incest usually occurs between a man and a young girl who is related to him. Women are also known to commit incest with younger members of their families.

Incest is committed against infants, young children, teenagers, and young adults. Older children may allow themselves to be victimized to protect a younger sibling from being victimized. In many cases, mothers know what is happening when fathers or stepfathers are the offenders and their daughters are the victims, but they may remain silent because they believe they are unable to intervene. These relationships often cause profound shame and guilt and can seriously affect children for the rest of their lives.

In most states, sexual contact or marriage between blood relatives is against the law. But some states allow marriage between first cousins.

Pedophilia is a psychological condition in which an adult is sexually aroused only by children. Using children for sexual arousal is a crime in every state. Most pedophiles are men who were sexually abused as children. It is very difficult for them to control their urges. Therapy is not always successful, and repeat offenses are common.

Many pedophiles control their sexual urges with **chemical castration.** They receive weekly injections of Depo-Provera® to reduce sexual desire. California offers this option to any first time sex offender who has molested a child under 13. If the man commits a second offense, the law *requires* either chemical or surgical castration. Removing the testicles stops nearly all testosterone production. Although it is not a foolproof way of preventing further sexual abuse, it permanently reduces sexual desire. Chemical castration is used in some parts of Europe and has decreased the rate of repeated sex offenses by treated men from 100 percent to 2 percent.

A new federal law, called **Megan's Law,** went into effect in 1997. It requires convicted pedophiles who have been released from jail to register with the police every 90 days. They must provide a blood sample for identification. Police must contact citizens to alert them to the presence of a pedophile in their community. Lifetime supervision by parole officials is mandatory.

Seven states now allow prison authorities to put dangerous sex offenders in mental hospitals without their consent after they have served their full sentences. This has raised legal questions about whether people who have already been punished for sexual crimes and who are not considered officially "mentally ill" should continue to be held in this way. The U.S. Supreme Court will rule on this matter in 1997.

Sexual Harassment

Sexual harassment is a newly defined sex offense that gives the victim the right to sue for monetary damages or other forms of relief such as job reinstatement or back pay. As more women have entered the workforce, college, the military, and other institutions, the incidence of unwanted sexual attention from men in authority has increased.

One-third to one-half of workingwomen have reported some kind of sexual harassment on the job. Now that people have become more aware of this behavior, we have begun to consider how women may sexually harass men, although this is less common.

Sexual harassment is considered a form of sex discrimination under the Civil Rights Act of 1964 because the victim is being singled out for different treatment based on his or her gender. Sexual harassment typically occurs in two forms. The first form of sexual harassment is called *quid pro quo* harassment. This occurs when an employee is told she or he will gain or lose a job or benefits depending on whether sexual favors are granted or refused.

The second form of sexual harassment is called hostile work environment. This occurs in the workplace when the members of one gender are subjected to some form of conduct that is so "pervasive and severe" that it makes it substantially more difficult for a member of the targeted gender to do her or his job. If the perpetrator is proved liable, the company can also be liable if it did nothing to stop a reported harassment.

The 1972 Educational Amendment law gives some protection against sexual harassment to students, but it does not allow a student to sue. Schools, colleges, and universities continue to develop their own policies on sexual harassment. Charges that could not be heard in court are sometimes treated by special committees appointed by university administrators. Some college professors who teach human sexuality courses and use explicit sexual materials or include frank discussions in their classrooms have faced charges of "harassment" from students who feel uncomfortable.

Commercial Sex

Prostitution

Prostitution is the performance of sexual acts for pay, including money, drugs, or other rewards. It has occurred throughout history. Women and men in ancient Babylon who worked as "sacred harlots" in the temples were greatly respected. Secular prostitution, though, has been much more common. Some prostitutes have enjoyed a high social status as courtesans—companions to wealthy men, kings, popes, and emperors.

Brothels, or houses of prostitution, were legal and regulated in many European cities during the Middle Ages. Prostitution continued to be legal in the frontier towns and mining camps of the American West and the Yukon in the late 1800s.

Prostitution continues to be legally tolerated in a few European countries today, including the Netherlands, Germany, and England. Nevada is the only state in the United States that has continued to allow legalized prostitution; however, it is allowed there only in counties with fewer than 250,000 people.

Most industrial societies have laws against prostitution because of concerns about public morals and the spread of sexually transmitted infections. Interestingly, the incidence of sexual infections among prostitutes in Nevada is virtually nonexistent because of increased condom use and frequent, mandated medical examinations.

In most states, prostitution is a misdemeanor. The penalty is usually a short jail term and payment of a fine. The charge under which most prostitutes are arrested is solicitation, which means openly offering sex to a potential client. Clients, called johns or tricks, are rarely arrested or prosecuted. They are usually white, middle-aged, middle-class, and married.

The more serious crimes in the sex industry include "pandering," "procurement," and "pimping"—recruiting prostitutes and living off their earnings. These are typically felonies punishable with significant jail sentences. A pimp is most often a man who takes care of the prostitute, offers clothes, shelter, and food, but takes most of the prostitute's earnings.

Prostitutes can be women or men. Many were sexually abused as children. They often refer to themselves as sex workers and serve heterosexual, bisexual, and homosexual clients. Some are teenagers, many of whom are runaways. There are more than 2 million teen sex workers in the United States. Streetwalkers or hustlers work the streets in urban areas. Many are drug addicts. Bar girls and boys, hotel prostitutes, call girls and boys, and "escorts" are often more independent than streetwalkers, who usually work for pimps.

There are groups working to decriminalize or legalize prostitution. They were formed by sex workers to offer assistance to others "in the life" and to promote social tolerance for this profession. These groups include COYOTE (Call Off Your Old Tired Ethics), which is based in California, and PONY (Prostitutes of New York) and Scapegoat, which are both based in New York.

Decriminalizing prostitution would eliminate penalties for prostitution but would retain penalties for procurement or pimping. Legalizing prostitution would legalize all aspects of the business. However, many people fear that suspending penalties for prostitution would increase organized crime, street crime, drug use, and pornography. But this has not been the case in European countries where prostitution is tolerated.

Through restrictive zoning and other local laws, many cities and towns try to limit commercial sex in areas for "adult entertainment." These areas can include pornography stores and theaters, peep shows, massage parlors, saunas, strip and lap dance clubs, and sexually explicit video arcades. These businesses often include prostitution services.

Pornography and Erotica

The word "pornography" means "the writing of prostitutes." The word comes from the way prostitutes advertised their services by writing their names and addresses on walls in ancient Rome and Greece. Pornography refers to any picture or writing that is meant to be sexually arousing. To many people, pornography is offensive and indecent. However, some people distinguish between pornography and erotica, which are sexually arousing pictures or writings that do not offend the average consumer.

"Soft-core" pornography is also distinguished from "hard-core" pornography. Soft-core pornography depicts naked bodies, including genitals, and limited sexual activity. Hard-core pornography depicts sexual intercourse and sex organs more graphically and more exclusively. It may also include violent sexual acts or other unusual behavior, such as sex with animals. Hard-core pornography is more likely to be considered obscene.

Although the First Amendment to the U.S. Constitution protects the right of free speech, the U.S. Supreme Court has always stated that obscenity is not protected because obscenity is not speech. Over the years, the Supreme Court has struggled to define obscenity.

In the 1973 case of *Miller v. California,* the U.S. Supreme Court issued a legal definition of obscenity, which is the standard still used today. The court found that a writing or picture, when taken as a whole, is legally obscene if:

- it appeals to a prurient—lascivious or lustful—interest in sex
- it offends the standards of the community in which it appears
- it has no serious literary, artistic, political, educational, or scientific value

If materials are legally obscene, then laws that ban their sale can be constitutionally upheld. In 1969, the U.S. Supreme Court ruled that a person could *privately* possess obscene material without committing a crime. But in 1990, the court ruled that private possession of **child pornography** is illegal and is not protected by the U.S. Constitution. Child pornography depicts children in sexual poses or engaged in sexual activity.

This controversy concerning whether sexually explicit material can be banned grows out of the 1873 Comstock Act that made it illegal to transmit any "obscene, lewd, lascivious, indecently filthy, or vile article" through the U.S. mail. The **censorship** that Anthony Comstock imposed on American society has had long-lasting and far-reaching effects.

The Supreme Court definition of obscenity remains vague in many ways. It continues to be challenged by people who advocate complete, unrestricted freedom of speech, and it is challenged by people who want greater restrictions.

Cybersex—Sex on the Internet

The old Comstock laws came back to haunt us again in the debate about using the Internet to send and receive pictures and writing that are "indecent or patently offensive." The Internet links personal computers in homes, schools, libraries, museums, and other public places around the world. It also allows people to have sexually explicit conversations and exchange sexually explicit pictures and stories very quickly and with great freedom.

In June 1995, as a response to public concerns about children viewing pornographic materials on their home computers, the U.S. Congress passed the Communications Decency Act. The act was an attempt to regulate obscene language and images on the World Wide Web. The penalty for sending any "indecent" or "patently offensive" information over the Internet was two years in jail and a $250,000 fine.

In June 1996, the American Civil Liberties Union, Planned Parenthood Federation of America, and other organizations challenged the law and won a court injunction that postponed its enforcement. The federal court declared in its decision that existing laws that limit the kind of speech publicly broadcast over television or radio cannot be applied to electronic speech such as the Internet.

In June 1997, the U.S. Supreme Court delivered its decision in *ACLU and Others v. Reno/Communications Act* and found that restrictions on Internet communication were unconstitutional.

HIV/AIDS Discrimination

People with HIV/AIDS need special protection in our society because of the serious social stigma attached to the disease. Many people have lost jobs, been evicted from apartments, been denied life and health insurance, or have experienced other disabling discriminations because they tested positive for HIV or developed AIDS.

These are the four laws that, taken together, provide some protection to people with HIV/AIDS:

- *The Civil Rights Act of 1964.* The Civil Rights Act protects all Americans from discrimination on grounds of race, gender, religion, and ethnic background.

- *The Rehabilitation Act of 1973.* The Rehabilitation Act extends the protections of the Civil Rights Act of 1964 to disabled citizens.
- *Fair Housing Amendments Act of 1988.* The Fair Housing Act protects against discrimination in public and private residential housing based on race, gender, religion, ethnic background, and disabled status.
- *Americans with Disabilities Act of 1990.* The Americans with Disabilities Act extends the Rehabilitation Act to apply to all public and private businesses with 15 or more employees. It requires removal of all physical and policy barriers to employment, shopping, transportation, entertainment, telephone use, and access to public places, including schools and colleges, for the nation's 43 million disabled citizens, including people with HIV/AIDS. However, the employer may reject a job applicant or dismiss an employee if the employer can prove that the person poses a "direct threat" to the health and safety of others on the job or if the person cannot perform the functions of the job even when the employer makes "reasonable accommodations."

Laws to protect people with HIV/AIDS against discrimination have not prevented discrimination in all cases. People with AIDS continue to be treated unfairly, despite the law. In some instances, attorneys have purposely delayed cases so that those who were very sick died before their lawsuits could be settled.

Testing for HIV

Mandatory testing for HIV has been controversial since HIV was first discovered in 1985. The Americans with Disabilities Act does not permit mandatory testing in civilian employment settings. But the government is allowed to test for HIV in certain programs. These include the military, the Peace Corps, the Diplomatic Service, state National Guard units, and the Job Corps. Any applicant with HIV is rejected for government service, even if that person is still healthy. Active-duty military personnel are tested regularly. If found infected, they are reassigned to limited duty and can be court-martialed if it is determined that they have not complied with strict guidelines to prevent transmission. Confidentiality is often violated.

Some government officials and health care providers want to mandate HIV testing for all pregnant women. However, the Centers for Disease Control and Prevention, which monitors the AIDS epidemic, suggests that all pregnant women be *offered* HIV testing. Many hospitals, especially in urban areas, routinely test newborn babies, although test results may not be given to the mothers. Donated body tissues, such as blood, semen, and eggs, and human organs for transplantation are routinely tested in every state.

With this brief summary of the laws that affect our sex lives, we close the last chapter of *All About Sex*. In these eight chapters, we have provided our readers with the basic information about our sexuality within the context of our society. We hope that this information will help readers understand and enjoy their sexuality in ways that are responsible and personally rewarding.

For information about the fascinating subject of human sexuality, please refer to the resource and reading lists that follow. Many of the books and journals we suggest were used as references by the writers who prepared the text for *All About Sex*.

Afterword

At different times of our lives, many of us may wonder if we are as sexually healthy as we might be. We may have also wondered what being a sexually healthy adult is all about. Planned Parenthood hopes that reading *All About Sex* has given you some clear ideas about sexual health, and we have a brief list to offer as a reminder. It was compiled by the Sexuality Information and Education Council of the United States and published in its *Guidelines for Comprehensive Sexuality Education: Grades K-12*. We think it provides a worthwhile inventory for ourselves and a good summary for our book.

For their own human development, sexually healthy adults:
- appreciate their own bodies
- enjoy a sense of self-esteem
- seek information about reproduction as needed
- recognize that human development includes sexual development, and that it may or may not include genital sexual experiences or reproduction
- interact with people of both genders in respectful and appropriate ways
- accept their own sexual orientation and respect the sexual orientation of others

In their relationships, sexually healthy adults:
- view their families as valuable sources of support
- express love and intimacy in appropriate ways
- develop and maintain meaningful relationships
- avoid exploitive or manipulative relationships
- make informed choices about family options and relationships
- develop skills that enhance personal relationships
- understand how cultural heritage affects ideas about family, interpersonal relationships, and ethics

In the development of personal skills, sexually healthy adults:
- identify and live according to their own values

- take responsibility for their behaviors
- practice effective decision making
- communicate effectively with family, peers, and partners

In their sexual behaviors, sexually healthy adults:
- enjoy and express their sexuality throughout life
- express their sexuality in ways that reflect their values
- enjoy sexual feelings without necessarily acting on them
- discriminate between life-enhancing sexual behaviors and those that are harmful to themselves and/or others
- express their sexuality while respecting the rights of others
- seek new information to enhance their sexuality
- engage in sexual relationships that are consensual, nonexploitive, honest, pleasurable, and protected against infection and unintended pregnancy

To preserve their sexual health, sexually healthy adults:
- use contraception effectively to avoid unintended pregnancy
- prevent sexual abuse
- act consistent with their own values in dealing with an unintended pregnancy
- seek early prenatal care
- avoid contracting or transmitting sexually transmitted infections
- practice health-promoting behaviors, such as regular checkups, breast and testicular self-exams, and early identification of potential problems

To benefit their society and culture, sexually healthy adults:
- assess the impact of family, cultural, religious, media, and societal messages on their thoughts, feelings, values, and behaviors related to sexuality
- promote the rights of all people to acquire accurate sexuality information
- demonstrate respect for people with different sexual values
- avoid behaviors that exhibit prejudice and bigotr.
- educate others about sexuality

Now it may be time to loan *All About Sex* to a friend!

The History of Planned Parenthood Federation of America

Planned Parenthood Federation of America, Inc., is the world's oldest and largest voluntary reproductive health care organization. Tracing its origins to the first birth control clinic in America, founded in 1916 by Margaret Sanger, Planned Parenthood is dedicated to the principle that every individual has the fundamental right to choose when or whether to have children.

On October 16, 1916, in the Brownsville section of Brooklyn, New York, Margaret Sanger, her sister, Ethel Byrne, and an associate, Fania Mindell, opened the first family planning clinic in America. They provided contraceptive advice to desperately poor, immigrant women.

A month later, all three women were charged with violating New York's antiobscenity statutes. Their arrest focused attention on federal and local Comstock laws that defined contraceptives and **abortifacients** as "obscene." To protest the laws, Sanger refused to pay the fine and chose instead to spend 30 days in prison.

Aided by Sanger's leadership, the birth control movement grew rapidly in size and impact during the years before and after World War I. In 1936, after two decades of reproductive rights activism, the U.S. Circuit Court of Appeals found that birth control could no longer be classified as obscene. In the years that followed, Sanger's controversial ideas ceased to be shocking and gradually became a part of American public life.

In 1942, the organization that Sanger founded took the name Planned Parenthood Federation of America (PPFA). Since then, PPFA has provided family planning counseling and reproductive health care in hundreds of communities nationwide.

In 1965, the right of all *married* couples to use contraception was finally upheld when the U.S. Supreme Court ruled, in *Griswold v. Connecticut,* that laws prohibiting the use of birth control by married couples violated the right of marital privacy. The Supreme Court's decision bears the name of Planned Parenthood of Connecticut's executive director of the time, Estelle Griswold, who was sued by the state for dispensing contraceptives and contraceptive information.

The right of *unmarried* people to use contraceptives was won only 25 years ago, when the U.S. Supreme Court, in *Eisenstadt v. Baird* (1972), struck down a Massachusetts statute that barred the distribution of contraceptives to unmarried people.

On January 22, 1973, the U.S. Supreme Court handed down its landmark decision *Roe v. Wade,* which struck down restrictive abortion laws throughout the nation and declared that U.S. women had a constitutional right to choose abortion.

An anti-choice constituency of about 20 percent of the American public has begun to wield considerable political influence in U.S. legislative and judicial systems. The terrorist arm of the anti-choice movement uses increasingly violent methods to prevent women from exercising their constitutional rights. The majority of Americans, however, continue to believe that individuals should be able to make their own reproductive health decisions without government interference.

Despite alarming threats from religious and political extremists, Planned Parenthood's 21,000 volunteers and staff members nationwide continue to provide medical, educational, and counseling services to meet the family planning needs of more than 5 million Americans each year. Supported by the gifts of 400,000 donors, Planned Parenthood also serves as a vigorous advocate for reproductive freedom for every individual.

Planned Parenthood Federation of America comprises 144 affiliates with more than 900 health centers in 48 states and the District of Columbia; a national office in New York City; a legislative and public information office in Washington, D.C.; and three U.S. affiliate service centers (Atlanta, San Francisco, and Chicago). PPFA's international family planning efforts maintain three regional offices (Nairobi, Kenya, for Africa; Bangkok, Thailand, for Asia and the Pacific; and Miami, for Latin America and the Caribbean).

For more than three-quarters of a century, Planned Parenthood has pursued its history-making tradition, advocating reproductive rights for women and men around the world. Providing health services to American women and their families is the foundation of that heritage and has earned Planned Parenthood its reputation as America's most trusted name in women's health. To make an appointment at the Planned Parenthood health center nearest you, call 800-230-PLAN.

Resources: Organizations, Hot Lines, and Web Sites

This is a short list of some of the national and regional resources available about sex, sexuality, and sexual health. While not exhaustive, it is a starting point for finding sexual health services and for gathering further information about sex and sexuality.

Academic Programs in Human Sexuality

Undergraduate Program in Human Sexuality
Department of Family Environmental Science
California State University
Northridge, CA 91330
818-885-4830

Graduate Programs: Sexuality Counseling, Marriage and Family
 Counseling
New College
130 **Hofstra University**
Hempstead, NY 11550-1090

Graduate Program: Minor in Human Sexuality
Department of Applied Health Sciences
Indiana University
Bloomington, IN 47405
812-855-7974
E-mail: yarber@indiana.edu

Graduate Program in Human Sexuality
Institute for the Advanced Study of Human Sexuality
1523 Franklin St.
San Francisco, CA 94109
415-928-1133

Graduate Program Health Education: Human Sexuality
Department of Health Studies
New York University
35 W. 4th St.
New York, NY 10012
212-998-5780
http://www.nyu.edu/education/

Graduate Program in Families and Sexuality
   Department of Family Social Science
290 McNeal Hall
University of Minnesota
St. Paul, MN 55108
612-624-1281
E-mail: jmaddock@che2.che.umn.edu

Graduate Programs in Human Sexuality
   Education
Graduate School of Education: Human
   Sexuality Education Program
University of Pennsylvania
3700 Walnut St.
Philadelphia, PA 19104-6216
215-898-7394
E-mail: AndyB@nwfs.gse.upenn.edu

Human Sexuality Program
University of Rhode Island
West Exchange Center, Ste. 307
260 W. Exchange St.
Providence, RI 02903
401-331-9120

Child Rights, Youth Services, and Family Counseling

Advocates for Youth
125 Vermont Ave.
Washington, DC 20005
202-237-5700

**Boston Alliance of Gay and Lesbian
   Youth (BAGLY)**
P.O. Box 814
Boston, MA 02103
800-42-BAGLY

Children's Defense Fund
25 E St.
Washington, DC 20001
202-628-8787

Family Service America
1170 W. Lake Park Dr.
Milwaukee, WI 53224
800-221-2681
National Information Center: 414-359-2111

Hetrick Martin Institute
2 Astor Pl.
New York, NY 10003
212-674-2400
Support and educational services for gay, lesbian, bisexual, transgender, questioning youth

Horizons Community Services, Inc.
961 W. Montana
Chicago, IL 60614
773-472-6469
Help line: 773-929-4357
Support and educational services for gay, lesbian, bisexual, transgender, questioning youth

Los Angeles Gay and Lesbian Center
Youth Services Department
1625 Schader Blvd.
Hollywood, CA 90028
213-993-7450
Talk line: 800-773-5540
Drop-in center, rap groups, clinic

LYRIC Youth Talkline
415-863-3636
Talk line for gay, lesbian, bisexual, transgender, questioning youth

Mothers without Custody
P.O. Box 56762
Houston, TX 77256-6762

**National Clearinghouse on Child
   Abuse and Neglect and Family
   Violence Information**
P.O. Box 1182
Washington, DC 20013
703-385-7565
800-FYI-3366

National Runaway Hotline
800-621-4000
TDD: 800-621-0394
Crisis intervention; offers referrals to local suicide hot lines

Runaway Hotline
P.O. Box 12428
Austin, TX 78711
800-231-6946

Childbirth and Maternal Care

Alcohol, Drug and Pregnancy Helpline
National Center for Prenatal Addiction,
Research and Education
200 N. Michigan Ave., Ste. 300
Chicago, IL 60601
800-638-2229

American College of Nurse-Midwives
1522 K St. NW, Ste. 1120
Washington, DC 20005
202-347-5445

American Foundation for Maternal and Child Health, Inc.
30 Beekman Pl.
New York, NY 10022

Association for Childbirth at Home International (ACHI)
P.O. Box 430
Glendale, CA 91209
213-667-0839

Maternity Center Association
48 E. 92nd St.
New York, NY 10128
212-369-7300

National Association of Childbearing Centers (NACC)
3123 Gottschall Rd.
Perkiomenville, PA 18074
215-234-8068

National Maternal and Child Health Clearinghouse
8201 Greensboro Dr., Ste. 600
McLean, VA 22102
703-821-8955, ext. 254 or 265
703-821-2098

Civil Rights and Sexual Discrimination

AIDS Law Project, Gay and Lesbian Advocates and Defenders
P.O. Box 218
Boston, MA 02112
617-426-1350

American Civil Liberties Union (ACLU)
AIDS-Related Discrimination Unit
132 W. 43rd St.
New York, NY 10036
212-944-9800

Fund for the Feminist Majority
1600 Wilson Blvd., Ste. 801
Arlington, VA 22209
703-522-2214

Human Rights Campaign
1101 14th St. NW, Ste. 200
Washington, DC 20005
202-628-4166
http://www.hrcusa.org

Lambda Legal Defense and Education Fund
120 Wall St.
New York, NY 10005-3904
212-995-8585

Ms. Foundation
120 Wall St.
New York, NY 10005
212-742-2300

National Center for Lesbian Rights
1663 Mission St.
San Francisco, CA 94103
415-621-0674

National Coalition against Censorship
275 7th Ave.
New York, NY 10001
212-807-6222

National Gay and Lesbian Task Force (NGLTF)
2320 17th St. NW
Washington, DC 20009
202-332-6483

People for the American Way
2000 M St. NW, Ste. 400
Washington, DC 20036
202-467-4999

Women's Legal Defense Fund (WLDF)
1875 Connecticut Ave. NW, Ste. 710
Washington, DC 20009
202-986-2600

Disabilities

Clearinghouse on Disability Information
Office of Special Education and
Rehabilitative Services
U.S. Department of Education
330 C St. SW
Washington, DC 20202-2524
202-205-8241

Coalition on Sexuality and Disability, Inc.
132 Holbrook Rd.
Holbrook, NY 11741

Committee on Sexuality: Advocating for People with Developmental Disabilities
P.O. Box 9216
Berkeley, CA 94709-0216

Health Resource Center
Hot line (V/TDD): 800-544-3284

Information Center for Individuals with Disabilities
Fort Point Pl., 1st floor
27-43 Wormwood St.
Boston, MA 02210-1606
800-462-5015

National Clearinghouse on Women and Girls with Disabilities
Educational Equity Concepts, Inc.
114 E. 32nd St.
New York, NY 10016
212-725-1803

National Information Center for Children and Youth with Disabilities
P.O. Box 1492
Washington, DC 20013
703-893-6061
Hot line: 800-999-5599

National Organization on Disability
Hot line: 800-248-ABLE

National Rehabilitation Information Clearinghouse
8455 Colesville Rd., Ste. 935
Silver Spring, MD 20910
301-588-9284
800-346-2742

Project on Women and Disability
One Ashburton Pl., Rm. 1305
Boston, MA 02108
617-727-7440
800-322-2020

Through the Looking Glass
801 Peralta Ave.
Berkeley, CA 94707
510-525-8138

Eating Disorders

American Anorexia-Bulimia Association
133 Cedar La.
Teaneck, NJ 07066
201-836-1800

Anorexia Nervosa and Related Disorders, Inc.
P.O. Box 5102
Eugene, OR 97405
503-344-1144

National Anorexic Aid Society
1925 E. Dublin-Granville Rd.
Columbus, OH 43229
614-436-1112

National Association for Advancement of Fat Acceptance
P.O. Box 188620
Sacramento, CA 95818
916-443-0303

National Eating Disorders Organization
6655 S. Yale Ave.
Tulsa, OK 74136
918-481-4044

Family Planning, Fertility, and Reproductive Rights

Alan Guttmacher Institute
120 Wall St.
New York, NY 10005
212-248-1111
http://www.agi-usa.org
Research, statistics, information

American College of Obstetricians and Gynecologists (ACOG)
409 12th St. SW
Washington, DC 20024-2188
202-638-5577
http:www.acog.com

American Society for Reproductive Medicine
1209 Montgomery Hwy.
Birmingham, AL 35216-2809
205-978-5000
http://www.asrm.com

Association of Reproductive Health Professionals (ARHP)
2401 Pennsylvania Ave. NW
Washington, DC 20037-1718
202-466-3825

Access to Voluntary Safe Contraception, International (AVSC)
79 Madison Ave.
New York, NY 10016
212-561-8000
http://www.avsc.org

Catholics for a Free Choice
1436 U St. NW, Ste. 301
Washington, DC 20009-3916
202-986-6093

Center for Reproductive Law and Policy
120 Wall St.
New York, NY 10005
212-514-5534

Center for Surrogate Parenting
8393 Wilshire Blvd., Ste. 750
Beverly Hills, CA 909211
213-655-1974
800-696-4664
Private organization; matches prospective parents with surrogate mothers for a fee

Emergency Contraception Hotline
888-NOT-2-LATE

Family Life Information Exchange
P.O. Box 37299
Washington, DC 20013-7299
301-585-6636

**Federation of Feminist Women's
   Health Centers**
633 E. 11th Ave.
Eugene, OR 97401
503-344-0966

**National Abortion and Reproductive
   Rights Action League (NARAL)**
1156 15th St. NW, Ste. 700
Washington, DC 20005
202-973-3000

National Abortion Federation
1436 U St. NW, Ste. 103
Washington, DC 20009
202-667-5881
Hot line: 800-772-9100

**National Organization for Women
   (NOW)**
1000 16th St. NW, Ste. 700
Washington, DC 20036
202-331-0066

**Planned Parenthood Federation of
   America, Inc.**
810 Seventh Ave.
New York, NY 10022
212-541-7800
800-230-PLAN for Planned Parenthood
health center nearest you
http://www.ppfa.org/ppfa

**Religious Coalition for Reproductive
   Choice**
1025 Vermont Ave. NW, Ste. 1130
Washington, DC 20005
202-628-7700

RESOLVE
1310 Broadway
Somerville, MA 02144
617-623-1156
http://www.resolve.org
Peer support for infertile couples

Right to Choose Education Fund
P.O. Box 65
Lincroft, NJ 07738
908-758-1182
http://www.righttochoose.org

Third Wave
185 Franklin St., 3rd floor
New York, NY 10013
212-388-1898

Gay, Lesbian, and Bisexual Issues

Bisexual Resource Center
http://www.qrd.org/qrd/www/orgs/brc/brl
   -toc.html

Custody Action for Lesbian Mothers
P.O. Box 281
Narberth, PA 19072

**Domestic Partnerships and Same Sex
   Marriages**
http://www.cs.cmu.edu/afs/cs.cmu.edu/user
   /scotts/domestic-partners/mainpage.html

**Gay and Lesbian Alliance against
   Defamation**
150 W. 26th St.
New York, NY 10001
212-807-1700

Gay and Lesbian National Hot Line
888-843-4564
http://www.glnh.org

**National Lesbian and Gay Health
   Foundation**
1638 R St. NW, Ste. 2
Washington, DC 20009
202-797-3708

**New York City Gay and Lesbian
  Anti-Violence Project**
Mailing address for National Coalition of
Anti-Violence Projects:
647 Hudson St.
New York, NY 10014
Hot line: 212-807-0197
General: 212-807-6761

**Parents, Friends, and Families of
  Lesbians and Gays (PFLAG)**
1101 14th St. NW, Ste. 1030
Washington, DC 20005
202-638-4200
http://www.pflag.org

**SAGE (Senior Action in a Gay
  Environment)**
208 W. 13th St.
New York, NY 10011
212-741-2247

Men's Sexual Health

Impotence Information Center
Hot line: 800-843-4315

**National Organization of Circumcision
  Information Resource Centers
  (NOCIRC)**
P.O. Box 2512
San Anselmo, CA 94970
415-488-9883
Provides information about circumcision as
well as female genital mutilation; opposes
routine hospital circumcision of newborns

Recovery of Male Potency
Hot line: 800-835-7667

Mental Health

**American Association for Counseling
  and Development**
5999 Stevenson Ave.
Alexandria, VA 22304
703-823-9800

**American Mental Health Council
  Association**
1021 Prince St.
Alexandria, VA 22314-2971
703-548-6002

American Psychological Association
750 1st St. NE
Washington, DC 20002-4242
202-336-5541

**Association of Gay and Lesbian
  Psychiatrists**
1439 Pineville Rd.
New Hope, PA 18938

National Alliance for the Mentally Ill
2101 Wilson Blvd., Ste. 302
Arlington, VA 22201
703-524-7600
800-950-6264

**National Clearinghouse on Family
  Support and Children's Mental Health**
Portland State University
P.O. Box 751
Portland, OR 97202-0751
800-628-1696

National Institute of Mental Health
9000 Rockville Pike
Bldg. 10, Rm. 3, D41
Bethesda, MD 20892
301-496-3421

National Mental Health Association
Hot line: 800-969-NMHA

Obsessive Compulsive Foundation
P.O. Box 9573
New Haven, CT 06535
203-722-0565

Self-Abuse Finally Ends (SAFE)
Hot line: 800-DONTCUT

United Way
Information Referral and Crisis Line
800-233-4357

Minority Health Issues

Asian Health Project
3860 W. King Blvd.
Los Angeles, CA 90008
213-295-6571

National Black Women's Health Project
1211 Connecticut Ave. NW, Ste. 301
Washington, DC 20036
202-835-0117
202-833-8790

National Latina Health Organization
P.O. Box 7567
1900 Fruitvale Ave.
Oakland, CA 94601
510-534-1362

Native American Women's Health Education Resource Center
P.O. Box 572
Lake Andes, SD 57356
605-487-7072

Office of Minority Health Resource Center
P.O. Box 37337
Washington, DC 20013-7337
800-444-6472

3X3 Bisexual People of Color
P.O. Box 10436
Oakland, CA 94610

Older Adults

American Association of Retired People
601 E St. NW
Washington, DC 20049
202-434-2277

Gray Panthers
1424 16th St. NW, Ste. 602
Washington, DC 20036
202-387-3111

National Association for Lesbian and Gay Gerontology
1853 Market St.
San Francisco, CA 94103
415-626-7000

National Caucus and Center on the Black Aged
1424 K St. NW
Washington, DC 20005

National Citizens Coalition for Nursing Home Reform
1825 Connecticut Ave. NW, Ste. 417B
Washington, DC 20009
202-797-0657

National Coalition on Older Women's Issues
2401 Virginia Ave. NW
Washington, DC 20037
202-466-7834

National Council on the Aging
409 3rd St. SW, 3rd floor
Washington, DC 20024
202-479-1200
800-424-9046

National Eldercare Institute on Health Promotion
601 E St. NW, 5th floor
Washington, DC 20049
202-434-2200

National Institute on Aging
800-222-2225
TDD: 800-222-4225

National Pacific/Asian Resource Center on Aging
811 1st Ave., Ste. 210
Seattle, WA 98104
206-624-1221

National Senior Citizens Law Center
1302 18th St. NW, Ste. 701
Washington, DC 20036
202-887-5280

Older Women's League
666 11th St. NW, Ste. 700
Washington, DC 20001-4512
202-783-6686

Sex Therapy

American Association of Sex Educators, Counselors, and Therapists (AASECT)
P.O. Box 238
Mount Vernon, IA 53214-0238
319-895-8407
Provides listing of certified sex therapists

Impotence Anonymous
119 S. Ruth St.
Maryville, TN 37801
615-983-6064

Sexual Compulsives Anonymous
Check for local newspaper listings.

Society for Sex Therapy and Research (SSTAR)
University Hospital of Cleveland
2074 Abington Rd.
Cleveland, OH 44106

Sexual Assault, Sexual Abuse, Incest, and Domestic Violence

Abused Women's Aid in Crisis
GPO Box 1699
New York, NY 10116
212-686-3628

Child Help U.S.A. Hot Line
800-422-4453

Clearinghouse on Family Violence Information
P.O. Box 1182
Washington, DC 20013
703-385-7565
800-FYI-3366

Feminist Alliance against Rape
P.O. Box 21033
Washington, D.C. 20009

Frequently Asked Questions about Sexual Assault and Rape
University of Wisconsin, Madison
http://linear.chsra.wisc.edu/chsra/chen-fu/QASEX.HTM

Incest Survivors Anonymous (ISA)
P.O. Box 1653
Long Beach, CA 90805

National Clearinghouse for the Defense of Battered Women
125 S. 9th St., Ste. 302
Philadelphia, PA 19107
215-351-0010

National Clearinghouse on Marital and Date Rape (NCOMDR)
Women's History Research, Inc.
2325 Oak St.
Berkeley, CA 94708
415-524-1582

National Coalition against Domestic Violence
2401 Virginia Ave. NW, Ste. 306
Washington, DC 20037
202-638-6388

National Coalition against Sexual Assault
125 N. Enola Dr.
Enola, PA 17025
717-232-7460
E-mail: ncasa@redrose.net

National Council on Child Abuse and Family Violence
1155 Connecticut Ave. NW, Ste. 300
Washington, DC 20036
800-222-2000

National Council on Safe Families
My Sister's Place
Yonkers, NY
914-969-5800

National Domestic Violence Hotline
Texas Council on Family Violence
3616 Far West Blvd., Ste. 101-297
Austin, TX 78731-3074
Hot line: 800-799-SAFE
TDD/deaf access line: 800-787-3224
http://www.inetport.com/~ndvh

National Gay and Lesbian Domestic Violence Victims' Network
3506 S. Curay Circle
Aurora, CO 80013
303-266-3477

National Woman Abuse Prevention Center
1112 16th St. NW, Ste. 920
Washington, DC 20036
202-857-0216

Parents United
Daughters and Sons United
Adults Molested as Children United
232 E. Gish Rd.
San Jose, CA 95112
408-453-7616
Crisis counseling: 408-279-8228
Referrals for self-help groups nationwide for family members affected by incest and child sexual abuse

Rape, Abuse, Incest National Network (RAINN)
Hot line: 800-656-HOPE
http://feminist.com/rainn.htm

Rape and Sexual Assault—National Victim Center Library Catalog: Bibliography
http://www.nvc.org/ldir/rape.htm

Survivors of Incest Anonymous
P.O. Box 21817
Baltimore, MD 21222
301-282-3400

Violence against Women Act Task Force
NOW Legal Defense and Education Fund
99 Hudson St.
New York, NY 10013
212-925-6635

VOICES in Action, Inc.
P.O. Box 148309
Chicago, IL 60614
Information on self-help groups

Sexual Enhancement

Betty Dodson Workshops
P.O. Box 1933
Murray Hill Station
New York, NY 10156
Sex for One and *Self-Loving*

Body Electric School
6527-A Telegraph
Oakland, CA 94609
510-653-1594
Workshops on erotic spirituality

E-Sensuals
http://www.tantra.com
Directory of Tantra teachers and workshops

Eve's Garden International, Ltd.
119 W. 57th St.
New York, NY 10019
800-848-3837

Good Vibrations
1210 Valencia St.
San Francisco, CA 94110
415-550-7399
http://www.goodvibes.com/books/books.htm

Sexuality Library
938 Howard St.
San Francisco, CA 94103
415-974-8990

Sexuality Information

History of Sexuality Resources at Duke University
http://odyssey.lib.duke.edu/women
/hist-sex.html#20th

Institute for the Scientific Study of Human Sexuality
Advanced Study of Human Sexuality
1523 Franklin St.
San Francisco, CA 94109
415-928-1133

The Kinsey Institute for Research in Sex, Gender, and Reproduction
313 Morrison Hall
Indiana University
Bloomington, IN 47405
812-855-7686
http://www.indiana.edu/~kinsey/

Masters and Johnson Institute
2 S. Kings Hwy.
St. Louis, MO 63108
314-361-2377

San Francisco Sex Information
Hot line: 415-989-SFSI
http://www.sfsi.org

Sexuality Bytes—On-Line Encyclopedia of Sexuality
http://www.sexualitybytes.com.au/

Society for Human Sexuality
University of Washington, Seattle
http://weber.u.washington.edu/~sfpse/

Society for the Scientific Study of Sexuality (SSSS)
P.O. Box 208
Mt. Vernon, IA 52314
319-895-8407
http://www.ssc.wisc.edu/ssss/

World Association of Sexology
1300 S. 2nd St., Ste. 180
Minneapolis, MN 55454-1015

Yahoo—Society and Culture: Sexuality
http://www.yahoo.com/Society_and_Culture
/Sexuality

Sexuality Education

American Association of Sex Educators, Counselors, and Therapists (AASECT)
P.O. Box 238
Mt. Vernon, IA 53214-0238
319-895-8407

Coalition for Positive Sexuality: Sex Ed for Teens
http://www.positive.org/

Eric Clearinghouse on Teacher Education
One Dupont Circle NW, Ste. 610
Washington, DC 20036
202-293-2450

New Jersey Network for Family Life Education
Rutgers University, Livingston Campus
New Brunswick, NJ 08903-5062
908-445-7929

Sex Information and Education Council of the United States (SIECUS)
130 W. 42nd St.
New York, NY 10036
212-819-9770
http://www.siecus.org

Sexually Transmitted Infections

Adolescent AIDS Program
Montefiore Medical Center
111 E. 120th St.
Bronx, NY 10467
212-920-2179

AIDS Action Council
729 8th St. SE, Ste. 200
Washington, DC 20003
202-547-3101

AIDS Clinical Trials Service
Hot line: 800-TRIALS-A,
   M–F 9 a.m.–7 p.m. EST
English and Spanish

AIDS Information
U.S. Public Health Services
Office of Public Affairs, Rm. 721-H
200 Independence Ave. SW
Washington, DC 20201
202-245-6867

AIDS Public Education Campaign
American Red Cross
1730 D St. NW
Washington, DC 20003
202-639-3223

AIDS Treatment Data Network
259 W. 30th St.
New York, NY 10001
212-268-4196

**American Foundation for AIDS
   Research**
1515 Broadway, Ste. 3601
New York, NY 10036
212-719-0033

**American Red Cross, Orange County
   Chapter**
105 W. Main St.
Carrboro, NC 27510
HIV/AIDS Teen Hot Line: 800-440-TEEN

**American Social Health Association
   (ASHA)**
P.O. Box 13827
Research Triangle Park, NC 27709
919-361-8400
National Herpes Hot Line: 919-361-8488
National STD Hot Line: 800-227-8922

National AIDS Hot Line: 800-342-AIDS
   Spanish: 800-344-SIDA
   Hearing-impaired: 800-AIDS-TTY

Cafe Herpe
http://www.cafeherpe.com
Herpes information sponsored by
SmithKline Beecham Pharmaceuticals

Gay Men's Health Crisis
129 W. 20th St.
P.O. Box 274
New York, NY 10011-3629
212-807-6655
HIV education and services

Hepatitis Hot Line
800-223-0179 (GO-LIVER)
e-mail: info@liver-foundation.org

**HIV/AIDS Treatment Information
   Service**
Sponsored by the U.S. Public Health Service
P.O. Box 6303
Rockville, MD 20849-6303
301-738-6616
Hot line: 800-HIV-0440
TDD/deaf access line: 800-243-7012

Lesbian AIDS Project
212-337-3532

**National Association of People with
   AIDS**
1413 K St. NW, Ste. 700
Washington, DC 20005
202-898-0414

**National Institute of Allergy and
   Infectious Diseases**
Office of Communications
Bldg. 31, Rm. 7A32
9000 Rockville Pike
Bethesda, MD 20892
301-496-5717
301-402-0120

National Minority AIDS Council
Hot line: 800-544-0586

New Friends Dating Service
P.O. Box 1235
Capitola, CA 95010
For people with herpes

New Jersey Women and AIDS Network
5 Elm Row, Ste. 112
New Brunswick, NJ 08901
908-846-4462

Project Inform
1965 Market St.
San Francisco, CA 94103
800-822-7422

Prototypes/Women's AIDS Risk Network
5601 W. Slauson Ave., Ste. 200
Culver City, CA 90230
213-641-7795

Rural Center for the Study and Promotion of HIV/STD Prevention
Indiana University
801 E. 7th St.
Bloomington, IN 47405-3085
800-566-8644
http://www.indiana.edu/~aids

Ryan White National Teen Education Program
Hot line: 800-933-KIDS

San Francisco AIDS Foundation
10 United Nations Plaza
San Francisco, CA 94102
415-487-3000
Safer-sex hot line: 800-FOR-AIDS

Unspeakable: The Naked Truth about STDs
http://www.unspeakable.com
Information about sexually transmitted infections sponsored by Pfizer Pharmaceuticals

U.S. Centers for Disease Control and Prevention (CDC)
Division of STD/HIV Prevention
U.S. Public Health Service
1600 Clifton Rd. NE
Atlanta, GA 30333
404-639-3311
http://www.cdc.gov/nchstp/hiv_aids/dhap.htm

Women and AIDS Resource Network (WARN)
718-596-6007

Sex Workers

CAL-PEP
630 20th St., Ste. 305
Oakland, CA 94612
415-874-7850
Safer-sex workshops for sex workers

COYOTE (Call Off Your Old Tired Ethics)
2269 Chestnut St., Ste. 452
San Francisco, CA 94123
415-474-3037
Support services

Genesis House
911 W. Addison St.
Chicago, IL 60613
773-281-3917

PONY (Prostitutes of New York)
212-713-5678
Support services

Transgender Issues

Harry Benjamin International Gender Dysphoria Association
18333 Egret Bay Blvd., Ste. 560
Houston, TX 77058

International Foundation for Gender Education
Box 367
Wayland, MA 01778
617-894-8340

Renaissance Education Association, Inc.
987 Old Eagle School Rd., Ste. 719
Wayne, PA 19087
610-975-9119
  or
P.O. Box 1263
King of Prussia, PA 19406

Uncommon Sex Practices

Center for Support
P.O. Box 460126
San Francisco, CA 94146
Parents of pedophiles

ETVC
P.O. Box 6486
San Francisco, CA 94101
Transvestites and transsexuals

The Eulenspiegel Society (TES)
Box 2483
Grand Central Station
New York, NY 10163
Dominance and submission

Foot Fetish and Fantasy Society
P.O. Box 24866
Cleveland, OH 44124

Girth and Mirth
176-B Page St.
San Francisco, CA 94102
415-552-1143
Obese partners referrals

Human Awareness Institute
1720 S. Amphlett Blvd., #128
San Mateo, CA 94402
Stan Dale intimacy workshops

Lifestyles
2641 W. La Palma, Ste. A
Anaheim, CA 92801
Swing organization with national events

National Leather Association
National Headquarters
Box 17463
Seattle, WA 98107
Dominance and submission

National Sexuality Symposium
P.O. Box 620123
Woodside, CA 94062

QSM
P.O. Box 882242
San Francisco, CA 94188-2242
415-550-7776
S and M lectures and classes

Society of Janus
P.O. Box 6794
San Francisco, CA 94101
415-85-7117
Dominance and submission

Tantra Workshops
c/o S. Wadel and D. Coleman
1470 DeHaro St.
San Francisco, CA 94107

TRI-ESS
Box 194
Tulare, CA 93275
Sorority for heterosexual cross-dressers;
publisher of *Femme Mirror,* a quarterly

Women's Health

Breast Cancer Action
P.O. Box 460185
San Francisco, CA 94146
415-922-8279

Center for Research on Women
Memphis State University
339 Clement Hall
Memphis, TN 38152
901-678-2770

Center for Women's Policy Studies
2000 F St. NW, Ste. 508
Washington, DC 20036
202-872-1770

Encore
Check phone book for local listings.
YWCA support groups for women with
breast cancer

**Hysterectomy Educational Resources
and Services (HERS)**
422 Bryn Mawr Ave.
Bala Cynwyd, PA 19004
215-667-7757

**Melpomene Institute for Women's
Health Research**
2125 Hennepin Ave.
Minneapolis, MN 55413
612-378-0545

**National Alliance of Breast Cancer
Organizations (NABCO)**
1180 Ave. of the Americas, 2nd floor
New York, NY 10036
212-221-3300

**National Association of Public Health
Policy (NAPHP)**
c/o Marin Institute
24 Belvedere St.
San Rafael, CA 94901
415-456-5692

National Cancer Institute
NIH/Office of Cancer Communications
Cancer Information Service
Bldg. 31
9000 Rockville Pike
Bethesda, MD 20892
Hot line: 800-4-CANCER

**National Council for Research on
Women**
530 Broadway, 10th floor
New York, NY 10012-3900
212-274-0730

National Council on Women's Health
1300 York Ave.
New York, NY 10021
212-535-0031

**National Women Health Resource
Center**
2425 L Street NW
Washington, DC 20037
202-293-6045

National Women's Health Network
1324 G St. NW
Washington, DC 20005-2052
202-347-1140

Office of Women's Health
Department of Health and Human Services
200 Independence Ave. NW, 730B
Washington, DC 20201
202-619-0257

**Planned Parenthood Federation of
America**
810 Seventh Ave.
New York, NY 10022
212-541-7800
800-230-PLAN for the Planned Parenthood
health center nearest you
http://www.ppfa.org/ppfa

Women's Cancer Resource Center
P.O. Box 11235
Oakland, CA 94611
415-548-WCRC

**Women's Health Action Mobilization
(WHAM)**
P.O. Box 733
New York, NY 10009
212-713-5966

Women's Health Information Center
Boston Women's Health Book Collective
47 Nichols Ave.
West Somerville, MA 02172
617-625-0271

Y-ME Breast Cancer Support Group
Hot line: 800-221-2141

Suggested Reading

For the last 15 years, there has been an enormous outpouring of writing on the subject of human sexuality. This brief listing includes some of the important publications that went into the research for this book.

BOOKS

Biology and Anthropology of Human Sexuality

Fisher, H. E. *The Sex Contract: The Evolution of Human Behavior.* New York: William Morrow, 1983.

———. *Anatomy of Love: The Natural History of Monogamy, Adultery, and Divorce.* New York: W. W. Norton, 1992.

Hrdy, S. B. *The Woman That Never Evolved.* Cambridge, MA: Harvard University Press, 1981.

Maxwell, K. *The Sex Imperative: An Evolutionary Tale of Sexual Survival.* New York: Plenum Press, 1994.

Perper, T. *Sexual Signals: The Biology of Love.* Philadelphia, PA: ISI Press, 1985.

Symons, D. *The Evolution of Human Sexuality.* New York: Oxford University Press, 1979.

Children and Adolescents

Bass, E., and Kaufman, K. *Free Your Mind: The Book for Gay, Lesbian, and Bisexual Youth and Their Allies.* New York: HarperPerennial, 1996.

Bell, R. *Changing Bodies, Changing Lives: A Book for Teens on Sex and Relationships.* New York: Vintage, 1988.

Gecas, V., and Seff, M. *Contemporary Families: Looking Forward, Looking Back.* Minneapolis, MN: National Council on Family Relations, 1991.

Harris, R. *It's Perfectly Normal: Changing Bodies, Growing Up, Sex, and Sexual Health.* Cambridge, MA: Candlewick Press, 1994.

Herdt, G., and Boxer, A. *Children of Horizons: How Gay and Lesbian Children Are Leading a New Way Out of the Closet.* Boston: Beacon Press, 1993.

Klein, M. *Ask Me Anything.* New York: Simon and Schuster, 1992.

Martin, A. *The Lesbian and Gay Parenting Handbook: Creating and Raising Families.* New York: HarperCollins, 1993.

Pipher, M. *Reviving Ophelia: Saving the Selves of Adolescent Girls.* New York: Ballantine Books, 1994.

Voydanoff, P., and Donnelly, B. W. *Adolescent Sexuality and Pregnancy.* Newbury Park, CA: Sage Publications, 1990.

Commercial Sex

Delacoste, F., and Alexander, P., eds. *Sex Work: Writings by Women in the Sex Industry.* Pittsburgh, PA: Cleis Press, 1987.

Ridgeway, J. *Red Light: Inside the Sex Industry.* Eng: Power House Books, 1996.

Steward, S. M. *Understanding the Male Hustler.* New York: Haworth Press, 1992.

Vanwesenbeeck, I. *Prostitutes' Well-Being and Risk.* Amsterdam, Neth.: VU University Press, 1994.

Disabilities

Burger, E. *Sexuality and Disability: Personal Perspectives.* St. Louis, MO: Mosby, 1981.

Ferreyra, S., and Hughes, K. *Table Manners: A Guide to the Pelvic Examination for Disabled Women and Health Care Providers.* San Francisco: Planned Parenthood Alameda/San Francisco, 1991.

Frank, R., and Edwards, J. *Building Self-Esteem in Persons with Developmental Disabilities.* Portland, OR: Ednick Communications, 1988.

Kempton, W. *Sex Education for Persons with Disabilities That Hinder Learning: A Teachers Guide.* Santa Monica, CA: Stanfield, 1988.

Klein, E., and Kroll, K. *Enabling Romance: A Guide to Love, Sex, and Relationships for the Disabled.* New York: Harmony Books, 1992.

Mooney, T. O. *Sexual Options for Paraplegics and Quadraplegics.* Boston: Little, Brown, 1975.

Schover, L., and Jensen, S. *Sexuality and Chronic Illness.* New York: Guilford Press, 1988.

Senn, C. *Vulnerable: Sexual Abuse and People with Intellectual Handicap.* Ontario, Can.: G. Allen Roecher Institute, York University, 1987.

Eating Disorders

Shute, J. *Life-Size.* Boston: Houghton Mifflin, 1992.

Family Planning and Birth Control

Hatcher, R. A., et al. *Contraceptive Technology.* New York: Irvington Publishers, 1994.

Weschler, T. *Taking Charge of Your Fertility: The Definitive Guide to Natural Birth Control and Pregnancy Achievement.* New York: HarperCollins, 1995.

History of Human Sexuality

Anderson, M. M. *Hidden Power: The Palace Eunuchs of Imperial China.* Buffalo, NY: 1990.

Blundell, S. *Women in Ancient Greece.* Cambridge, MA: Harvard University Press, 1995.

Boswell, J. *Same-Sex Unions in Premodern Europe.* New York: Villard Books, 1994.

Brodie, J. F. *Contraception and Abortion in 19th Century America.* Ithaca, NY: Cornell University Press, 1994.

Bullough, V. *Sexual Variance in Society and History.* New York: Wiley, 1976.

Burg, B. R. *Sodomy and the Pirate Tradition: English Sea Rovers in the Seventeenth-Century Caribbean.* New York: New York University Press, 1983.

Carnes, M. C. *Secret Ritual and Manhood in Victorian America.* New Haven, CT: Yale University Press, 1989.

Chesler, E. *Woman of Valor: Margaret Sanger and the Birth Control Movement in America.* New York: Simon and Schuster, 1992.

Coontz, S. *The Way We Never Were: American Families and the Nostalgia Trap.* New York: BasicBooks, 1992.

Danielou, A., trans. *The Complete Kama Sutra: The First Unabridged Modern Translation of the Classic Indian Text.* Rochester, VT: Park Street Press, 1994.

D'Emilio, J., and Freedman, E. B. *Intimate Matters: A History of Sexuality in America.* New York: Harper and Row, 1988.

Dover, K. J. *Greek Homosexuality.* Cambridge, MA: Harvard University Press, 1989.

Gay, P. *The Bourgeois Experience: Victoria to Freud: Education of the Senses.* New York: Oxford University Press, 1984.

————. *The Bourgeois Experience: Victoria to Freud: The Tender Passion.* New York: Oxford University Press, 1986.

Grimal, P. *Love in Ancient Rome.* Norman, OK: University of Oklahoma Press, 1986.

Hardman, P. D., *Homoaffectionalism: Male Bonding from Gilgamesh to the Present.* San Francisco: GLB Publishers, 1993.

Hunt, L., ed., *The Invention of Pornography.* New York: Zone Books, 1993.

Jones, J. H. *The Tuskegee Syphilis Experiment: A Tragedy of Race and Medicine Revisited.* New York: The Free Press, 1993.

Katz, J. *Gay American History.* New York: Harper Colophon, 1985.

Kertzer, D. I. *Sacrificed for Honor: Italian Infant Abandonment and the Politics of Reproductive Control.* Boston: Beacon Press, 1994.

Keuls, E. C. *The Reign of the Phallus: Sexual Politics in Ancient Athens.* Los Angeles: University of California Press, 1993.

Knight, C. *Blood Relations: Menstruation and the Origins of Culture.* New Haven, CT: Yale University Press, 1991.

Marcus, E. *Making History: The Struggle for Gay and Lesbian Equal Rights: 1945–1990; An Oral History.* New York: HarperCollins, 1992.

Pomeroy, S. B. *Goddesses, Whores, Wives, and Slaves: Women in Classical Antiquity.* New York: Schocken Books, 1975.

Ranke-Heinemann, U. *Eunuchs for the Kingdom of Heaven: Women, Sexuality, and the Catholic Church.* New York: Doubleday, 1990.

Reed, J. *The Birth Control Movement and American Society: From Private Vice to Public Virtue.* Princeton, NJ: Princeton University Press, 1984.

Richards, J. *Sex, Dissidence, and Damnation: Minority Groups in the Middle Ages.* New York: Routledge, 1991.

Riddle, J. M. *Contraception and Abortion from the Ancient World to the Renaissance.* Cambridge, MA: Harvard University Press, 1992.

Ruggerio, G. *The Boundaries of Eros: Sex Crime and Sexuality in Renaissance Venice.* New York: Oxford University Press, 1989.

Stanley, J. *Bold in Her Breeches: Women Pirates across the Ages.* San Francisco: Pandora, 1995.

Tannahill, R. *Sex in History: United States of America.* New York: Scarborough House, 1992.

Watanabe, T., and Iwata, J. *The Love of the Samurai: A Thousand Years of Japanese Homosexuality.* Boston: Alyson Publications, 1989.

Law and Sexuality

Green, R. *Sexual Science and the Law.* Cambridge, MA: Harvard University Press, 1992.

Strossen, N. *Defending Pornography: Free Speech, Sex, and the Fight for Women's Rights.* New York: Scribner, 1995.

Men's Health

Morgentaler, M. D. *The Male Body: A Physician's Guide to What Every Man Should Know about His Sexual Health.* New York: Simon and Schuster, 1993.

Zilbergeld, B. *The New Male Sexuality.* New York: Bantam Books, 1992.

Sexual Assault and Sexual Abuse

Bass, E., and Davis, L. *The Courage to Heal: A Guide for Women Survivors of Child Sexual Abuse.* New York: Harper and Row, 1988.

Brownmiller, Susan. *Against Our Will: Men, Women, and Rape.* New York: Simon and Schuster, 1975.

Powell, E. *Talking Back to Sexual Pressure.* Minneapolis, MN: CompCare Publishers, 1991.

Prentky, R. A. and Quinsey, V. L., eds. *Human Sexual Aggression: Current Perspectives.* New York: New York Academy of Sciences, 1988.

Strauss, M. A. *Beating the Devil out of Them: Corporal Punishment in American Families.* New York: Macmillan, 1994.

Sexual Enhancement and Relationships

Allgeier, E. R. and A. R. *Sexual Interactions.* Lexington, MA: D. C. Heath, 1984.

Blank, J. *Good Vibrations: The Complete Guide to Vibrators.* Burlingame, CA: Down There Press, 1989.

Branden, N. *The Psychology of Romantic Love.* New York: J. P. Tarcher, 1980.

Comfort, A. *The Joy of Sex.* New York: Crown, 1972.

———. *More Joy: A Lovemaking Companion to "The Joy of Sex."* New York: Crown, 1985.

Dodson, B. *Sex for One: The Joy of Self-Loving.* New York: Harmony Books, 1987.

Friday, N. *My Secret Garden: Women's Sexual Fantasies.* New York: Pocket Books, 1973.

———. *Forbidden Flowers: More Women's Sexual Fantasies.* New York: Delacorte, 1975.

Heiman, J. R., and LoPiccolo, J. *Becoming Orgasmic: A Sexual and Personal Growth Program for Women.* New York: Prentice-Hall, 1988.

Isensee, R. *Love between Men: Enhancing Intimacy and Keeping Your Relationship Alive.* New York: Prentice-Hall, 1990.

Kaufman, G., and Raphael, L. *Coming Out of Shame: Transforming Gay and Lesbian Lives.* New York: Doubleday, 1996.

Ladas, A. K., et al. *The G Spot and Other Recent Discoveries about Human Sexuality.* New York: Dell, 1983.

Loulan, J. *Lesbian Sex.* San Francisco: Spinsters Books, 1984.

Masters, W. H., and Johnson, V. E. *Human Sexual Response.* Boston: Little, Brown, 1966.

McWhirter, D. P., and Mattison, A. M. *The Male Couple: How the Relationships Develop.* Englewood Cliffs, NJ: Prentice-Hall, 1984.

Morin, J. *Anal Pleasure and Health.* San Francisco: Down There Press, 1987.

Rosenthal, S. H. *Sex over Forty.* New York: J. P. Tarcher, 1988.

Schwartz, P. *Peer Marriage: How Love between Equals Really Works.* New York: The Free Press, 1994.

Silverstein, C., and Picano, F. *The New Joy of Gay Sex.* New York: HarperCollins, 1992.

Sisley, E., and Harris, B. *The Joy of Lesbian Sex.* New York: Simon and Schuster, 1978.

Winks, C., and Semans, A. *The New Good Vibrations Guide to Sex.* San Francisco: Cleis Press, 1997.

Sexuality

Beauvoir, S. de. *The Second Sex.* New York: Knopf, 1952.

Borhek, M. V. *Coming Out to Parents: A Two-Way Survival Guide for Lesbians and Gay Men and Their Parents.* New York: Pilgrim Press, 1983.

Bozett, F. W., ed. *Gay and Lesbian Parents.* New York: Praeger, 1987.

Bullough, V. and B., eds. *Human Sexuality: An Encyclopedia.* New York: Garland, 1994.

Crooks, R., and Baur, K. *Our Sexuality.* New York: Benjamin/ Cummings Publishing, 1990.

D'Augelli, A. R., and Patterson, C. J., eds. *Lesbian, Gay, and Bisexual Identities over the Lifespan: Psychological Perspectives.* New York: Oxford University Press, 1995.

Davis, A. Y. *Women, Race, and Class.* New York: Random House, 1981.

Faludi, S. *Backlash: The Undeclared War against American Women.* New York: Crown, 1991.

Francoeur, R. T. *Becoming a Sexual Person.* 2nd ed. New York: Macmillan, 1991.

Friedan, B. *The Feminine Mystique.* New York: Norton, 1963.

Greer, G. *The Female Eunuch.* New York: McGraw-Hill, 1970.

Kelly, K., and Byrne, D. *Exploring Human Sexuality.* Old Tappan, NJ: Prentice-Hall, 1991.

Laumann, E. O., et al. *The Social Organization of Sexuality: Sexual Practices in the United States.* Chicago: University of Chicago Press, 1994.

Lorde, A. *Sister Outsider: Essays and Speeches.* Trumansburg, NY: Crossing Press, 1984.

McCammon, S. L., Knox, D., and Schacht, C. *Choices in Sexuality.* Minneapolis/St. Paul, MN: West Publishing Company, 1993.

McCormick, N. B. *Sexual Salvation.* New York: Greenwood Press, 1994.

Michael, R. T., et al. *Sex in America: A Definitive Survey.* New York: Little, Brown, 1995.

Millet, K. *Sexual Politics.* Garden City, NY: Doubleday, 1970.

Money, J. *Lovemaps.* Buffalo, NY: Prometheus Books, 1993.

Money, J., and Lamacz, M. *Vandalized Lovemaps.* Buffalo, NY: Prometheus Books, 1989.

Reiss, I. L. *An End to Shame: Shaping Our Next Sexual Revolution.* Buffalo, NY: Prometheus Books, 1990.

Strong, B., and DeVault, C. *Human Sexuality: Diversity in Contemporary America.* 2nd ed. Mountain View, CA: Mayfield Publishing, 1997.

Umans, M. *Like Coming Home: Coming Out Letters.* Austin, TX: Banned Books, 1988.

Westheimer, R. *Dr. Ruth's Encyclopedia of Sex.* New York: Continuum, 1994.

Sexually Transmitted Infections

Brandt, A. M. *No Magic Bullet: A Social History of Venereal Disease in the United States since 1880.* New York: Oxford University Press, 1987.

Ebel, C. *Managing Herpes: How to Live and Love with a Chronic STD.* Research Triangle Park, NC: American Social Health Association, 1994.

Hatcher, R. *Safely Sexual.* New York: Irvington Publishers, 1995.

Shilts, R. *And the Band Played On: People, Politics, and the AIDS Epidemic.* New York: St. Martin's Press, 1987.

Stine, G. J. *Acquired Immune Deficiency Syndrome: Biological, Medical, Social and Legal Issues.* Englewood Cliffs, NJ: Prentice Hall, 1993.

Transgender

Bolin, A. *In Search of Eve: Transsexual Rites of Passage.* South Hadley, MA: Bergin and Garvey, 1988.

Docter, R. F. *Transvestites and Transsexuals: Toward a Theory of Cross-Gender Behavior.* New York: Plenum Press, 1990.

Uncommon Sex Practices

Bartell, G. *Group Sex.* New York: Wyden, 1971.

Brame, G., et al. *Different Loving: An Exploration of the World of Sexual Dominance and Submission.* New York: Villard Books, 1993.

Califia, P. *The Lesbian S/M Safety Manual.* Boston: Alyson Publications, 1988.

Chia, M., and Winn, M. *Cultivating Male Sexuality: Taoist Secrets of Love.* Santa Fe, NM: Aurora Books, 1984.

————. *Cultivating Women's Sexuality: Healing Love Through Tao.* Huntington, NY: Healing Tao Books, 1986.

Colter, E., et al., eds. *Policing Public Sex: Queer Politics and the Future of AIDS Activism.* Boston: South End Press, 1996.

Dailey, D., ed. *The Sexually Unusual: A Guide to Understanding and Helping.* New York: Harrington Park Press, 1988.

Garber, M. *Vested Interests: Cross-Dressing and Cultural Anxiety.* New York: Routledge, 1992.

Gosselin, C., and Wilson, G. *Sexual Variations: Fetishism, Sadomasochism, Transvestism.* New York: Simon and Schuster, 1980.

Love, B. *Encyclopedia of Unusual Sex Practices.* Fort Lee, NJ: Barricade Books, 1992.

Mains, G. *Urban Aboriginals: A Celebration of Leather-Sexuality.* East Haven, CT: Gay Sunshine/Inland Book Company, 1988.

Suggs, D. N., and Miracle, A. *Culture and Human Sexuality.* Pacific Grove, CA: Brooks/Cole Publishing, 1993.

Women's Health

Ammer, C. *A to Z of Women's Health.* New York: Facts on File, 1995.

Barbach, L. *For Each Other: Sharing Sexual Intimacies.* Garden City, NY: Doubleday/Anchor, 1982.

———. *The Pause: Positive Approaches to Menopause.* New York: Penguin, 1993.

Barbach, L., and Levine, L. *Shared Intimacies: Women's Sexual Experiences.* New York: Anchor Press, 1980.

Boston Women's Health Collective. *The New Our Bodies, Ourselves.* New York: Simon and Schuster, 1992.

Doress-Worters, P. B., and Siegal, D. L. *The New Ourselves, Growing Older.* New York: Simon and Schuster, 1994.

Gilligan, C. *In a Different Voice: Psychological Theory and Women's Development.* Cambridge, MA: Harvard University Press, 1982.

Hepburn, C., and Gutierrez, B. *Alive and Well: A Lesbian Health Guide.* Freedom, CA: Crossing Press, 1988.

Hite, S. *The Hite Report on Female Sexuality.* New York: Macmillan, 1976.

Lark, S. *Premenstrual Syndrome Self-Help Book: A Woman's Guide to Feeling Good All Month.* Berkeley, CA: Celestial Arts, 1989.

Laundau, C., et al. *The Complete Book of Menopause: Every Woman's Guide to Good Health.* New York: G. P. Putnam's Sons, 1994.

Notelovitz, M., and Tonnessen, D. *Menopause and Midlife Health*. New York: St. Martin's, 1993.

Ogden, G. *Women Who Love Sex*. New York: Pocket Books, 1994.

The Planned Parenthood Women's Health Encyclopedia. New York: Crown, 1996.

Rako, S. *The Hormone of Desire: The Truth about Sexuality, Menopause, and Testosterone*. New York: Random House, 1996.

Villarosa, L., ed. *Body and Soul: The Black Women's Guide to Physical Health and Emotional Well-Being*. New York: HarperCollins, 1994.

Whipple, B., and Ogden, G. *Safe Encounters: How Women Can Say Yes to Pleasure and No to Unsafe Sex*. New York: McGraw-Hill, 1989.

White, E. C., ed. *The Black Women's Health Book: Speaking for Ourselves*. New York: Seal Press, 1994.

JOURNALS

Most of the following journals are published for the information of professionals in their fields, but general readers may also find them interesting.

Annual Review of Sex Research. Society for the Scientific Study of Sexuality, Box 208, Mt. Vernon, IA 52314-0208.

Archives of Sexual Behavior. Plenum Publishing Company, 233 Spring St., New York, NY 10013. 212-620-8495.

Family Planning Perspectives. The Alan Guttmacher Institute, 120 Wall St., New York, NY 10005. 212-248-1111.

Journal of Family History: Studies in Family, Kinship, and Demography. SAGE Publications, Inc., P.O. Box 5084, Thousand Oaks, CA 91359.

Journal of Homosexuality. The Haworth Press, Inc., 10 Alice St., Binghamton, NY 13904-1580.

Journal of Marriage and the Family. National Council on Family Relations, 3989 Central Ave. NE, Ste. 550, Minneapolis, MN 55421.

Journal of Sex Education and Therapy. American Association of Sex Educators, Counselors, and Therapists (AASECT), Box 208, Mt. Vernon, IA 52314-0208.

Journal of Sex Research. Society for the Scientific Study of Sexuality, Box 208, Mt. Vernon, IA 52314–0208.

Journal of the History of Sexuality. University of Chicago Press, Journals Division, P.O. Box 37005, Chicago, IL 60637.

Journal of Women in Culture and Society. University of Chicago Press, Journals Division, P.O. Box 37005, Chicago, IL 60637.

Sexuality and Disability. Human Sciences Press, Inc., 233 Spring St., New York, NY 10013–1578.

Sexual Well-Being. Sexual Health Resources, P.O. Box 60332, Palo Alto, CA 94306.

SIECUS Reports. Sexuality Information and Education Council of the United States, 130 W. 42nd St., Ste. 2500, New York, NY 10036.

Signs: Journal of Women in Culture and Society. University of Chicago Press, Journals Division, P.O. Box 37005, Chicago, IL 60637.

Glossary

Abortifacient: A drug, herb, or device that can cause an abortion.

Abortion: The termination of pregnancy before birth.

Abstinence: Not having sex play.

Abstinence-Only Curricula: Sexuality education programs that advocate sexual abstinence before marriage. They do not provide information about contraception, safer sex, or sexual orientation.

Acquaintance Rape: Sexual intercourse coerced by someone known to the victim.

Adolescence: The period of physical and emotional change between puberty and adulthood.

Adultery: Sexual intercourse between a married person and someone who is not his or her spouse.

Age of Consent: The age at which one is considered old enough to decide to have sexual intercourse.

Age of Majority: The age at which one becomes a legal adult.

AIDS (Acquired Immune Deficiency Syndrome): A set of conditions associated with the last stages of HIV disease.

Alveoli: Sacs inside the breast that produce milk.

Anal Intercourse: Sex play in which the penis enters the anus.

Androgens: Certain hormones that stimulate male sexual development and secondary male sex characteristics. They are most abundantly produced in the testicles of men but are also produced in small amounts in women's ovaries. The most common androgen is testosterone.

Androgyny: A gender identity that allows expression of both gender roles.

Anorexia: An eating disorder often caused by poor body image in which people, usually women, don't eat or eat very little to remain or become thin.

Anorgasmia: The inability to have an orgasm.

Anti-Choice: Opposed to the belief that women have the right to choose abortion.

Anus: The opening from the rectum from which solid waste (feces) leaves the body.

Aphrodisiac: A substance that is supposed to increase sexual desire.

Areola: The dark area surrounding the nipples of women and men.

Asphyxophilia: A paraphilia in which sexual arousal becomes dependent on being strangled up to the point of passing out.

Autoerotic: Providing sexual stimulation for one's self.

Autoerotic Asphyxiation: Self-strangulation for sexual arousal.

Autonomy: The ability to freely exercise one's own will.

Balanitis: An inflammation of the glans and foreskin of the penis that can be caused by infections—including sexually transmitted infections—irritations, drugs, or other factors.

Barrier Methods of Birth Control: Contraceptives that block sperm from entering the uterus. These are the condom, vaginal pouch, diaphragm, cervical cap, and spermicide.

Bartholin's Glands: Glands in the labia minora on each side of the opening to the vagina that provide lubrication during sexual excitement.

Basal Body Temperature Method: A method for predicting fertility in which women chart when ovulation occurs by taking their rectal temperature every morning before getting out of bed.

Biastophilia: A paraphilia in which sexual arousal becomes dependent on sexually attacking a nonconsenting, surprised, terrified, and struggling stranger. This is a kind of rape, but most rapes are committed by normophilic men.

Bimanual Exam: Physical examination of the internal reproductive organs of the pelvis.

Binge-Eating Disorder: Compulsive overeating.

Biology: The scientific study of life.

Bisexual: One who is attracted to people of both genders.

Bladder: The organ that collects and stores urine produced by the kidney. The bladder is emptied through the urethra.

Blue Balls: The genital aching that may occur when men do not have an ejaculation following sexual stimulation. Women may experience similar aches if they do not reach orgasm, but because of sexist influences in development of our language about sex, there is no common expression to describe a woman's symptoms.

Body Image: One's attitudes and feelings about one's own body and appearance.

Bondage and Discipline (B and D): Sexual role play or behavior that includes elements of sadism or masochism. Often one partner is bound or leashed.

Breasts: Two glands on the chests of women. Men also have breast tissue. Breasts are considered sex organs because they are often sexually sensitive and may inspire sexual desire. They produce milk during and after pregnancy.

Bubo: A swollen gland and sore caused by chancroid.

Bulimia: An eating disorder in which binge eating is followed by purging with laxatives or self-induced vomiting.

BV (Bacterial Vaginosis): An inflammation of the vagina—vaginitis —that is caused by a change in the balance of vaginal bacteria.

Calendar Method: A method for predicting fertility for women with regular menstrual cycles to attempt to predict their fertility by charting their menstrual cycles on a calendar.

Candida: A type of yeast and the most common cause of vaginitis.

Celibacy: Not having sex play.

Censorship: The official suppression of information or expression.

Cerebral Cortex: The area of the brain associated with higher functions, including learning and perception.

Cervical Cap: A firm rubber cap intended to fit securely on the cervix. Used with contraceptive jelly, the cervical cap is a barrier method of birth control that is reversible and available only by prescription.

Cervical Mucus Method: A method for predicting a woman's fertility by observing changes in her cervical mucus.

Cervix: The narrow lower part of the uterus (womb), with an opening connecting the uterus to the vagina.

Chancroid: A sexually transmitted bacterium that causes open genital sores.

Chastity Belts: A variety of devices designed to prevent women, men, or children from having sex. Used from medieval to modern times, these devices were also supposed to preserve morality. Some were meant to ensure fidelity in women in the absence of their husbands. Others were designed to prevent masturbation and nocturnal emissions in men and boys.

Chemical Castration: The use of Depo-Provera to decrease sexual desire and arousal.

Child Abuse: Sexual assault against a child by an older person.

Child Pornography: Images of children designed to be sexually arousing.

Chlamydia: A common sexually transmitted organism that can cause sterility in women and men.

Circumcision: An operation to remove the foreskin of the penis. See also **Female Circumcision.**

Climacteric: The time of change that leads to menopause. The physiological midlife changes for women and men.

Climax: An orgasm or to have orgasm.

Clinician: A qualified health care professional, such as a doctor, nurse practitioner, or physician assistant.

Clitoral Hood: A small flap of skin that covers and protects the clitoris.

Clitoris: The female sex organ that is very sensitive to the touch—located between the labia at the top of the vulva.

Cohabitation: Living together in a sexual relationship.

Colposcope: A viewing instrument with a bright light and magnifying lens that is used to examine the vagina and cervix.

Combined Oral Contraceptives: Birth control pills that contain the hormones estrogen and progestin.

Coming Out: The process of accepting and being open about one's sexual orientation.

Companionate Love: Affection and deep emotional attachment that may be erotic.

Comstock Act: An 1873 law that made it a federal crime to use the U.S. mail to distribute anything considered "obscene, lewd, lascivious, indecently filthy, or vile," including information about contraception, abortion, and sexual health.

Conception: The moment when the pre-embryo attaches to the lining of the uterus and pregnancy begins; term also used to describe the fertilization of the egg.

Condom: A sheath of thin rubber, plastic, or animal tissue that is worn on the penis during sexual intercourse. It is an over-the-counter, reversible barrier method of birth control, and it also provides protection against the most serious sexually transmitted infections.

Continuous Abstinence: Having no sex play for long periods of time—months or years.

Contraception: The prevention of pregnancy; birth control.

Contraceptive Creams and Jellies: Substances containing spermicide, which immobilizes sperm, preventing it from joining with the egg; used with diaphragms or cervical caps. These are over-the-counter, reversible barrier methods of birth control.

Contraceptive Film: Inserted deep into the vagina, a square of tissue that melts into a thick liquid and blocks the entrance to the uterus with a spermicide to immobilize sperm, preventing it from joining with an egg; an over-the-counter, reversible barrier method of birth control. Most effective when used with a condom.

Contraceptive Foam: Inserted deep into the vagina, a substance that blocks the entrance to the uterus with bubbles and contains a spermicide to immobilize sperm, preventing it from joining with an egg; an over-the-counter, reversible barrier method of birth control. Most effective when used with a condom.

Contraceptive Suppository Capsule: Inserted deep into the vagina, a solid that melts into a fluid liquid to immobilize sperm, preventing it from joining with an egg; an over-the-counter, reversible barrier method of birth control. Most effective when used with a condom.

Corporal Punishment: A form of discipline that inflicts pain on one's body.

Corpus Cavernosa: Two strips of tissue that lie on each side of the urethra in the penis. During sexual excitement, they fill with blood to create an erection.

Corpus Spongiosum: The tissue that surrounds the urethra inside the penis and is responsible, like the corpus cavernosa, for an erection; also the type of tissue that forms the glans of the clitoris and the penis.

Cowper's Glands: The glands beneath the prostate gland that are attached to the urethra. They produce a substance that makes seminal fluid sticky.

Cremaster Reflex: An automatic response to stimulation—for example, cold temperature or touching the inside of the thigh—in which the cremaster muscle pulls the scrotum and testes closer to the body.

Cross-Dressers: Women and men who like to occasionally wear various articles of clothing associated with the other gender for the fun of it—not for sexual excitement.

Cryptorchidism: The condition in which one or both of the testicles do not descend from the lower abdomen before puberty.

Cultural Norm: An activity, belief, or value that is shared by members of a particular culture. Deviation from cultural norms often invites scorn, ridicule, punishment, or banishment.

Culture: The shared beliefs, values, heritage, customs, norms, art, food, language, and rituals of a community.

Cystitis: An infection of the bladder.

Cytomegalovirus: An infection that may be transmitted through sexual or intimate contact that may cause permanent disability, including hearing loss and mental retardation for infants and blindness and mental disorders for adults.

Date Rape: Coerced sexual intercourse during a dating relationship.

Delayed Ejaculation: Commonly used term for inhibited orgasm in men.

Depo-Provera®: A progestin that is injected into the buttock or arm every 12 weeks to prevent pregnancy. It is a reversible method of birth control available only by prescription.

Depression: The feeling of great sadness that takes control over one's life.

Desire: A feeling of sexual attraction or arousal. The first stage of the sexual response cycle.

Diaphragm: A soft rubber dome intended to fit securely over the cervix. Used with contraceptive cream or jelly, the diaphragm is a reversible barrier method of birth control available only by prescription.

Diversity: The presence of many different kinds of people, including people of various racial and ethnic backgrounds, sexual orientations, and social classes.

Domestic Partnership: The committed, long-term relationship of two unmarried people who live together.

Dominance and Submission (D and S): Erotic activities that play out fantasies of power and powerlessness.

Dominant Culture: The group that holds political, ideological, and economic power in a diverse society.

Don Juanism: The desire by a man to have sex very frequently with many different partners.

Double Standard: An unequal set of moral standards, rules, or expectations that allows one group to have more privileges than another group within a society. A sexual double standard, for example, usually places more restrictions on women than on men.

Douche: A spray of water or solution of medication into the vagina.

Dyspareunia: Painful intercourse for women that may be caused by hormonal imbalances, especially those that happen after menopause.

Early Ejaculation: Ejaculation occurring before a man wants it to occur.

Ectopic Pregnancy: A life-threatening pregnancy that develops outside the uterus, often in a fallopian tube.

Egg: The reproductive cell in women; the largest cell in the human body.

Ejaculation: The moment when semen spurts out of the opening of the urethra in the glans of the penis.

Ejaculatory Inevitability: The moment during sexual excitement when a man cannot stop his ejaculation. The prostate begins contracting and pulsing out seminal fluid.

Emancipated Minor: A minor who has legal autonomy and usually lives on her or his own without financial support from parents or guardians.

Embryo: The organism that develops from the pre-embryo and begins to share the woman's blood supply about nine days after fertilization.

Emergency Contraception: The use of oral contraceptives or IUDs to prevent pregnancy after unprotected intercourse.

Emergency Hormonal Contraception: The use of oral contraceptives to prevent pregnancy after unprotected intercourse.

Endometrium: The lining of the uterus that develops every month in order to nourish a fertilized egg. The lining is shed during menstruation if there is no fertilization.

Epididymis: The tube in which sperm mature. It is tightly coiled on top of and behind each testis. The plural of epididymis is epididymides.

Epididymitis: An inflammation of the epididymis.

Erectile Dysfunction: The inability to become erect or maintain an erection with a partner.

Erection: A "hard" penis when it becomes full of blood and stiffens.

Erogenous Zone: Any area of the body very sensitive to sensual touch.

Erotic: That which is sexually arousing.

Erotica: Sexually arousing imagery that is not considered pornographic, obscene, or offensive to the average person.

Erotophilia: Appreciation of the erotic.

Erotophobia: Fear and anxiety about the erotic.

Estrogen: A hormone commonly made in a woman's ovaries. Estrogen's major effects are seen during puberty, menstruation, and pregnancy.

Estrus: The period of fertility and sexual arousal in the female animal.

Ethnocentric: The belief that one's own country, culture, or ethnic group is superior to others'.

Excitement: The body's physical response to desire and to stimulation. The second stage of the sexual response cycle.

Exhibitionism: A paraphilia in which sexual arousal becomes dependent on exposing the sex organs to those who will be surprised.

Exhibitionists: Women or men who expose their sex organs to other people without their consent, usually in public places.

External Sex and Reproductive Organs: The sex organs and structures on the outside of the body that are primarily used during sexual activity. These include the vulva in a woman and the penis and scrotum in a man.

Extramarital Sex: Sexual intercourse by a married person with someone other than his or her spouse.

Fake Orgasm: The pretense of having reached climax in order to end sex play or please a partner.

Fallopian Tube: One of two narrow tubes that carry the egg from the ovary to the uterus.

FAM (Fertility Awareness Methods): Barrier methods of birth control for vaginal intercourse during the "unsafe days" of a woman's fertile phase.

Fantasy: A sexually arousing thought and mental image.

Feces: Solid waste that leaves the body through the anus.

Female Circumcision: The practice of removing a girl's clitoral hood, clitoris, and/or the labia; often called female genital mutilation. This is practiced in some African, Near Eastern, and Southeast Asian cultures.

Female Genital Mutilation: Female circumcision.

Feminine: Characteristics and ways of behaving that a culture associates with being a girl or a woman.

Feminism: The belief that women and men have equal social, economic, sexual, and political rights.

Fertilization: The joining of an egg and sperm.

Fetal Alcohol Effects: Fetal abnormalities caused by alcohol during pregnancy that may not be as severe as those associated with fetal alcohol syndrome.

Fetal Alcohol Syndrome: Fetal abnormalities affecting growth, the central nervous system, and facial features that are caused by women drinking alcohol during pregnancy.

Fetishism: A paraphilia in which certain objects, substances, or parts of the body become necessary for sexual arousal.

Fetus: The organism that develops from the embryo at the end of about seven weeks of pregnancy and receives nourishment through the placenta.

Fidelity: Strict observance of promises, especially of sexual faithfulness.

Foreplay: Physical and sexual stimulation—kissing, touching, stroking, and massaging—that often happens in the excitement stage of sexual response; often occurs before intercourse, but can lead to orgasm without intercourse, in which case it can be called outercourse.

Foreskin: A retractable tube of skin that covers and protects the glans of the penis.

Formal Values: Socially sanctioned ideals for human behavior that may or may not be consistent with actual behaviors that are sanctioned.

Fornication: Sexual intercourse between unmarried people.

Gamete: The reproductive cell—egg or sperm.

Gang Rape: Sexual assault committed by two or more people; also known as fraternity or party rape.

Gay: Homosexual.

Gay-Bashing: Physical or verbal assaults on people who are perceived to be lesbian, gay, bisexual, or transgender.

Gay Liberation Movement: The movement to establish civil rights for lesbian, gay, bisexual, and transgender women and men.

Gay Rights: Civil rights for lesbian, gay, bisexual, and transgender people that are equal to those guaranteed to straight people.

Gender: One's biological, social, or legal status as male or female.

Gender Assignment: Medical and legal description of one's gender that is given at birth.

Gender Dysphoria: Conflicted feelings about one's gender, gender assignment, and gender identity.

Gender Identity: Feelings about one's gender and gender role.

Gender Norms: Social standards about appropriate feminine and masculine behavior.

Gender Roles: Social norms about behaving feminine or masculine.

Gender Scripting: The socialization process by which one is conditioned to adopt certain behaviors, preferences, and attitudes considered appropriate for her or his gender.

Gender Stereotypes: Unrealistic expectations based on gender.

Genitals: External sex and reproductive organs—the penis and scrotum in men, the vulva in women. Sometimes the internal reproductive organs are also called genitals.

Glans: The soft, highly sensitive tip of the clitoris or penis. In men, the urethral opening is located in the glans.

Gonadotropins: Hormones secreted by the pituitary gland that trigger puberty by stimulating the gonads.

Gonads: The organs that produce reproductive cells—the ovaries of women, the testes of men.

Gonorrhea: A sexually transmitted bacterium that can cause sterility, arthritis, and heart problems.

Guilt: Remorse at believing one has done something wrong.

Gynecology: Sexual and reproductive health care for women.

Gynecomastia: A usually temporary condition during puberty in which the breasts of boys become larger.

HBV (Hepatitis B Virus): An infection that can be sexually transmitted and may cause severe liver disease and death.

Hermaphrodite: Someone with both female and male sex organs.

Heterosexism: The bias that everyone is or should be heterosexual.

Heterosexual: Someone who has sexual desire for people of the other gender.

HIV (Human Immunodeficiency Virus): An infection that weakens the body's ability to fight disease and can cause AIDS.

Homophobia: Fear and hatred of people who are gay, lesbian, or bisexual.

Homosexual: Someone who has sexual desire for people of the same gender.

Homosocial: Including only one gender.

Hormonal Contraceptives: Prescription methods of birth control that use hormones to prevent pregnancy. These include the Pill, implants, and injectables.

Hormones: Chemicals that guide the changes in our bodies and influence how glands and organs work.

HPV (Human Papilloma Virus): Any of 90 different types of infection, some of which may cause genital warts. Others may cause cancer of the cervix, vulva, or penis.

HSV (Herpes Simplex Virus): An infection that can be sexually transmitted and cause a recurring rash with clusters of blistery sores on the vagina, cervix, penis, mouth, anus, buttocks, or elsewhere on the body.

Hymen: A thin fleshy tissue that stretches across part of the opening to the vagina.

Hyperfemininity: The exaggeration of gender-stereotyped behavior that is believed to be feminine.

Hypermasculinity: The exaggeration of gender-stereotyped behavior that is believed to be masculine.

Hyperphilia: Having sex more often than most people.

Hypoactive Sexual Desire: The lack of sexual desire.

Hypophilia: Having sex very infrequently, or not at all.

Hypothalamus: A small area in the brain that regulates basic animal functions.

Implantation: The attachment of the pre-embryo to the lining of the uterus.

Incest: Sexual activity between members of the same family.

Infatuation: Impulsive, usually short-lived, emotional and erotic attachment to another person.

Informal Values: Social sanctions for behaviors that may or may not be consistent with socially sanctioned ideals for behavior.

Inhibited Arousal: The inability to become sexually aroused and enjoy sex play, despite one's sexual desire.

Inhibited Orgasm: Inability to have an orgasm.

Inhibited Sexual Desire: The lack of sexual desire.

Inhibition: Feeling restraint due to fear or guilt.

Intercourse: Sexual activity between two people in which insertion of the penis occurs. This includes vaginal intercourse, oral intercourse, and anal intercourse.

Internalized Homophobia: The fear of homosexuality within one's self.

Internal Sex and Reproductive Organs: The organs inside the body that are responsible for producing, moving, and nourishing human reproductive cells. Because internal organs may be sensitive or respond to sexual stimulation, these organs are also called sex organs.

Intimacy: The closeness and familiarity we feel as we share our private and personal selves with someone else.

Introitus: The tissue of the inner vulva that frames the opening to the vagina.

IUD (Intrauterine Device): A small device made of plastic, which may contain copper or a natural hormone, that is inserted into the uterus by a clinician. A reversible method of birth control available only by prescription.

Jealousy: Anxiety about a partner's love and commitment.

Jock Itch: A very common fungal skin infection in the genital area of men that is caused by wearing tight clothing, sweating, or not drying the genitals carefully after bathing. It can cause a reddish, scaly rash that can become inflamed, very itchy, and painful.

Kleptophilia: A paraphilia in which sexual arousal becomes dependent on stealing.

Labia Majora: The larger, outer lips of the vulva.

Labia Minora: The smaller, inner lips of the vulva.

Lactobacilli: Bacteria present in healthy vaginas of women. They help relieve vaginitis by limiting the growth of candida, a yeast.

LAM (Lactational Amenorrhea Method): Breast-feeding as birth control for up to six months after childbirth.

Lesbian: A homosexual woman.

Leukorrhea: A white, sticky vaginal discharge that is normal during adolescence.

Levonorgestrel: A synthetic progestin similar to the hormone progesterone, which is produced by the body to regulate the menstrual cycle; the active ingredient in Norplant®.

Libido: The sex drive.

Limerance: A powerful and constantly distracting and obsessive infatuation.

Lobes: Groups of alveoli sacs in women's breasts.

Long-Term Reorganization Phase: The second phase of rape trauma syndrome, in which the victim tries to regain control of life.

Love: A strong caring for someone else. It comes in many forms. There can be love for romantic partners and also for close friends, for parents and children, for God, and for humankind.

Lovemap: A blueprint of one's adult sexual appreciations and preferences that develops while one is growing up.

Lust: The desire for sexual pleasure.

Mammogram: X-ray photographs of the breasts that can detect cancerous tumors before they can be felt.

Marital Rape: Coerced sexual intercourse within marriage.

Masculine: Characteristics and ways of behaving that a culture associates with being a boy or a man.

Masochism: A paraphilia in which sexual arousal becomes dependent on sexual role play or fantasy that includes receiving punishment, discipline, or humiliation.

Masturbation: Touching one's own sex organs for pleasure.

Megan's Law: Federal and state laws that require police to notify citizens of the presence of convicted pedophiles in their communities.

Menarche: The time of a girl's first menstruation.

Menopause: The time at "midlife" when menstruation stops; a woman's last period; usually occurs between the ages of 45 and 55. "Surgical" menopause, however—which results from removal of the ovaries—may occur earlier.

Menstrual Cycle: The time from the first day of one period to the first day of the next period; a repeating pattern of fertility and infertility.

Menstrual Flow: Blood, fluid, and tissue that are passed out of the uterus during the beginning of the menstrual cycle.

Menstruation: The flow of blood, fluid, and tissue out of the uterus and through the vagina that usually lasts from three to five days.

Method-Effectiveness: The reliability of a contraceptive method itself—when it is always used consistently and correctly.

Milk Ducts: The passages in women's breasts through which milk flows from the alveoli to the nipple.

Mini-Pills: Birth control pills that contain only the hormone progestin.

Miscegenation: Marriage or sexual relations between people of different races.

Molluscum Contagiosum: A virus that can be sexually transmitted, causing small, pinkish-white, waxy, round, polyplike growths in the genital area or on the thighs.

Monogamous Relationship: A relationship in which both people date or have sex only with one another and no one else.

"Morning-After" Pills: Emergency hormonal contraception that is taken within 72 hours of unprotected intercourse.

Multiple Orgasms: More than one orgasm occurring within the same sexual encounter.

Mutuality: Reciprocating equally with feelings and behavior.

Myths: Unfounded or false stories or ideas.

Nipple: The dark tissue in the center of the areola of each breast in women and men that can stand erect when stimulated by touch or cold. In a woman's breast, the nipple may release milk that is produced by the breast.

Normophilia: Sexual preferences that are considered common or "normal" according to social norms.

Norplant®: A contraceptive system of six small soft capsules containing the hormone levonorgestrel that is inserted under the skin of the upper arm. A reversible method of birth control that is available only by prescription.

Nymphomania: The desire by a woman to have sex very frequently with many different partners.

Obscenity: Sexually arousing imagery that is considered socially offensive.

Oedipal Conflict: The Freudian theory that children have an unconscious sexual attachment to the parent of the other gender, causing them to be hostile toward the parent of the same gender.

Open Relationship: A relationship in which both partners are free to date or have sex with other people.

Oral Contraceptive: The birth control pill.

Oral Sex: Sex play involving the mouth and sex organs.

Orgasm: The peak of sexual arousal when all the muscles that were tightened during sexual arousal relax, causing a very pleasurable feeling that may involve the whole body. The fourth stage of the sexual response cycle.

Outercourse: Sex play that does not include inserting the penis in the vagina or anus.

Ovaries: The two organs that store eggs in a woman's body. Ovaries also produce hormones, including estrogen, progesterone, and testosterone.

Over-the-Counter: Available without a prescription.

Ovulation: The time when an ovary releases an egg.

Ovulation Method: See **Cervical Mucus Method.**

Pap Test: A procedure used to examine the cells of the cervix in order to detect infection and hormonal conditions. It can also detect precancerous and cancerous cells.

ParaGard® (Copper T-380 A): An IUD that contains copper and can be left in place for 10 years.

Paraphilia: A sex practice that becomes necessary for sexual arousal but that is not approved by social norms.

Parental Consent: Requirement that one or both parents give written permission for a minor child to receive medical attention or to enter into a legal contract.

Passionate Love: Powerfully intense feelings of erotic attachment.

Pedophilia: A paraphilia in which sexual arousal for an adult becomes dependent on having sexual contact or fantasies of sexual contact with a child.

Peer Pressure: The efforts of a group of equals to maintain conformity to the group's social norms.

Pelvic Exam: Physical examination of the vulva, vagina, cervix, uterus, and ovaries—usually includes taking cervical cells for a Pap test and a manual exam of the internal pelvic organs.

Pelvic Girdle: A bony and muscular structure inside a woman's body that supports her internal sex and reproductive organs.

Penis: A man's reproductive and sex organ that is formed of spongy tissue and fills with blood during sexual excitement, a process known as erection. Urine and seminal fluid pass through the penis.

Perfect Use: The contraceptive effectiveness for women and men whose use is consistent and always correct.

Performance Anxiety: The fear of being unable to please a partner.

Perimenopause: The period of change leading to menopause.

Period: The days during menstruation.

Periodic Abstinence: Not having vaginal intercourse during the "unsafe days" of a woman's fertile phase in order to prevent pregnancy.

Peyronie's Disease: A rare condition that is caused by fibrous growths inside the penis.

Pheromones: Odors given off by animals that attract the other gender.

Physical Fitness: A condition of good health that results from healthful foods, exercise, and regular medical checkups.

Pictophilia: A paraphilia in which sexual arousal becomes dependent on viewing pornographic pictures, movies, or videos with or without a partner.

PID (Pelvic Inflammatory Disease): An infection of a woman's internal reproductive system that can lead to sterility, ectopic pregnancy, and chronic pain. It is often caused by sexually transmitted infections such as gonorrhea and chlamydia.

Pill, The: Common expression for oral hormonal contraception.

Plateau: The stage of sexual arousal in which a person has been sexually excited and may approach orgasm. The third stage of the sexual response cycle.

Polygamy: Having more than one spouse.

Pornography: Erotic imagery that is considered obscene and offensive.

Post-Ovulation Method: A method of contraception using periodic abstinence or FAMs from the beginning of menstruation until the morning of the fourth day after predicted ovulation—more than half of the menstrual cycle.

Pre-Ejaculate: The liquid that oozes out of the penis during sexual excitement before ejaculation; produced by the Cowper's glands.

Pre-Embryo: The ball of cells that develops from the fertilized egg until after about nine days, when it attaches to the lining of the uterus and the embryo is formed.

Premarital Sex: Sexual intercourse between people before marriage.

Premature Ejaculation: Ejaculation occurring before a man wants it to occur—often before his partner reaches orgasm.

Priapism: A continuous partial erection without sexual stimulation that is caused by dysfunctional blood flow into the corpus cavernosa.

Primary Sex Characteristics: The body organs and reproductive structures and functions that differ between women and men. The differences include the external and internal sex and reproductive organs. It also includes a woman's ability to produce eggs and a man's ability to produce sperm.

Pro-Choice: The belief that women have the right to choose abortion.

Progestasert®: An IUD containing natural hormones that must be replaced every year.

Progesterone: A hormone produced in the ovaries of women that is important in puberty, menstruation, and pregnancy.

Progestin: A synthetic progesterone.

Prophylactic: A device used to prevent infection; the condom.

Prostate: An internal reproductive organ below the bladder that produces a fluid that helps sperm move.

Prostatitis: An enlargement and inflammation of the prostate gland that results in a dull persistent pain in the lower back, testes, scrotum, and glans of the penis. There may also be a thin mucus discharge from the penis, especially in the morning.

Prostitution: The performance of sexual acts for pay.

Psychology: The study of the mind and its processes.

Puberty: A time in life when a girl is becoming a woman and a boy is becoming a man. Puberty is marked by physical changes of the body such as breast development and menstruation in girls and facial hair growth and ejaculation in boys.

Pubic Hair: Hair that grows in the genital area of women and men. Pubic hair is a secondary sex characteristic appearing at puberty.

Pubic Lice: Tiny insects that can be sexually transmitted. They live in pubic hair and cause intense itching in the genitals or anus.

Puritans: Early American Protestant colonists who established English laws and social and sexual mores in the northeastern United States. Though actually less sexually restrictive than commonly believed, the Puritan is now the symbol of sexual suppression.

Rape: Coerced sexual intercourse.

Rape Trauma Syndrome: The emotional and physical consequences one experiences after being sexually assaulted.

Rapid Orgasm: When a woman climaxes more quickly than her partner and loses interest in continued sex play.

Reality-Based Sexuality Education: Age-appropriate, culturally sensitive sexuality education programs that include open, nonjudgmental information about all aspects of sexuality; they encourage critical thinking, self-actualization, and behavioral changes through the empowerment of holistic knowledge about the body, sex, relationships, birth control, safer sex, gender role, and so on, by being realistic about people's lives. Also referred to as comprehensive sexuality education.

Rectovaginal Exam: Physical examination of the reproductive organs and the tissues that separate the vagina and rectum.

Rectum: The lowest end of the intestine before the anus, where solid waste (feces) is stored.

Refractory Period: The time after ejaculation during which a man is not able to have an erection.

Reproductive Cell: The unique cell—egg in women, sperm in men—that can join with its opposite to make reproduction possible.

Resolution: The period after orgasm in which the body returns to a nonstimulated state. The last stage in the sexual response cycle.

Retarded Ejaculation: Commonly used term for inhibited orgasm in men.

Retrograde Ejaculation: An ejaculation from the prostate into the bladder.

"Rhythm" Method: See **Calendar Method.**

Roe v. Wade: The 1973 U.S. Supreme Court decision that legalized abortion.

Role Play: Acting out a fantasy with a partner.

Romantic Love: An idealized love relationship that is often as unrealistic as it is passionate. In courtship, romance may have elements of flattery, excitement, and the feeling of being "swept away," as in a fairy tale.

Rut: The period of sexual arousal in male animals that is a response to estrus.

Sacred: Devoted to religious purpose.

Sadism: A paraphilia in which sexual arousal becomes dependent on sexual role play or fantasy that includes giving punishment, discipline, or humiliation.

Sadomasochism (S and M): The consensual use of domination and/or pain for sexual stimulation in sex play. The "sadist" is the partner who dominates and inflicts pain. The "masochist" is the partner who is dominated and receives pain.

Safer Sex: Ways in which people reduce the risk of getting sexually transmitted infections, including HIV.

Safe Word: A previously agreed upon signal that means a partner is no longer enjoying a sexual activity and it must stop.

Sample: The group of people or subjects studied in a research project.

Sanitary Pad: An absorbent "napkin" made of cotton or similar fibers that is worn against the vulva to absorb menstrual flow.

Satyriasis: The desire by a man to have sex very frequently with many different partners.

Scabies: Tiny mites that can be sexually transmitted. They burrow under the skin, causing intense itching—usually at night—and small bumps or rashes that appear in dirty-looking, small curling lines, especially on the penis, between the fingers, on buttocks, breasts, wrists, and thighs, and around the navel.

Scrotum: A sac of skin, divided into two parts, enclosing the testes, epididymides, and a part of the vasa deferentia.

Secondary Sex Characteristics: Characteristics of the body that are caused by hormones, develop during puberty, and last through adult life. For women, these include breast development and widened hips. For men, they include facial hair development. Both genders develop pubic hair and underarm hair.

Secular: Devoted to human purpose.

Self-Esteem: Self-respect; worthwhile feeling.

Semen: Fluid containing sperm that is ejaculated during sexual excitement. Semen is composed of seminal fluid from the seminal vesicles, fluid from the prostate, and fluid from the Cowper's glands.

Seminal Fluid: A fluid that nourishes and helps sperm to move. Seminal fluid is made in the seminal vesicles.

Seminal Vesicle: One of two small organs located beneath the bladder that produce seminal fluid.

Seminiferous Tubules: A network of tiny tubules in the testes that constantly produce sperm. Seminiferous tubules also produce androgens, the "male" sex hormones.

Sex: Gender; the act of sex play.

Sex Cell: A reproductive cell.

Sex Drive: Our natural urge and desire to have sex.

Sexism: Bias against a certain gender—especially against women.

Sexology: The scientific study of sex and sexuality through many disciplines including, but not limited to, anthropology, biology, sociology, history, psychology, medicine, and law.

Sex Play: Any voluntary sexual activity, with or without a partner.

Sex Therapy: Treatment to resolve a sexual problem or dysfunction such as premature ejaculation, inability to have orgasm, or low level of sexual desire.

Sexual Abuse: Sexual activity that is harmful or not consensual.

Sexual Addiction: The compulsive search for having very frequent sex.

Sexual Assault: The use of force or coercion, physical or psychological, to make a person engage in sexual activity.

Sexual Aversion Disorder: The fear of sexual contact.

Sexual Compulsion: An obsession with having very frequent sex, often with many different sex partners.

Sexual Compulsives Anonymous: A self-help recovery group for women and men who want to control what they believe to be sexual addictions.

Sexual Conflict: The clash between sex drive and sexual inhibition.

Sexual Desire: A strong physically arousing attraction.

Sexual Discomfort: Feelings of sexual inhibition that are not as severe as dysfunctions.

Sexual Double Standard: See **Double Standard.**

Sexual Dysfunction: A psychological or physical disorder of sexual function.

Sexual Harassment: Unwanted sexual advances with suggestive gestures, language, or touching.

Sexual Identity: Feelings about one's own sexual orientation, gender, gender role, and gender identity.

Sexuality: The interplay of gender, gender role, gender identity, sexual orientation, sexual preference, and social norms as they affect physical, emotional, and spiritual life.

Sexually Transmitted Infections (STIs): Infections that are often or usually passed from one person to another during sexual or intimate contact.

Sexual Norm: A cultural norm regarding sex or sexuality.

Sexual Orientation: The term used to describe the gender of the objects of our sexual desires. People who feel sexual desire for members of the other gender are heterosexual, or straight. People who feel sexual desire for people of the same gender are homosexual, or gay. Gay women are called lesbians. People who are attracted to both genders are bisexuals.

Sexual Repression: The suppression of sexual activities, ideas, or identities that are perceived to be harmful or morally wrong.

Sexual Response Cycle: The pattern of response to sexual stimulation. The five stages of the cycle are desire, excitement, plateau, orgasm, and resolution.

Sexual Seduction: Legally, the encouragement of a younger or less mature person into an illegal sexual situation.

Sexual Stereotype: An overly simplified judgment or bias regarding the sexuality of a person or group.

Sex Worker: One who is paid for providing sex or sexually arousing conditions, including prostitution, striptease, lap dancing, commercial phone sex, and erotic massage.

Shaft: A part of the penis and clitoris.

Smegma: A sticky, white, unpleasant-smelling substance produced at the glans of the penis. It is formed by bacteria and body oils.

Social Stigma: Severe disapproval for behavior that is not within cultural norms.

Sociology: The study of human relationships, interactions, beliefs, values, behaviors, and their meanings.

Sodomy: Oral or anal intercourse.

Somatotropin: The human growth hormone secreted by the pituitary gland.

Spectatoring: The habit of thinking about, comparing, grading, and monitoring one's sexual performance while having sex.

Speculum: A plastic or metal instrument used to separate the walls of the vagina so the clinician can examine the vagina and cervix.

Speculum Exam: Physical examination of the walls of the vagina and cervix that is accomplished by using a speculum.

Sperm: The reproductive cells in men, produced in the seminiferous tubules of the testes.

Spermarche: The time when sperm is first produced by the testes of a boy.

Spermatogenesis: The process of producing sperm. Spermatogenesis occurs in the seminiferous tubules of the testes.

Spermicides: Chemicals used to immobilize sperm and protect against certain sexually transmitted infections.

Spirochete: Organism that causes syphilis.

Squeeze Technique: A method for postponing early ejaculation.

Statutory Rape: Sexual intercourse between an adult and anyone who is below the age of consent, whether or not it is voluntary.

STD (Sexually Transmitted Disease): A sexually transmitted infection that has developed symptoms.

Stereotype: An overly simplified judgment or bias regarding a person or group.

Sterilization: Surgical methods of birth control that are intended to be permanent—blocking of the fallopian tubes for women or the vasa deferentia for men.

Stimuli: Things that excite response or action.

Straight: Heterosexual.

Stranger Rape: Coerced sexual intercourse by an assailant unknown to the victim.

Stress: Being made to feel threatened or challenged in some way.

Syphilis: A sexually transmitted organism that can lead to disfigurement, neurological disorders, or death.

Taboo: Behavior that is beyond the moral limits of cultural norms.

Tampon: A firm roll of absorbent cotton or other fiber that is worn inside the vagina to absorb menstrual flow.

Tenting: The expansion of the inner vagina during sexual excitement.

Testes: Two ball-like glands inside the scrotum that produce sperm.

Testicles: The testes.

Testosterone: An androgen that is produced in the testes of men and in smaller amounts in the ovaries of women.

Thelarche: The time when a girl's breasts begin to develop.

Toxic Shock Syndrome: A rare but very dangerous overgrowth of bacteria in the vagina. Symptoms include vomiting, high fever, diarrhea, and a sunburn-type rash.

Transgender: Women and men who dress in the clothing associated with the other gender because they enjoy being treated as if they were of the other gender—not for sexual pleasure.

Transsexuals: Women and men who fully identify themselves as the gender other than their biological one.

Transvestites: Women and men who dress in clothing associated with people of the other gender because it gives them sexual pleasure.

Transvestophilia: A paraphilia in which sexual arousal becomes dependent on wearing clothing, especially underwear, associated with the other gender.

Tubal Sterilization: Surgical blocking of the fallopian tubes that is intended to provide permanent birth control.

Typical Use: Contraceptive effectiveness for women and men whose use is not consistent or always correct.

Uncircumcised: Description of a penis that has a foreskin.

Ureters: The two tubes that lead from the kidneys to the bladder.

Urethra: The tube and opening from which women and men urinate. The urethra empties the bladder and carries urine to the urethral opening. In men, the urethra runs through the penis and also carries ejaculate and pre-ejaculate during sex play.

Use-Effectiveness: The reliability of a contraceptive method as it is usually used—when it is *not* always used consistently or correctly.

Uterus: The pear-shaped, muscular reproductive organ from which women menstruate and where normal pregnancy develops; the womb.

UTI (Urinary Tract Infection): A bacterial infection of the bladder (also called cystitis), the ureters, or the urethra; can be sexually transmitted.

Vagina: The stretchable passage that connects a woman's outer sex organs—the vulva—with the cervix and uterus.

Vaginal Intercourse: Sex play in which the penis enters the vagina.

Vaginal Pouch (Female Condom): A polyurethane sheath with flexible rings at each end that is inserted deep into the vagina like a diaphragm. It is an over-the-counter, reversible barrier method of birth control that may provide protection against many sexually transmitted infections.

Vaginismus: Painful intercourse for a woman that occurs when her fear and anxiety about vaginal intercourse cause the muscles around her vagina to go into spasm when her partner tries to insert a penis or dildo.

Vaginitis: An inflammation of the vagina that is caused by a change in the normal balance of vaginal bacteria.

Values: Ideas of what is right, worthwhile, or moral.

Varicocele: An enlargement of the spermatic vein, which supplies blood to the testis. It can reduce blood flow and increase the temperature of the testicle, thereby causing infertility.

Vas Deferens: A long, narrow tube that carries sperm from each epididymis to the seminal vesicles. The plural of vas deferens is vasa deferentia.

Vasectomy: Surgical blocking of the vasa deferentia in men that is intended to provide permanent birth control.

Venereologist: One who studies sexually transmitted infections.

Viability: The ability of a fetus to survive outside a woman's body.

Victorians: People who lived during and after the reign of Britain's Queen Victoria (1837-1901)—especially those who shared her fears about human sexuality.

Virginity: Never having had sexual intercourse.

Voluntary Sterilization: Surgically implemented contraception that is intended to be permanent and that is freely chosen.

Voyeurism: A paraphilia in which sexual arousal becomes dependent on watching people undress or have sex play unaware that they are being watched.

Voyeurs: Women or men who become aroused by secretly watching another person undress or engage in sexual behavior.

Vulva: A woman's external sex organs, including the clitoris, the labia (majora and minora), the opening to the vagina (introitus), and two Bartholin's glands.

Wet Dreams: Erotic imaging during sleep that causes ejaculation.

Withdrawal: Pulling the penis out of the vagina before ejaculation in order to avoid pregnancy.

Index

defined, 25, 163, 328
effects, 163
laws, 278–279
Incontinence. *See* Stress incontinence;
Urine loss
Infatuation, defined, 121, 328
Informal values, defined, 260, 328
Information hot lines, U.S. Centers for
Disease Control and Prevention, 213
Inhibition, defined, 144, 328
Initiation rituals, cultural norms, 31,
35–36
Intercourse. *See also* Anal intercourse;
Axillary intercourse; Interfemoral
intercourse; Mammary intercourse;
Oral intercourse; Sexual intercourse;
Vaginal intercourse
defined, 1, 328
painful. *See* Dyspareunia; Vaginismus;
Vaginitis
Interfemoral intercourse, defined, 90
Internet, Supreme Court decisions, 284
Interracial relationships, effects, 41
Intimacy
defined, 1, 329
incest and, 163
older adults and, 137
sexual abuse in children and, 163
sexual inhibition and, 149
young adults and, 119–121
Intrauterine device (IUD). *See* IUD
Introitus, defined, 69, 329
IUD
defined, 45, 234, 329
emergency insertion, 256–258
ParaGard® (Copper T-380 A), 235, 332
Progestasert®, 235, 333
pros/cons, 217, 234–239, 256–258

J
Jealousy
defined, 121, 329
sexual inhibition and, 147–148
Jock itch, defined, 185–186, 329
Johnson, Virginia, 58–59

K
The *Kama Sutra,* sexuality and, 36–37
Kegel exercises, effects, 131, 132
Kinsey, Alfred, 58
Kleptophilia, defined, 162, 329

L
Labia majora
defined, 67, 68, 329
sexual response and, 88, 91
Labia minora
defined, 67, 68, 329
sexual response and, 88, 91
Lactational amenorrhea method. *See* LAM
Lactobacilli, defined, 184, 329
LAM
defined, 223, 329
pros/cons, 223–224
Laws, sexuality and, 29–30, 33–34,
263–286
Lesbians, defined, 9, 329
Leukorrhea, defined, 80, 329
Levodopa, effects, 96
Levonorgestrel, defined, 243, 329
Libido, defined, 143, 329
Limerance, defined, 121, 329
Living arrangements, young adults and,
117–118
Lobes, defined, 70, 329
Long-term reorganization phase, defined,
168, 329